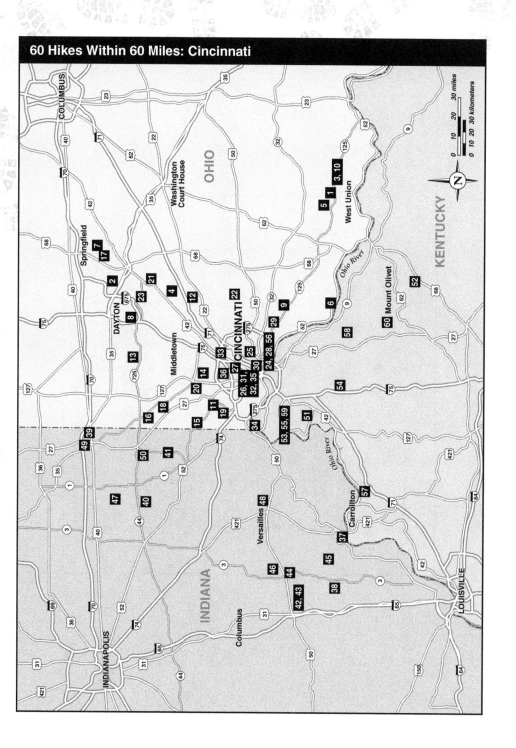

Directional arrows   Off-map pointer

Featured trail   Alternate trail   Park/forest

Interstate   Major road   Minor road

Boardwalk   Dirt road   Railroad

Borderline   Water body   River/creek

Amphitheater	• General point of interest	Playground
Archery range	⑦ Information	Restroom
Bench	Marina	RV campsite
Bicycle trail	Marsh	Scenic view
Boat launch	Monument/sculpture	Shelter
Bridge	Office	Spring
Camping	Overlook	Tower
Cemetery	P Parking	Trailhead
Dam	Peak	Tunnel
Garden	Picnic area	Viewing platform
Gate	Picnic shelter	Waterfall

Overview-Map Key

Ohio

1 Adams Lake SP and Adams Lake Prairie State NP (p. 18)
2 Beaver Creek Wildlife Area: Siebenthaler Fen (p. 23)
3 Buzzardroost Rock Preserve (p. 28)
4 Caesar Creek Gorge State NP: Gorge Loop Trail (p. 33)
5 Chaparral Prairie State NP (p. 38)
6 Chilo Lock 34 Park and Crooked Run NP (p. 43)
7 Clifton Gorge State NP (p. 49)
8 Cox Arboretum MetroPark (p. 55)
9 East Fork SP: South Trail (p. 60)
10 Edge of Appalachia Preserve: The Wilderness Trail (p. 65)
11 Fernald Preserve (p. 70)
12 Fort Ancient State Memorial (p. 76)
13 Germantown MetroPark (p. 82)
14 Gilmore MetroPark (p. 87)
15 Governor Bebb MetroPark and Pioneer Village (p. 92)
16 Hueston Woods SP (p. 97)
17 John Bryan SP (p. 102)
18 Miami University Natural Areas (p. 107)
19 Miami Whitewater Forest: Shaker Trace Outer Loop (p. 112)
20 Pyramid Hill Sculpture Park & Museum (p. 117)
21 Spring Valley Wildlife Area (p. 122)
22 Stonelick SP (p. 127)
23 Sugarcreek MetroPark (p. 132)
24 Withrow NP (p. 138)

Cincinnati

25 Ault Park (p. 146)
26 Buttercup Valley Preserve and Parkers Woods (p. 151)
27 Caldwell Preserve (p. 157)
28 California Woods NP (p. 162)
29 Cincinnati Nature Center's Rowe Woods (p. 167)
30 Eden Park (p. 173)
31 Mount Airy Forest: Furnas, Twin Bridge, Beechwood, Red Oak, and Ponderosa (p. 178)
32 Mount Airy Forest: West Fork Road, Diehl Ridge, and Elm Ravine (p. 184)
33 Sharon Woods (p. 188)
34 Shawnee Lookout (p. 193)
35 Spring Grove Cemetery (p. 198)
36 Winton Woods (p. 204)

Indiana

37 Clifty Falls SP and Clifty Canyon NP (p. 210)
38 Hardy Lake State Recreation Area (p. 215)
39 Hayes Arboretum (p. 220)
40 Mary Gray Bird Sanctuary (p. 225)
41 Mounds State Recreation Area (p. 230)
42 Muscatatuck National Wildlife Refuge: Chestnut Ridge Trail (p. 235)
43 Muscatatuck National Wildlife Refuge: Hunt–Richart Lake Trail (p. 240)
44 Muscatatuck Park (p. 244)
45 Pennywort Cliffs Preserve (p. 249)
46 Selmier State Forest (p. 253)
47 Shrader–Weaver NP (p. 258)
48 Versailles SP (p. 263)
49 Whitewater Gorge: Cardinal Greenway (p. 268)
50 Whitewater Memorial SP (p. 273)

Kentucky

51 Big Bone Lick State Historic Site (p. 282)
52 Blue Licks Battlefield State Resort Park (p. 287)
53 Boone Cliffs State NP (p. 292)
54 Curtis Gates Lloyd Wildlife Management Area (p. 297)
55 Dinsmore Homestead and Dinsmore Woods State NP (p. 303)
56 Fort Thomas Landmark Tree Trail (p. 308)
57 General Butler State Resort Park (p. 313)
58 Kincaid Lake SP (p. 318)
59 Middle Creek Park (p. 323)
60 Quiet Trails State NP (p. 328)

NP = Nature Preserve   SP = State Park

Other cities in the 60 Hikes Within 60 Miles series:

Albuquerque	*New York City*
Atlanta	*Philadelphia*
Baltimore	*Phoenix*
Boston	*Pittsburgh*
Chicago	*Richmond*
Cleveland	*Sacramento*
Dallas and Fort Worth	*Salt Lake City*
Denver and Boulder	*San Antonio and Austin*
Harrisburg	*San Diego*
Houston	*San Francisco*
Los Angeles	*Seattle*
Madison	*St. Louis*
Minneapolis and St. Paul	*Washington, D.C.*
Nashville	

60 HIKES WITHIN 60 MILES

CINCINNATI

**INCLUDING Southwest Ohio,
Southeast Indiana,
and Northern Kentucky**

SECOND EDITION

Tamara York

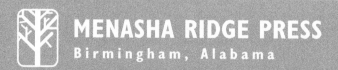

MENASHA RIDGE PRESS
Birmingham, Alabama

60 Hikes Within 60 Miles: Cincinnati

Copyright © 2014 by Tamara York
All rights reserved
Published by Menasha Ridge Press
Printed in the United States of America
Distributed by Publishers Group West
Second edition, first printing

Library of Congress Cataloging-in-Publication Data

York, Tamara.
  60 hikes within 60 miles, Cincinnati : including Clifton Gorge, Southeast Indiana, and Northern
Kentucky / Tammy York.
    pages cm
  ISBN 978-0-89732-510-3 (paperback) — ISBN 0-89732-510-9 — ISBN 978-0-89732-511-0 (ebook)
  ISBN 978-1-63404-161-4 (hardcover)
  1. Hiking—Ohio—Cincinnati Region—Guidebooks. 2. Cincinnati Region (Ohio)—Guidebooks.
  3. Hiking—Indiana—Guidebooks. 4. Indiana—Guidebooks. 5. Hiking—Kentucky—Guidebooks.
  6. Kentucky—Guidebooks. I. Title. II. Title: Sixty hikes within sixty miles, Cincinnati.
  GV199.42.O32C528 2014
  796.5109771—dc23
                          2014016132

Cover design, cartography, and elevation profiles: Scott McGrew
Text design: Annie Long
Front cover: Cox Arboretum MetroPark. *Back cover, left to right:* Pyramid Hill Sculpture Park & Museum,
Shawnee Lookout, Thistlethwaite Falls at Whitewater Gorge, and Withrow Nature Preserve.
Cover photo © Texas141/Wikimedia Commons/CC-BY-SA-3.0
Back cover and interior photos, unless otherwise noted on page, by Tamara York

 MENASHA RIDGE PRESS
An imprint of AdventureKEEN
2204 1st Ave., S., Suite 102
Birmingham, Alabama 35233
menasharidge.com

Disclaimer

This book is meant only as a guide to select trails in the Cincinnati area and does not guarantee hiker safety in any way—you hike at your own risk. Neither Menasha Ridge Press nor Tamara York is liable for property loss or damage, personal injury, or death that result in any way from accessing or hiking the trails described in the following pages. Please be aware that hikers have been injured in the Cincinnati area. Be especially cautious when walking on or near boulders, steep inclines, and drop-offs, and do not attempt to explore terrain that may be beyond your abilities. To help ensure an uneventful hike, please read carefully the introduction to this book, and perhaps get further safety information and guidance from other sources. Familiarize yourself thoroughly with the areas you intend to visit before venturing out. Ask questions, and prepare for the unforeseen. Familiarize yourself with current weather reports, maps of the area you intend to visit, and any relevant park regulations.

Table of Contents

To my husband, who demanded that I mention him by name
—thanks for always believing in me.

To my daughters for being my hiking buddies, cheerleaders,
and comedy team.

To my mom for taking me hiking in the woods near
Grandma and Grandpa's farm.

To my brother, who answers all of my weird questions.

To all of my fabulous readers and hikers—thanks!

Acknowledgments

I wouldn't have been able to write this book without the continuous and overflowing support from my family. My husband, Allen, is a tremendous support; without his devotion to my success, I'd still be using a typewriter. My daughters, Margaret and Madaelynne, never fail to show me the lighter side of life and provided comic relief in the midst of thunderstorms, simmering hot days, and 16 inches of snow.

Thanks to my mother, who discovered some of the trails less traveled and took care of the girls while I hiked the more difficult trails. My brother, Michael, who graciously provided GPS, Google Earth, and mapping tech support—even though I tend to call in the middle of the night.

I owe a tremendous amount of gratitude to so many behind-the-scenes people who help bring a book from an idea to a reality. The second edition is no less of an undertaking than the first, and I would like to thank Amber Kaye Henderson and Molly Merkle for their support; Kara Pelicano for simply rocking; Richard Hunt for guiding the way; and Jack Heffron—his enthusiasm for writing is contagious and delightful. Thanks to Molly Merkle and Holly Cross for patiently leading me through the maze of writing my first book; Tanya Sylvan, Liliane Opsomer, Jim Nunn, Howard Cohen, and Darcy Lathrop for helping market the book; Kerry Smith for his magical copyediting; Annie Long for her incredible graphic design work; cartographer Scott McGrew for creating easy-to-read maps; and Russell Helms for answering my mapping questions.

Special thanks to Great Parks of Hamilton County naturalists, especially Amy Roell and Jerry Lippert; naturalist John Cimarosti; Keith Robinson of Clermont County Parks; Erin Morris of Cincinnati Parks; Chris Bedel of The Edge of Appalachia; and Bernadette Harawa of Five Rivers MetroParks. Thanks to Kevin Snyder and Dick Davis at Clifty Falls State Park; David Whitehouse of Boone County Parks; Rob McGriff and Darrel Breedlove at Selmier State Forest; Joyce Bender and Daniel Cox of Kentucky Nature Preserves and Natural Areas; and Quinton Tyree at Blue Licks Battlefield State Resort Park. Thanks to Scotty Richards and John Cunningham for their dedication to the Tri-State Hiking Club and their top picks for hiking trails.

I owe much gratitude to the incredible women of the Mom's Club, especially Dayna Brown, Kim Johnson, and Nicole Eckert. Thanks to naturalist Bonnie Martens for her from-the-trenches advice on hiking with young children and her top picks for kid-friendly hiking trails.

Along the trail I've met many incredible people, but special thanks to my hiking buddies Allen York, Margaret York, Madaelynne York, Kathy Keller, Mike Keller, Renee McBride, Kiersten McBride, Chris Bedel, and Bonnie, Samantha, Josh, and Clay Martens for joining me.

Thanks to all of the naturalists, maintenance staff, law-enforcement officers, and land managers who take care of the natural areas. And thanks to all of the people who in one way or another had a hand in preserving these natural spaces.

If by some chance I haven't acknowledged your contributions, I am truly sorry and will make amends by buying you a soda pop and joining you for a hike.

To everyone who reads this book and is encouraged to take a hike, I owe you a debt of gratitude, especially if you share the wonders of nature with your children or a friend or—better yet—both!

—*Tamara York*

PS: Connect with me and other hikers at **cincyhikes.com** and **facebook.com/6060CincyHikes.**

Foreword

Welcome to Menasha Ridge Press's 60 Hikes Within 60 Miles, a series designed to provide hikers with the information they need to find and hike the very best trails surrounding metropolitan areas.

Our strategy is simple: First, find a hiker who knows the area and loves to hike. Second, ask that person to spend a year researching the most popular and very best trails around. And third, have that person describe each trail in terms of difficulty, scenery, condition, elevation change, and other categories of information that are important to hikers. "Pretend you've just completed a hike and met up with other hikers at the trailhead," we told each author. "Imagine their questions; be clear in your answers."

An experienced hiker and writer, Tamara York has selected 60 of the best hikes in and around the Greater Cincinnati area. From the urban hikes at Mount Airy Forest and Spring Grove Cemetery to the more surreal hikes of Clifty Falls State Park and Clifton Gorge State Nature Preserve, York provides hikers and walkers, as well as parents with young children, a variety of fun and interesting excursions—all within roughly 60 miles of the I-275 loop around Cincinnati.

You'll get more out of this book if you take a moment to read the Introduction, which explains how to read the trail listings. The "Topo Maps" section (pages 4–5) will help you understand how useful topos are on a hike and also will tell you where to get them. And though this is a where-to, not a how-to, guide, readers who have not hiked extensively will find the Introduction of particular value.

As much for the opportunity to free the spirit as to free the body, let these hikes elevate you above the urban hurry.

All the best,
The Editors at Menasha Ridge Press

Preface

*"Because how we spend our days is, of course,
how we spend our lives."*
—Annie Dillard

I'm not what you would expect for a hiker. I'm not a lean-mean-hiking machine, and my point is you don't need to be either to enjoy time outdoors. You just need a good pair of hiking boots, a bottle of water, this book, and time.

That is the important part—time. We all are so busy with the many tasks of daily life that we tend to put aside what is most important to us—our connections with our family, our health, and our little slice of sanity. Hiking not only burns off those chocolate chip cookies you couldn't resist, but also burns off all the electronic flotsam cluttering your mind and bogging you down. And if you hike with a loved one, it gives you time to talk and connect.

But it's hard to find the time, find the right place, find a hiking buddy, have good weather (which doesn't guarantee a great hike), or just get up the courage to try something you've never done before—even if it is something as simple as a new trail. In *60 Hikes Within 60 Miles: Cincinnati,* I've done the legwork and covered the places to go, how to get there, and how long it will take to do the hike. I also have included a list of hiking clubs so you can find hiking friends.

You'll also be happy to know that I have a severe inability to sugarcoat anything. I'll tell you exactly what to expect of the hike because that is what I would want in a guidebook. Plus, Cincinnati really isn't that big, and our paths may cross, and I won't want you chasing me down the trail yelling, "You could have mentioned the TICKS!"

Defining 60 Miles

As the crow flies, the hikes are within a 60-mile radius of I-275. Some hikes will take longer than an hour to reach.

Cincinnati Rocks

The Cincinnati area has everything from flat hikes to incredible gorge hikes and urban pathways to rugged trails. The trails pass over a unique geological formation—the

Cincinnati Arch, which is world renowned for Ordovician fossils. You'll find it is easy to get to most of the trails because Cincinnati has many major roads radiating out from the center of town, like the spokes on a bicycle wheel. Cincinnati is also the epicenter of two enormous grassroots movements: Leave No Child Inside—Greater Cincinnati and the Great Outdoor Weekend. Both are aimed at getting more people, especially kids, outdoors and enjoying the benefits of fresh air and exercise. For contact information, see Appendix C: Hiking with Children and Outdoor Programs.

Handpicked Hikes

In selecting the hikes, I used the simple criteria of "I would recommend this to my friend." I asked naturalists, parents, avid hikers, and land managers what their favorite places to hike were and why. And then I hiked the trails. Some hikes didn't make it into the book for various reasons. The 60 that did make the cut provide an opportunity for you to pack your water bottle and a snack, lace up your favorite pair of hiking boots, and reconnect with nature.

The Cincinnati area offers plenty of activities and destinations for families to enjoy. You'll find that several of the trails are easy enough to be done with little ones. Some of my family's favorite places near Cincinnati include Sharon Woods, California Woods Nature Preserve, and Cincinnati Nature Center.

In the region, Clifty Falls State Park and Clifty Canyon Nature Preserve in Indiana; Clifton Gorge State Nature Preserve in Ohio; and Blue Licks Battlefield State Resort Park in Kentucky offer incredible views and glimpses of the history of the land. You'll learn about the time when the entire area was under a great sea; when it was under a mile-thick sheet of ice; more current times when battles were fought over landownership, salt, and freedom; and about entrepreneurs who built mills along raging rivers or attempted to blast tunnels through hillsides.

The hikes range from urbanized jaunts such as Cox Arboretum MetroPark, Sugarcreek MetroPark, and Eden Park to the more rugged, less-used trails such as Wilderness Trail, Quiet Trails State Nature Preserve, and Pennywort Cliffs Preserve (which verges on woods wandering).

What Bad Weather?

In regard to the weather, I'd like to dispel the myth that you can't hike in "bad" weather. As long as it isn't dangerous weather, hiking during "bad" weather, such as a mild rain or light snowfall, provides some of the best times to hike because there are fewer people to bump into and more wildlife to see. Snow? So what? Bundle up and head out the door on any one of these hikes.

In the winter of 2008, I hiked "all alonely" (my daughter's phraseology) at Shrader–Weaver Nature Preserve and Mary Gray Bird Sanctuary when there were about 8 inches of snow on the ground and more snow was falling. These were two of my most memorable hikes. Shrader–Weaver was perfectly still, peaceful, and serene, which was only amplified by the falling snow dampening any noise. It was literally so quiet that I could hear my heart beating. Later in the day, at Mary Gray, my heart skipped a few beats when I came around a blind corner and was about 30 feet from two coyotes taking turns pouncing on something beneath the snow. Both were so busy diving into the snow and sending up plumes of snowflakes that neither noticed me for several moments. Once the coyotes spotted me, they turned and cautiously trotted away.

Oh, Find Me A Trail . . .

The hikes in this book cover three states and 25 counties. On the next page, I've divided them into smaller sections of hikes that are located close together. "60 Hikes by Category," on page xvi, sorts the hikes by their attributes and is a quick place to look for a hike that suits your needs.

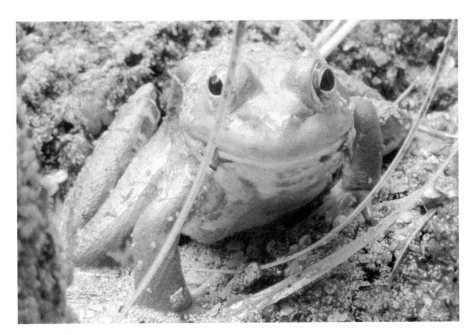

This bullfrog is guarding his territory.

Near I-275

Although the trails in and near Cincinnati are more urban, some places (such as trails at California Woods Nature Preserve, Mount Airy Forest, Caldwell Preserve, Cincinnati Nature Center, Gilmore MetroPark, and Shawnee Lookout) are fun romps through woods and wetlands. Pushing a stroller? Dragging a wagon? Eden Park, Winton Woods, Sharon Woods, and Miami Whitewater Forest have trails that are mostly paved, and sections that aren't paved are small and easily passable.

Gorgeous Little Miami River

Feel like stepping into a children's storybook? The gorge trails of Clifton Gorge State Nature Preserve and John Bryan State Park follow along the rough waters at the head of the Little Miami River. Several species of plants not typically found in this region of Ohio flourish in the gorge's cool, wet climate and add to the feel of stepping into another world—perhaps one with hobbits. Farther along the Little Miami River corridor, you'll find birding hot spots at Spring Valley Wildlife Area and Caesar Creek Gorge State Nature Preserve. Nearby, Fort Ancient's earthworks, mounds, and stone serpent effigy take you back in time a few thousand years to when the Hopewell American Indians lived in this area.

Edge of Appalachia

Step into another world at Chaparral Prairie State Nature Preserve, Adams Lake State Park, and Adams Lake Prairie State Nature Preserve. The plants found in Chaparral are remnants of what the glacier dragged in, and at Adams Lake Prairie State Nature Preserve, the scoured prairie landscape is busy with the comings and goings of thousands and thousands of Allegheny mound ants. Buzzardroost Rock Trail and Wilderness Trail weave through the woods, climb cliffs, and provide incredible vistas.

Brookville Lake Area

Seep springs, mounds, and miles of trails await at Whitewater Memorial State Park and Mounds State Recreation Area in rural Indiana. Travel a few miles north and hike the paved Cardinal Greenway through Richmond, Indiana, or head over to Hayes Arboretum and take your time strolling through the woods preferably thinking about nothing. A little to the west of Brookville Lake, you'll find my favorite hike, Shrader–Weaver Nature Preserve, near Connersville, Indiana. To the south of Connersville is birding central at Mary Gray Bird Sanctuary.

Southern Indiana

Need to recharge? Reboot? Restore? Wow! You really do need to hit the trail. To clear your mind of all the clutter, there is no better prescription than the visual therapy of the cliffs and waterfalls at Clifty Falls State Park and Clifty Canyon Nature Preserve. Muscatatuck Park, Muscatatuck National Wildlife Refuge, Hardy Lake, Versailles State Park, and Selmier State Forest are all nearby. (I'd plan on at least a day to romp around Muscatatuck National Wildlife Refuge.) If you are really looking to get lost (figure of speech), Pennywort Cliffs Preserve pushes the limits on what could be considered a trail, and maybe that is why it is a delightful hike to literally get away from it all. (Just be sure to bring a compass.)

Kentucky

In Boone County, Kentucky, trails in Middle Creek Park, Dinsmore Woods State Nature Preserve, Boone Cliffs State Nature Preserve, and Big Bone Lick State Historic Site meander through forests and back to the time of glaciers and giant sloths, and to the time of pioneers and early homesteaders. Blue Licks Battlefield State Resort Park's history includes historic battles, making salt, and bottling spring water. Nearby Quiet Trails State Nature Preserve is everything its name says it is. And for those of you who appreciate quirky humor and old-growth trees, try out the meandering nature trail at Curtis Gates Lloyd Wildlife Management Area.

Now it's time to hike! Thumb through the "60 Hikes by Category," select a hike that appeals to you, pack your water bottle, lace up your boots, and head for the trail. Who knows? We might pass each other along the way. I'll be the mom running after the two darling little girls! After all, what you decide is important is what you'll find time for.

60 Hikes by Category

Hike Categories

✓ < 2 Miles   ✓ 4–6 Miles   ✓ Kid-Friendly*   ✓ Dogs Allowed**
✓ 2–4 Miles*   ✓ >6 Miles   ✓ Portions
                                   Accessible

REGION HIKE NUMBER/HIKE NAME	page	< 2 Miles	2–4 Miles	4–6 Miles	>6 Miles	Kid-Friendly	Portions Accessible	Dogs Allowed
OHIO								
1 Adams Lake State Park and Adams Lake Prairie State Nature Preserve	18	✓				✓		
2 Beaver Creek Wildlife Area: Siebenthaler Fen	23	✓				✓	✓	✓
3 Buzzardroost Rock Preserve	28			✓				
4 Caesar Creek Gorge State Nature Preserve: Gorge Loop Trail	33	✓				✓		
5 Chaparral Prairie State Nature Preserve	38	✓				✓		
6 Chilo Lock 34 Park and Crooked Run Nature Preserve	43	✓	✓			✓		
7 Clifton Gorge State Nature Preserve	49		✓					
8 Cox Arboretum MetroPark	55		✓			✓	✓	
9 East Fork State Park: South Trail	60		✓			✓		✓
10 Edge of Appalachia Preserve: The Wilderness Trail	65		✓					
11 Fernald Preserve	70			✓		✓		
12 Fort Ancient State Memorial	76		✓					
13 Germantown MetroPark	82				✓			✓
14 Gilmore MetroPark	87		✓			✓		✓
15 Governor Bebb MetroPark and Pioneer Village	92	✓				✓		✓
16 Hueston Woods State Park	97			✓				
17 John Bryan State Park	102		✓					✓
18 Miami University Natural Areas	107			✓		✓		✓
19 Miami Whitewater Forest: Shaker Trace Outer Loop	112				✓	✓	✓	✓
20 Pyramid Hill Sculpture Park & Museum	117		✓					

REGION HIKE NUMBER/HIKE NAME	page	<2 Miles	2–4 Miles	4–6 Miles	>6 Miles	Kid-Friendly	Portions Accessible	Dogs Allowed
OHIO *(continued)*								
21 Spring Valley Wildlife Area	122		✓			✓		✓
22 Stonelick State Park	127				✓			✓
23 Sugarcreek MetroPark	132			✓		✓	✓	✓
24 Withrow Nature Preserve	138	✓	✓			✓		✓
CINCINNATI								
25 Ault Park	146		✓			✓		✓
26 Buttercup Valley Preserve and Parkers Woods	151		✓					✓
27 Caldwell Preserve	157		✓			✓		✓
28 California Woods Nature Preserve	162		✓			✓		
29 Cincinnati Nature Center's Rowe Woods	167			✓		✓	✓	✓
30 Eden Park	173		✓			✓	✓	✓
31 Mount Airy Forest: Furnas, Twin Bridge, Beechwood, Red Oak, and Ponderosa	178			✓				✓
32 Mount Airy Forest: West Fork Road, Diehl Ridge, and Elm Ravine	184	✓						✓
33 Sharon Woods	188			✓		✓	✓	✓
34 Shawnee Lookout	193		✓			✓		✓
35 Spring Grove Cemetery	198			✓			✓	
36 Winton Woods	204		✓			✓	✓	✓
INDIANA								
37 Clifty Falls State Park and Clifty Canyon Nature Preserve	210			✓				
38 Hardy Lake State Recreation Area	215		✓			✓		✓
39 Hayes Arboretum	220		✓			✓	✓	✓
40 Mary Gray Bird Sanctuary	225		✓			✓		
41 Mounds State Recreation Area	230				✓			✓
42 Muscatatuck National Wildlife Refuge: Chestnut Ridge Trail	235	✓				✓	✓	
43 Muscatatuck National Wildlife Refuge: Hunt–Richart Lake Trail	240	✓				✓		
44 Muscatatuck Park	244		✓					✓
45 Pennywort Cliffs Preserve	249		✓			✓		

Hike Categories *(continued)*

✓ < 2 Miles	✓ 4–6 Miles	✓ Kid-Friendly*	✓ Dogs Allowed**
✓ 2–4 Miles*	✓ >6 Miles	✓ Portions Accessible	

REGION HIKE NUMBER/HIKE NAME	page	< 2 Miles	2–4 Miles	4–6 Miles	>6 Miles	Kid-Friendly	Portions Accessible	Dogs Allowed
INDIANA *(continued)*								
46 Selmier State Forest	253		✓			✓		✓
47 Shrader–Weaver Nature Preserve	258		✓			✓		
48 Versailles State Park	263			✓		✓		✓
49 Whitewater Gorge: Cardinal Greenway	268				✓		✓	✓
50 Whitewater Memorial State Park	273			✓				✓
KENTUCKY								
51 Big Bone Lick State Historic Site	282			✓		✓	✓	✓
52 Blue Licks Battlefield State Resort Park	287		✓			✓		
53 Boone Cliffs State Nature Preserve	292	✓						
54 Curtis Gates Lloyd Wildlife Management Area	297	✓				✓		
55 Dinsmore Homestead and Dinsmore Woods State Nature Preserve	303	✓				✓		
56 Fort Thomas Landmark Tree Trail	308	✓				✓		
57 General Butler State Resort Park	313				✓	✓		✓
58 Kincaid Lake State Park	318		✓			✓		✓
59 Middle Creek Park	323			✓				✓
60 Quiet Trails State Nature Preserve	328	✓				✓		

More Hike Categories

✓ Geologically Rich ✓ Streams, Wet- ✓ Hills, Cliffs, and ✓ Nearly Flat
✓ Historic Interest lands, Ponds, Ravines ✓ Great Nature Centers
and Lakes ✓ Waterfalls*

REGION Hike Number/Hike Name	page	Geologically Rich	Historic Interest	Streams, Wetlands, Ponds, and Lakes	Hills, Cliffs, and Ravines	Waterfalls	Nearly Flat	Great Nature Centers
OHIO								
1 Adams Lake State Park and Adams Lake Prairie State Nature Preserve	18	✓		✓			✓	
2 Beaver Creek Wildlife Area: Siebenthaler Fen	23	✓		✓			✓	
3 Buzzardroost Rock Preserve	28	✓			✓	✓		
4 Caesar Creek Gorge State Nature Preserve: Gorge Loop Trail	33	✓		✓	✓			✓
5 Chaparral Prairie State Nature Preserve	38	✓					✓	
6 Chilo Lock 34 Park and Crooked Run Nature Preserve	43		✓	✓			✓	✓
7 Clifton Gorge State Nature Preserve	49	✓	✓	✓	✓	✓		
8 Cox Arboretum MetroPark	55	✓		✓			✓	✓
9 East Fork State Park: South Trail	60		✓	✓				
10 Edge of Appalachia Preserve: The Wilderness Trail	65	✓			✓	✓		
11 Fernald Preserve	70		✓	✓	✓			✓
12 Fort Ancient State Memorial	76		✓		✓			✓
13 Germantown MetroPark	82			✓	✓	✓		✓
14 Gilmore MetroPark	87		✓	✓			✓	
15 Governor Bebb MetroPark and Pioneer Village	92		✓	✓				
16 Hueston Woods State Park	97			✓	✓			✓
17 John Bryan State Park	102	✓	✓	✓	✓	✓		
18 Miami University Natural Areas	107			✓	✓			
19 Miami Whitewater Forest: Shaker Trace Outer Loop	112			✓			✓	✓
20 Pyramid Hill Sculpture Park & Museum	117		✓					

More Hike Categories *(continued)*

✓ Geologically Rich ✓ Streams, Wet- ✓ Hills, Cliffs, and ✓ Nearly Flat
✓ Historic Interest   lands, Ponds,   Ravines   ✓ Great Nature Centers
                      and Lakes   ✓ Waterfalls*

REGION Hike Number/Hike Name	page	Geologically Rich	Historic Interest	Streams, Wetlands, Ponds, and Lakes	Hills, Cliffs, and Ravines	Waterfalls	Nearly Flat	Great Nature Centers
OHIO *(continued)*								
21 Spring Valley Wildlife Area	122			✓			✓	
22 Stonelick State Park	127			✓				
23 Sugarcreek MetroPark	132	✓		✓	✓			
24 Withrow Nature Preserve	138		✓	✓				
CINCINNATI								
25 Ault Park	146	✓		✓	✓			
26 Buttercup Valley Preserve and Parkers Woods	151			✓	✓			
27 Caldwell Preserve	157			✓	✓			
28 California Woods Nature Preserve	162			✓	✓			✓
29 Cincinnati Nature Center's Rowe Woods	167		✓	✓	✓	✓		✓
30 Eden Park	173			✓				
31 Mount Airy Forest: Furnas, Twin Bridge, Beechwood, Red Oak, and Ponderosa	178			✓	✓			
32 Mount Airy Forest: West Fork Road, Diehl Ridge, and Elm Ravine	184			✓	✓			
33 Sharon Woods	188	✓		✓	✓	✓		✓
34 Shawnee Lookout	193	✓	✓		✓			
35 Spring Grove Cemetery	198		✓					
36 Winton Woods	204			✓				✓
INDIANA								
37 Clifty Falls State Park and Clifty Canyon Nature Preserve	210	✓	✓	✓	✓	✓		✓
38 Hardy Lake State Recreation Area	215			✓				
39 Hayes Arboretum	220			✓	✓			✓

REGION Hike Number/Hike Name	page	Geologically Rich	Historic Interest	Streams, Wetlands, Ponds, and Lakes	Hills, Cliffs, and Ravines	Waterfalls	Nearly Flat	Great Nature Centers
INDIANA *(continued)*								
40 Mary Gray Bird Sanctuary	225			✓	✓			
41 Mounds State Recreation Area	230	✓	✓	✓	✓			
42 Muscatatuck National Wildlife Refuge: Chestnut Ridge Trail	235			✓			✓	✓
43 Muscatatuck National Wildlife Refuge: Hunt–Richart Lake Trail	240			✓			✓	✓
44 Muscatatuck Park	244	✓		✓	✓			
45 Pennywort Cliffs Preserve	249			✓			✓	
46 Selmier State Forest	253						✓	
47 Shrader–Weaver Nature Preserve	258		✓	✓			✓	
48 Versailles State Park	263	✓		✓	✓			
49 Whitewater Gorge: Cardinal Greenway	268		✓	✓				
50 Whitewater Memorial State Park	273	✓		✓	✓			
KENTUCKY								
51 Big Bone Lick State Historic Site	282	✓	✓	✓	✓			
52 Blue Licks Battlefield State Resort Park	287		✓		✓			
53 Boone Cliffs State Nature Preserve	292	✓	✓		✓			
54 Curtis Gates Lloyd Wildlife Management Area	297			✓				
55 Dinsmore Homestead and Dinsmore Woods State Nature Preserve	303		✓		✓			
56 Fort Thomas Landmark Tree Trail	308				✓			
57 General Butler State Resort Park	313	✓	✓	✓	✓			
58 Kincaid Lake State Park	318			✓	✓			
59 Middle Creek Park	323			✓	✓			
60 Quiet Trails State Nature Preserve	328			✓	✓			

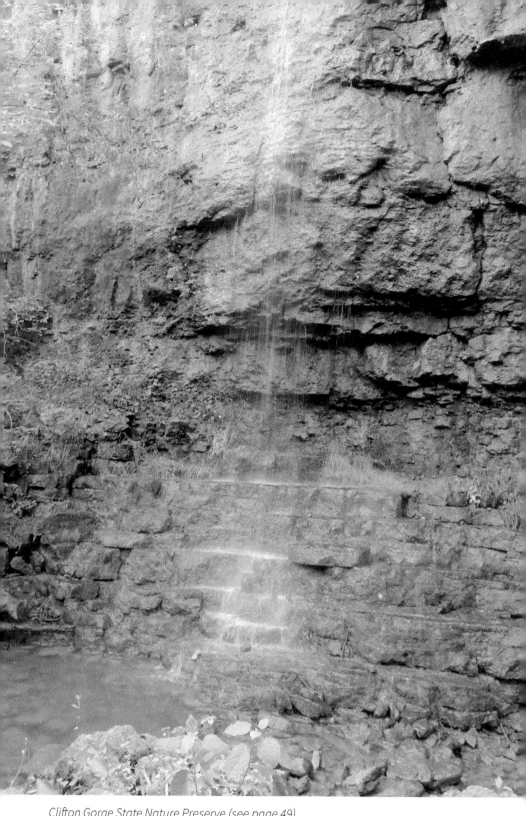

Clifton Gorge State Nature Preserve (see page 49)

Introduction

How to Use This Guidebook

Overview Map, Overview-Map Key, and Map Legend

Use the overview map on the inside front cover to assess the general locations of each hike's primary trailhead. Each hike's number appears on the overview map, on the map key facing the overview map, and in the table of contents. As you flip through the book, a hike's full profile is easy to locate by watching for the hike number at the top of each page. The book is organized by region, as indicated in the table of contents. A map legend that details the symbols found on trail maps appears on the inside back cover.

Regional Maps

The book is divided into regions. Prefacing each regional section is an overview map of that region. The regional map provides more detail than the overview map, bringing you closer to the hike.

GPS Information

To produce the highly accurate maps in this book, I used a handheld GPS unit to gather data while hiking each route, and then sent that data to Menasha Ridge Press's expert cartographers. Provided for each hike profile, the GPS coordinates—the intersection of latitude (north) and longitude (west)—will orient you from the trailhead. In some cases, you can park within viewing distance of a trailhead. Other hiking routes require a short walk to the trailhead from a parking area.

The latitude–longitude grid system is likely quite familiar to you, but here's a refresher, pertinent to visualizing the coordinates:

Imaginary lines of latitude—called *parallels* and approximately 69 miles apart from each other—run horizontally around the globe. The equator is established to be 0°, and each parallel is indicated by degrees from the equator: up to 90°N at the North Pole, and down to 90°S at the South Pole.

Imaginary lines of longitude—called *meridians*—run perpendicular to lines of latitude and are likewise indicated by degrees. Starting from 0° at the Prime Meridian in Greenwich, England, they continue to the east and west until they meet 180° later at the International Date Line in the Pacific Ocean. At the equator, longitude lines also are approximately 69 miles apart, but that distance narrows as the meridians converge toward the North and South Poles.

In this book, latitude and longitude are expressed in degree–decimal minute format. For example, the coordinates for Hike 1, Adams Lake State Park and Adams Lake Prairie State Nature Preserve (page 18), are as follows: N38° 48.794' W83° 31.296'. To convert GPS coordinates given in degrees, minutes, and seconds to degrees and decimal minutes, divide the seconds by 60. For more on GPS technology, visit **usgs.gov.**

Hike Profiles

Each hike contains seven or eight key items: an "In Brief" description of the trail, a "Key At-a-Glance Information" box, directions to the trail, GPS coordinates, a trail map, an elevation profile (if the elevation gain/loss exceeds 100 feet), and a trail description, and notes on things to see and do nearby. Combined, the maps and information provide a clear method to assess each trail from the comfort of your favorite reading chair.

Trail Maps

A detailed map of each hike's route appears with its profile. On each of these maps, symbols indicate the trailhead, the complete route, significant features, facilities, and topographic landmarks such as creeks, overlooks, and peaks.

Elevation Profiles

Each hike with an elevation gain/loss of more than 100 feet contains a detailed elevation profile that corresponds

directly to the trail map. This graphical element provides a quick look at the trail from the side, enabling you to visualize how the trail rises and falls. On the diagram's vertical axis, or height scale, the number of feet indicated between each tick mark lets you visualize the climb. To avoid making flat hikes look steep and steep hikes appear flat, varying height scales provide an accurate image of each hike's climbing challenge. Elevation profiles for loop hikes show total distance; those for out-and-back hikes show only one-way distance.

In Brief

A "taste of the trail." Think of this section as a snapshot focused on the historical landmarks, beautiful vistas, and other sights you may encounter on the hike.

Key At-a-Glance Information

The information in the "Key At-a-Glance Information" boxes gives you a quick idea of the statistics and specifics of each hike.

LENGTH & CONFIGURATION The length of the trail from start to finish (total distance traveled). There may be options to shorten or extend the hikes, but the mileage corresponds to the described hike. Consult the hike description to help decide how to customize the hike for your ability or time constraints. This line also provides a description of what the trail might look like from overhead. Trails can be loops, out-and-backs (trails on which one enters and leaves along the same path), figure eights, or a combination of shapes.

DIFFICULTY The degree of effort an "average" hiker should expect on a given hike. For simplicity, the trails are rated as "easy," "moderate," or "difficult."

SCENERY A short summary of the attractions offered by the hike and what to expect in terms of plant life, wildlife, natural wonders, and historic features.

EXPOSURE A quick check of how much sun you can expect on your shoulders during the hike.

TRAFFIC Indicates how busy the trail might be on an average day. Trail traffic, of course, varies from day to day and season to season. Weekend days typically see the most visitors. Other trail users that may be encountered on the trail are also noted here.

TRAIL SURFACE Indicates whether the trail surface is paved, rocky, gravel, dirt, boardwalk, or a mixture of elements.

HIKING TIME The length of time it takes to hike the trail. A slow but steady hiker will average 2–3 miles an hour, depending on the terrain.

DRIVING DISTANCE Indicates expected distance from an easily identified point.

SEASON Indicates whether a hike can be enjoyed year-round or only during certain times of the year.

ACCESS A notation of any fees or permits that may be needed to access the trail or park at the trailhead. Great Parks of Hamilton County, Cincinnati Nature Center, and Indiana state parks and recreation areas require a gate fee or an annual pass. If you plan to hike or visit the parks frequently each year, it is worth buying the annual pass. You can purchase the annual passes at the gates. City and county parks typically do not require any permits or parking fees. Access to the Muscatatuck National Wildlife Refuge is free. Here you'll also find information about when the trail is open.

MAPS Here you'll find a list of maps that show the topography of the trail, including site maps and USGS topo maps.

WHEELCHAIR ACCESSIBLE What to expect in terms of trail access and facilities.

FACILITIES What to expect in terms of restrooms, water, and other amenities at the trailhead or nearby.

CONTACTS Phone numbers and websites for up-to-date information on trail conditions.

COMMENTS These cover useful phone numbers and websites, advice, and tips.

GPS Trailhead Coordinates

These may be used, in conjunction with the directions to the trail, below, to ascertain exactly where the trailhead is.

Directions

Used in conjunction with the overview map, the driving directions will help you locate each trailhead. Once at the trailhead, park only in designated areas.

Description

The trail description is the heart of each hike. Here, the author provides a summary of the trail's essence and highlights any special traits the hike has to offer. The route is clearly outlined, including landmarks, side trips, and possible alternate routes along the way. Ultimately, the hike description will help you choose which hikes are best for you.

Nearby Activities

Look here for information on nearby activities or points of interest. This includes parks, museums, restaurants, or even a brewpub where you can get a well-deserved beer after a long hike. Note that not every hike has a listing.

Weather

There are two old jokes about the weather in Cincinnati. The first is that you can run the furnace and the air conditioner in the same day. The second is that if you don't like the weather—wait an hour.

Most of the year the weather is moderate—not too cold and not too hot. In early March, cold spring rains keep most people home, but this is the best time to look for wildflowers and tranquility. In summer, the temperature usually

behaves itself, and you can comfortably hike until late July. However, late July and August usually have a few sweltering days of 100°F with high humidity, which are good days to hike one of the gorge trails, especially Clifton Gorge. Fall temperatures range between 60°F and 70°F until late November, when the cold rains move in and strip off most of the leaves. Winter time—well who knows? It could be 70°F or -9°F in February but averages between 27°F and 44°F. Bad weather typically has a lead time, and if the forecasters are calling for snow, odds are 50/50 it'll snow, sleet, or rain—but not necessarily in that order.

Topo Maps

The maps in this book have been produced with great care and the assistance of a GPS unit. When used with the route directions present in each profile, the maps are sufficient to direct you to the trail and guide you on it. However, you will find superior detail and valuable information in the U.S. Geological Survey's (USGS) 7.5-minute series topographic maps.

AVERAGE DAILY TEMPERATURES BY MONTH						
	JAN	**FEB**	**MAR**	**APR**	**MAY**	**JUN**
HIGH	38°	44°	55°	66°	75°	83°
LOW	23°	27°	35°	43°	54°	62°
	JUL	**AUG**	**SEP**	**OCT**	**NOV**	**DEC**
HIGH	87°	86°	79°	67°	54°	43°
LOW	67°	65°	58°	46°	37°	27°

Topo maps are available online in many locations. At **MyTopo.com,** for example, you can view and print topos of the entire United States free of charge. Online services such as **Trails.com** charge annual fees for additional features such as shaded relief, which makes the topography stand out more. If you expect to print out many topo maps each year, it might be worth paying for shaded-relief topo maps. The downside to USGS topos is that most of them are outdated, having been created 20–30 years ago. But they still provide excellent topographic detail. Of course, **Google Earth (earth.google .com**) does away with topo maps and their inaccuracies—replacing them with satellite imagery and its inaccuracies. Regardless, what one lacks, the other augments. Google Earth is an excellent tool whether you have difficulty with topos or not.

If you're new to hiking, you might be wondering, "What's a topographic map?" In short, a topo indicates not only linear distance but also elevation, using contour lines. Contour lines spread across the map like dozens of intricate spiderwebs. Each line represents a particular elevation, and at the base of each topo a contour's interval designation is given. If the contour interval is 20 feet, then the distance between each contour line is 20 feet. Follow five contour lines up on the same map, and the elevation has increased by 100 feet.

Let's assume that the 7.5-minute series topo reads "Contour Interval 40 feet," that the short trail we'll be hiking is 2 inches in length on the map, and that it crosses five contour lines from beginning to end. What do we know? Well, because the linear scale of this series is 2,000 feet to the inch (roughly 2.75 inches representing 1 mile), we know our trail is approximately 0.8-mile long (2 inches are 4,000 feet). But we also know we'll be climbing or descending 200 vertical feet (five contour lines are 40 feet each) over that distance. And the elevation designations written on occasional contour lines will tell us if we're heading up or down.

In addition to the outdoor shops listed in Appendix A, you'll find topos at major universities and some public libraries, where you might try photocopying what you need. But if you want your own and can't find them locally, visit **national map.gov** or **store.usgs.gov.**

Water

How much is enough? Well, one simple physiological fact should convince you to err on the side of excess when deciding how much water to pack: a hiker working hard in 90-degree heat needs approximately 10 quarts of fluid per day. That's 2.5 gallons—12 large water bottles or 16 small ones. In other words, pack along one or two bottles even for short hikes.

Some hikers and backpackers hit the trail prepared to purify water found along the route. This method, while less dangerous than drinking it untreated, comes with risks. Purifiers with ceramic filters are the safest. Many hikers pack along the slightly distasteful tetraglycine–hydroperiodide tablets to debug water (sold under the names Potable Aqua, Coghlan's, and others).

Probably the most common waterborne "bug" that hikers face is *Giardia,* which may not hit until one to four weeks after ingestion. It will have you living in the bathroom, passing noxious rotten-egg gas, vomiting, and shivering with chills. Other parasites to worry about include *E. coli* and *Cryptosporidium,* both of which are harder to kill than *Giardia.*

For most people, the pleasures of hiking make carrying water a relatively minor price to pay to remain healthy. If you're tempted to drink "found water," do so only if you understand the risks involved. Better yet, hydrate prior to your hike, carry (and drink) 6 ounces of water for every mile you plan to hike, and hydrate after the hike.

Clothing

There is a wide variety of clothing from which to choose. Basically, use common sense and be prepared for anything. If all you have are cotton clothes when a sudden rainstorm comes along, you'll be miserable, especially in cooler weather. It's a good idea to carry along a light wool sweater or some type of synthetic apparel (polypropylene, Capilene, Thermax, and so on) as well as a hat.

Be aware of the weather forecast and its tendency to be wrong. Always carry

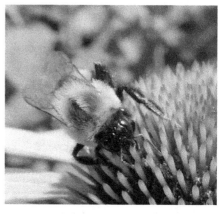

Bee on coneflower

raingear. Thunderstorms can come on suddenly in the summer. Keep in mind that rainy days are as much a part of nature as those idyllic ones you desire. Besides, rainy days really cut down on the crowds. With appropriate raingear, a normally crowded trail can be a wonderful place of solitude. Do, however, remain aware of the dangers of lightning strikes.

Footwear is another concern. Though tennis shoes may be appropriate for paved areas, some trails are rocky and rough; tennis shoes may not offer enough support. Waterproof or not, boots should be your footwear of choice. Sport sandals are more popular than ever, but these leave much of your foot exposed, leaving you vulnerable to hazardous plants and thorns or the occasional piece of glass.

The Ten Essentials

One of the first rules of hiking is to be prepared for anything. The simplest way to be prepared is to carry the "Ten Essentials." In addition to carrying the items listed below, you need to know how to use them, especially navigational items. Always consider worst-case scenarios such as getting lost, hiking back in the dark, broken gear (for example, a broken hip strap on your pack or a water filter getting plugged), a twisted ankle, or a brutal thunderstorm. The items listed below don't cost a lot of money, don't take up much room in a pack, and don't weigh much, but they might just save your life.

Water: durable bottles, and water treatment such as iodine or a filter

Map: preferably a topo map and a trail map with a route description

Compass: a high-quality compass

First-Aid Kit: a good-quality kit including first-aid instructions

Knife: a multitool device with pliers is best

Light: flashlight or headlamp with extra bulbs and batteries

Fire: windproof matches or lighter, and fire starter

Extra Food: you should always have food in your pack for when you've finished hiking

Extra Clothes: rain protection, warm layers, gloves, warm hat

Sun Protection: sunglasses, lip balm, sunblock, sun hat

First-Aid Kit

A typical first-aid kit may contain more items than you might think necessary.

These are just the basics. Prepackaged kits in waterproof bags (Atwater Carey and Adventure Medical Kits make a variety of kits) are available. Even though there are quite a few items listed here, they pack down into a small space:

➢ Ace bandages or Spenco joint wraps

➢ Antibiotic ointment (Neosporin or the generic equivalent)

➢ Aspirin or acetaminophen

➢ Band-Aids

➢ Benadryl or the generic equivalent diphenhydramine (in case of allergic reactions)

➢ Butterfly-closure bandages

➢ Epinephrine in a prefilled syringe (for people known to have severe allergic reactions to such things as bee stings)

➢ Gauze (one roll and a half dozen 4-by-4-inch pads)

➢ Hydrogen peroxide or iodine

➢ Insect repellent

➢ Matches or pocket lighter

➢ Dr. Scholl's Moleskin/Spenco 2nd Skin

➢ Sunscreen

➢ Whistle (it's more effective in signaling rescuers than your voice)

Hiking with Children

I hiked most of these hikes carrying a backpack full of supplies and a messenger bag with the GPS, equipment, and water while accompanied by my two daughters under the age of 5 (hence the full backpack). So, I know firsthand what it is like to be a busy mother trying to get her kids out in nature because it is good for them physically, mentally, and emotionally.

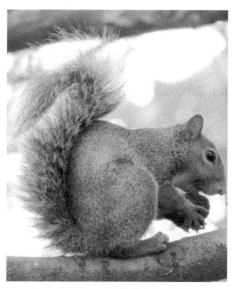

Squirrel! (Eastern gray squirrel that is.)

The benefits of children spending unstructured time in nature are enormous. By getting away from all the whiz-bang distractions of daily life, we're able to make connections with nature and, more importantly, with each other. Children who spend time in nature do better in math, science, and language arts, as well as socially. They're also typically a healthy weight. For more information on the connection between children and nature, read *Last Child in the Woods: Saving Our Children from Nature-Deficit Disorder* by Richard Louv.

My girls embrace nature and are curious about how it works. We've watched cicadas drying out on the undersides of leaves, listened to turkeys gobble, and spooked a deer or two (yes, I am convinced the deer must have been

deaf to not hear us coming). I hope my daughters have gained an appreciation for nature and someday will share their love for the outdoors with their children. And I hope you are able to share some of these simple joys with your children.

Another benefit of getting children outdoors is they gain a great deal of confidence, self-reliance, and esteem. Once, a friend's little boy tried to scare my youngest with a plastic snake. His mom laughed and said that's not going to work on her. And she was right. Madaelynne took one look at the snake and said in the I'm-not-impressed tone of a 3 year old, "That's not a *real* snake." Now my daughters are climbing trees, swinging on grapevines, walking along creek beds, and leading the hikes.

No one is too young for a hike in the outdoors. Be mindful, though. Flat, short, and shaded trails are best with an infant. Toddlers who have not quite mastered walking can ride along on an adult's back in a child carrier. Consider bringing a jogging stroller or wagon for little ones to ride in along the flat portions of the trail. Use common sense to judge a child's ability to hike a particular trail, and always plan on that child tuckering out and you carrying everything and everyone. Budget at least one hour per mile when hiking with children and opt for trails ranked easy or easy–moderate.

When packing for the hike, remember the child's needs as well as your own. Make sure children are adequately clothed for the weather, have proper shoes, and are protected from the sun and biting insects. Read the product labels and speak with your pediatrician to make sure the products are safe for children.

Kids dehydrate quickly, so have plenty of water for everyone. Make sure they drink the water slowly rather than gulping it all down at once, which can cause stomach pains.

Check into the programs at the Departments of Natural Resources in Ohio, Indiana, and Kentucky for identification guides, kids' activity pages, and clubs. Five Rivers MetroParks have a Passport to Nature program; Cincinnati Nature Center and Great Parks of Hamilton County have similar programs. Look into the area that interests you and check with the managing agency for upcoming events and programs.

So to all of the parents reading this book, I had you in mind when I selected the hikes and have included a list of hikes that are good to do with young children (see page xvi). I've also included a section on how to hike with young children (see Appendix C).

Trail Etiquette

Whether you're on a city, county, state, or national park trail, always remember that great care and resources (from nature as well as from your tax dollars) have gone into creating these trails. Treat the trail, wildlife, and fellow hikers with respect.

➢ *Hike only on open trails.* Respect trail and road closures (ask if not sure), avoid possible trespassing on private land, and obtain all permits and authorization as required. Also, leave gates as you found them or as marked.

➢ *Leave only footprints.* Be sensitive to the ground beneath you. This also means staying on the existing trail and not blazing any new trails. Be sure to pack out what you pack in. No one likes to see the trash someone else has left behind. If you do find trash and it is safe for you to remove, then pack it out.

➢ *Never spook animals.* An unannounced approach, a sudden movement, or a loud noise startles most animals. A surprised animal can be dangerous to you, to others, and to itself. Give plenty of space.

➢ *Plan ahead.* Know your equipment, your ability, and the area in which you are hiking—and prepare accordingly. Be self-sufficient at all times; carry necessary supplies for changes in weather or other conditions. A well-executed trip is a satisfaction to you and to others.

➢ *Be courteous to hikers,* bikers, equestrians, and others you encounter on the trails.

General Safety and Captain Cautious

No doubt, potentially dangerous situations can occur outdoors, but as long as you use sound judgment and prepare yourself before hitting the trail, you'll be much safer in the woods than in most urban areas of the country. Before you leave to go on a hike, always call the location first to access the trail conditions.

Trails might be closed due to damage from emerald ash borers, slides, flooding, or general maintenance. Here are a few tips to make your trip safer and easier.

- Be careful at overlooks. While these areas may provide spectacular views, they are potentially hazardous. Stay back from the edge of outcrops and be absolutely sure of your footing; a misstep can mean a nasty and possibly fatal fall.

- Standing dead trees and storm-damaged living trees pose a real hazard to hikers and tent campers. These trees may have loose or broken limbs that could fall at any time. When choosing a spot to rest, look up.

- Take along your brain. A cool, calculating mind is the single most important piece of equipment you'll ever need on the trail. Think before you act. Watch your step. Plan ahead. Avoiding accidents before they happen is the best recipe for a rewarding and relaxing hike.

- Ask questions. Park employees are there to help. It's a lot easier to gain advice beforehand and avoid a mishap away from civilization when it's too late to amend an error. Use your head out there and treat the place as if it were your own backyard.

- Always tell at least two "keepers" (people you trust) where you are hiking, and text them at regular intervals to let them know of your progress. Why two? One will likely get distracted and forget they are supposed to be your safety net.

- Never tell someone you meet on the trail that you are hiking alone. Always be hiking with "someone who is a little ahead of you or is catching up."

- Know when sundown and nightfall occur, and plan to be out of the woods prior to nightfall. If you get delayed and you are hiking in the dark, go slowly and use your flashlight intermittently to see the trail.

Animal and Plant Hazards

American Black Bears

American black bears have been seen in Kentucky and Ohio. The sightings are most likely bachelor bears (young males) finding their way to new territory. However, I feel it necessary to provide you with some practical advice on bears. If you see one, leave it alone and give it plenty of room to escape. Wild bears don't want to have contact with humans—that's why it is important not to feed a bear. Once a bear associates humans with food, conflicts arise, and the bear will need to be dispatched. For more information on black bears and sightings, review the information provided online by the Ohio Department of Natural Resources Division of Wildlife and the Kentucky Department of Fish and Wildlife Resources.

Ticks

Ticks like to hang out in the brush and tall grasses that grow along trails. Hot and damp summer months seem to explode their numbers, but you should be tick-aware year-round. Ticks, which are arthropods and not insects, need a host to feast on in order to reproduce. The ticks that attach to you while hiking will be very small, sometimes so tiny that you won't be able to spot them. Primarily of two varieties, deer ticks and dog ticks, both need a few hours of actual attachment before they can transmit any disease they may harbor. Ticks may settle in shoes, socks, clothing, and hats, and may take several hours to actually latch on. The best strategy is to do a tick check—a visual check—every half hour or so while hiking. Check the insides of pant legs, seam lines, waistbands, under straps, hairlines, and along the edges of hats. Complete another thorough check before you get in the car, put all of your gear into a trash bag and tie it shut, and then, when you take a post-hike shower, complete an even more thorough check of your entire body, including your navel and ears.

Ticks that haven't attached are easily removed but not easily killed. If you pick off a tick in the woods, just toss it aside. If you find one on your body at home, dispatch it and then send it down the toilet. For ticks that have embedded, removal with tweezers is best. Grasp the tick with the tweezers as close to the skin as possible. Apply steady pressure and pull the tick straight out. If you twist or jerk the tick, the mouthparts might remain under the skin. After removal, disinfect the bite mark, wash your hands with soap and water, and treat the bite mark with a topical antibiotic.

Once you are done with your shower, place your hiking clothes and the contents of the plastic trash bag in the bathtub. The post-shower heat of the tub will typically draw the ticks away from your stuff as you check through your belongings. The brown-colored ticks stand in sharp relief to a white bathtub, making them easy to spot and remove.

Mosquitoes

Although it's not a common occurrence, individuals can become infected with the West Nile virus by being bitten by an infected mosquito. *Culex* mosquitoes, the primary variety that can transmit West Nile virus to humans, thrive in urban rather than natural areas. They lay their eggs in stagnant water and can breed in any standing water that remains for more than five days. Most people infected with West Nile virus have no symptoms of illness, but some may become ill, usually 3–15 days after being bitten.

Anytime you expect mosquitoes to be buzzing around, you may want to wear protective clothing, such as long sleeves, long pants, and socks. Loose-fitting, light-colored clothing is best. Spray clothing with insect repellent. Remember to follow the instructions on the repellent and to take extra care with children.

Chiggers

Chiggers are parasitic mite larvae found on tall grass or other vegetation. They wait for passing hosts, attach themselves to a skin pore or hair follicle, and inject a digestive enzyme that ruptures the cells, causing itchy red bumps that last for several days. Chiggers are too small to be seen with the naked eye. They are most commonly found in damp areas with a lot of vegetation. On hosts they prefer to attach to skin under tight clothing, such as socks and underwear, or in concealed areas of the body, such as the groin and the armpits. One way to decrease the chance of chigger bites is to wear loose clothing when you're in the woods or other infested areas. You should also take a shower as soon as you get home from an outdoor expedition to remove any chiggers before they attach to your skin. Keep the irritated area clean and refrain from scratching. To relieve itching use a salve or cream that contains antihistamines (Caladryl or hydrocortisone salves are the most common). These will also help prevent infection. If the welts continue to irritate you for more than a couple of weeks, they might be infected and you should see a doctor.

Emerald Ash Borer

The emerald ash borer (*Agrilus planipennis*) is an exotic insect native to Asia that is currently threatening and killing thousands of ash trees. The pest can be spread inadvertently in infested firewood, and most parks have strict rules about what wood you can bring into the park. By following some simple rules, you can help prevent the spread of these destructive insects, as well as the spread of other wood-boring beetles. Purchase aged firewood near your campsite location; don't bring it from home. Many parks offer firewood at reasonable prices, and it is often available from private sellers just outside the parks. Firewood purchased at or near your destination should be used during your camping trip; don't take any to another destination. Buy wood that has no bark or loose bark (a sign the

wood is very dry). This will reduce the chances of infestation while also making your fire easier to start.

Snakes

Several snakes are found throughout the tristate region, but only three are poisonous. The northern copperhead is found in Kentucky and southern Indiana. The timber rattlesnake is found in southern Indiana. The eastern massasauga is found in a small region in Ohio.

Odds are you'll never see one of these snakes, and you can increase the chance of avoiding them by not reaching under or blindly stepping over logs or rocky outcrops. Don't go off-trail, and watch where you are stepping. If you do come across a

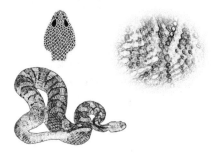

RATTLESNAKE

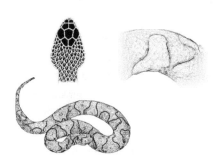

COPPERHEAD

rattlesnake, give it plenty of room to escape and don't hang around.

Poison Ivy

Leaves of three, leave it be. Poison ivy grows anywhere and on anything. The terminal buds of poison ivy are powdery looking and a mustard-yellow color. Leaves range from dark green to chartreuse. Be wary of the vines growing up the trunks of trees. The vines send out roots that appear hairy. The best way to prevent getting the itchy rash is to avoid contact with any part of the plant. If you do get into poison ivy, wash your skin immediately and repeatedly with cold water and soap. Urushiol, the oil in the sap of poison ivy, is responsible for the rash. Usually within 12–14 hours of exposure (but sometimes much later), raised lines and/or blisters will appear, accompanied by a terrible itch. Refrain from scratching because bacteria under fingernails can cause infection. Wash and dry the rash thoroughly, applying a calamine lotion or other product to help dry the rash. If you get the oil near your eyes, nose, or mouth, or the itching or blistering is severe, seek medical attention. Remember that oil-contaminated clothes,

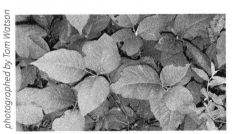

photographed by Tom Watson

pets, or hiking gear can easily cause an irritating rash on you or someone else, so wash not only any exposed parts of your body but also clothes, gear, and pets.

Stinging Nettles

Stinging nettles are common in disturbed areas, moist woodlands, and partially shaded trails. The toothed leaves are oval, ribbed, opposite, and covered with "hairs." When you brush past stinging nettles, sharp, tiny spines covering the leaves and stems penetrate your skin and release histamine and formic acid. The result is an itchy rash relieved only with hydrocortisone creams and cool compresses.

Tips For Enjoying Your Hike

Consider a couple tips that will make your hike enjoyable and more rewarding:

➢ Take your time along the trails. Pace yourself for the longer hikes. The forests, fields, and wetlands of the tristate region are filled with wonders both big and small. Keep watch on the ground for box turtles, blue-lined skinks, and butterflies. Stop and enjoy the delicate blooms of trout lilies. Imagine what the day was like when that enormous mass of stone fell into the valley. Enjoy listening to the banter of birds, the calm of a pine stand, or the wind at an overlook. Shorter hikes allow you to stop and linger more than long hikes. Take close notice of the elevation maps that accompany each hike. If you see many ups and down over large altitude changes, you'll obviously need more time. Inevitably you'll finish some of the hike times long before or after what is suggested. Nevertheless, leave yourself plenty of time for those moments when you simply feel like stopping and taking it all in and letting it all out.

➢ We can't always schedule our free time when we want, but try to hike during the week and avoid the traditional holidays if possible. Trails that are packed in the summer are often clear during the colder months. If you are hiking on a busy day, go early in the morning; it'll enhance your chances of seeing wildlife. The trails really clear out during rainy times; however, don't hike during a thunderstorm. Hiking in winter is also a good time to have the trail all to yourself. The best times to hike are after a snow and during a fall of fluffy snow, which muffles the noises of daily life and lets you enjoy a few moments of serenity. (Just remember to turn off the cell phone.)

➢ Participate in some online wildlife observation counts. Cornell Lab of Ornithology operates **ebird.org,** where you can log in for free and submit your bird lists from your hikes or find out what's being seen at some of the area's birding hot spots. A similar count is being done for butterflies by the North American Butterfly Association at **naba.org.** In Ohio, you can volunteer for the Frog and Toad Calling Survey at **ohioamphibians. com.** If you have a favorite hiking location, speak with the property manager or naturalist to see if they need assistance conducting counts.

Put Your Money Where Your Feet Go

People devoted to nature and sharing it with others are a unique group. They work for little compensation, often pay for supplies out of their own pockets, work extra hours (without pay) so the job is done right, and always strive to improve. Without their zest for all things outdoorsy, we wouldn't be so fortunate to have such wonderful hiking destinations.

If you enjoy hiking, I encourage you to support the parks, nature preserves, and natural areas you love. State and county nature preserves and parks are funded by general revenues. Each time the government decides to cut the budget, nature preserves and parks are first on the chopping block. The continual slashing of their budgets means that they're left working with ridiculously old equipment that they are unable to replace when it breaks. They also have less funding for maintenance, law enforcement, and naturalist personnel. Plus, they lack the funds to purchase critical habitat.

You are the key to helping parks and nature preserves become self-sufficient and immune to the general-revenue-funding decision makers. Besides telling lawmakers you don't want to see the budgets of natural areas, parks, or nature preserves cut, you can make a direct and most likely tax-deductible donation to the managing agency or join a "friends of" group. Talk to the area manager to find out more about how you can help the natural spaces you love.

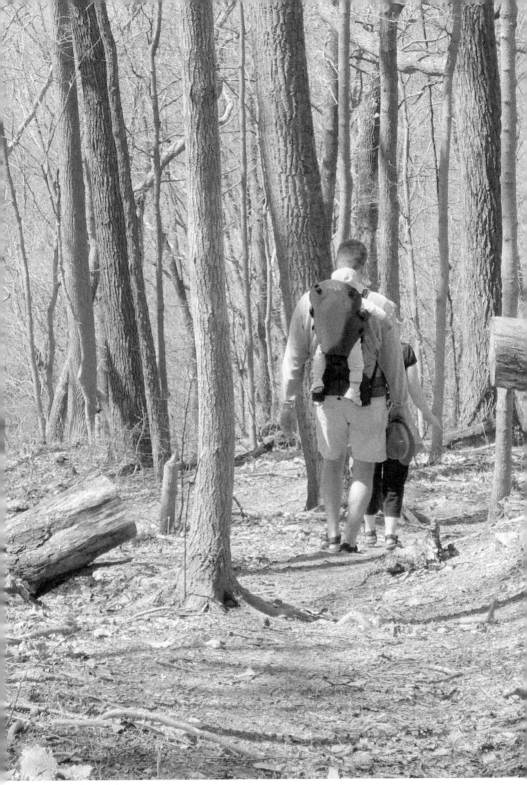

Family on hike

OHIO

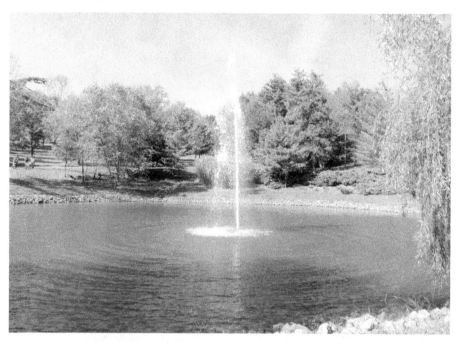

Pyramid Hill Sculpture Park & Museum (see page 117)

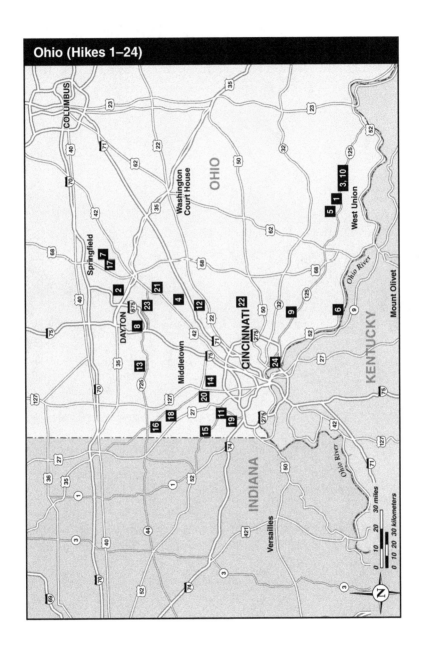

Ohio (Hikes 1–24)

1 Adams Lake State Park and Adams Lake Prairie State Nature Preserve

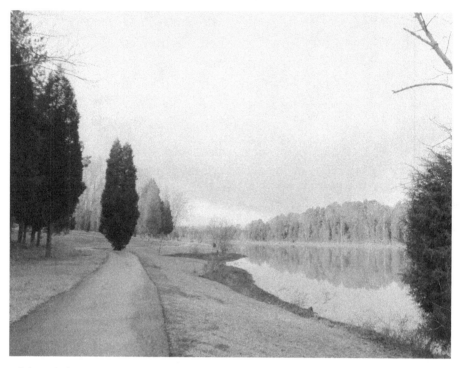

Adams Lake

In Brief

The hike starts lakeside and then enters the unique xeric prairie and oak forest. Adams County has a rich geological history, of which a small portion is visible on the nature preserve portion of the hike.

Description

This small state park offers a variety of activities, including hiking, fishing, picnicking, and enjoying the playground areas.

When you enter the park you'll see a small parking area to your right. Park in this area, secure your vehicle, and walk toward the boat ramp. On the other side of the ramp, a large boulder marks the beginning of the trail.

18

LENGTH & CONFIGURATION 1.9-mile balloon	**MAPS** USGS *West Union;* Adams Lake State Park map and Adams Lake Prairie State Nature Preserve map
DIFFICULTY Easy	
SCENERY Lake, xeric prairie, and Allegheny mound ants	**WHEELCHAIR ACCESSIBLE** Lake Trail
	FACILITIES Water fountains, restrooms, picnic benches, and shelters
EXPOSURE Sun	
TRAFFIC Moderate	**CONTACTS** Ohio Department of Natural Resources, Shawnee State Park, 740-858-6652; **parks.ohiodnr.gov/adamslake** or **tinyurl.com/adamslakenp**
TRAIL SURFACE Paved and gravel	
HIKING TIME 1–1.5 hours	
DRIVING DISTANCE Less than 10 minutes north of West Union	**COMMENTS** Don't mess with the ants! Bring sunscreen and identification books for trees and prairie plants. Includes Lake, Prairie Dock, and Post Oak hikes.
SEASON Year-round	
ACCESS Daily, sunrise–sunset; free	

Eastern red cedars do very well in the limestone soils abundant in Adams County. In fact, the eastern red cedar is the backbone of a thriving business community that uses the red cedar wood to create bird feeders and birdhouses.

The Adams Lake State Park Trail is the first trail on this hike. The paved trail borders the lake and is wide enough for two people to comfortably walk side by side. As at most parks in southern Ohio, Canada geese are everywhere. You'll readily see geese and other waterfowl species along the shoreline. Please do not feed the waterfowl; it is unhealthy for both birds and humans.

The paved trail was created in 1999 with Nature Works funding from the Ohio Department of Natural Resources (ODNR). Look for a playground area shortly after you start, at 0.1 mile. If you like to fish, consider an afternoon relaxing along the lake's edge on one of the many benches overlooking the water.

You'll find red oaks, horseshoe pits, and a pavilion area at 0.37 mile. Cross the bridge over a small creek at 0.45 mile. The trail exits into an open area that is the turnaround for the road. Continue to your left and walk along the edge of the woods. On the right side of the road at 0.6 mile, you'll see the trail that leads to the entrance of the nature preserve trail.

The Adams Lake Prairie State Nature Preserve's formal entrance, complete with an information kiosk, is at 0.87 mile. The gravel-covered trail leads uphill over several erosion-control steps. The ODNR Division of Natural Areas and Preserves maintains the xeric prairie area via prescribed burning every two to three years. The prescribed burns remove the plant competition for sunlight and other resources. The prairie plants in this

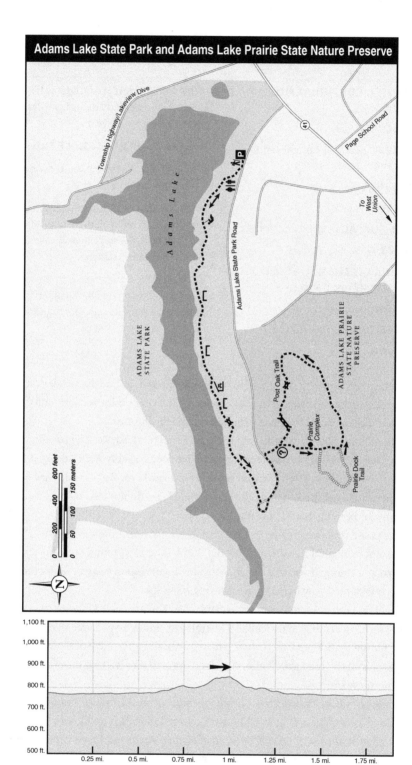

Adams Lake State Park and Adams Lake Prairie State Nature Preserve

area must have full sun to survive. Fire is simply used as a tool to remove saplings and brush that would shade out the sun-loving prairie plants, eventually killing them.

One of the most unusual things you'll see on this trail are Allegheny mound ants. When they bite, the ants' formidable mandibles (jaws) secrete formic acid. That's reason enough to stay on the trail. The mounds are impressive structures about 2.5 feet tall and 3 feet in circumference at the base. The ants typically won't bother people as long as their mound is not disturbed. I'm strongly in favor of erring on the side of caution though, so I don't stand too near an ant mound just in case the ants decide I'm disturbing it. But do spend some time watching these fascinating creatures go about their day.

The plants that you see in this area migrated to Ohio when the climate was much warmer and drier than it is today. Many are species of concern in Ohio and survive only in isolated areas where conditions favor drought-resistant species. Some of the plants in this unique prairie area include blazing star, American aloe, and rattlesnake master.

When you come to the trail junction a few feet beyond the kiosk, bear right onto Prairie Dock Trail. As you enter into the prairie area, you'll see plenty of prairie dock. This plant has large leaves and several yellow, daisylike flowers at the top of the naked stalk it sends up. You'll find a boardwalk 0.9 mile into the hike, after which the trail narrows to allow only single-file hiking. Look for the brilliant red blooms of blazing stars in this area. Within 200 feet of the first boardwalk is a second one.

This prairie area might look barren, but a complex system of life, death, and bartering occurs here. The small Edwards' hairstreak butterfly has an interesting relationship with the Allegheny mound ants. Edwards' hairstreak larvae produce a honeylike substance relished by Allegheny mound ants, so much so that the ants will act as bodyguards to protect the larvae from predators. The Edwards' hairstreak is susceptible to attack from a small parasitic insect, but with the ants on guard, the larvae can survive and eventually become butterflies.

The ant mounds can reach nearly a yard high, with summertime populations of 100,000 workers per mound. Some of the mounds on this prairie area are more than 20 years old. Once again, please do not disturb them.

At the next trail intersection, follow the Post Oak Trail to the right and into the woods. Ohio is home to 15 species of oaks, of which 14 can be found in Adams County, including blackjack, shingle, and post oak. The area where you're hiking was once heavily forested, but the need for weapons during the War of 1812 resulted in the iron industry consuming the trees. In fact, during that era, 1–2 acres of forest were cut down each day just to operate one iron furnace.

Be careful crossing the footbridges as some of them are exceedingly slippery, especially if there are fallen leaves covering the mossy wood. Cross a footbridge at 1.31 miles and slow down to enjoy the trail as it meanders through this beautiful oak forest.

You'll see a mix of young and older saplings, as well as canopy trees, but sugar maples are beginning to take over the forest.

Be careful of your footing as you cross several footbridges before crossing a bridge at 1.4 miles and heading uphill, where you will see a large white oak tree. When the trail joins itself turn right to follow it to the kiosk you encountered earlier. Cross the street and return to the paved trail that borders the lake and will lead you back to your vehicle.

Nearby Activities

The Adams County area has several Amish shops, which sell everything from well-crafted furniture to cinnamon rolls. If you go Saturday morning you can score some cinnamon-caramel donuts from the local Amish bakeries. You'll need to spend the remainder of the day hiking off the extra calories (completely worth it) so you might also like the Wilderness Trail and Buzzardroost Rock Trail.

GPS Trailhead Coordinates and Directions

N38° 48.794'   W83° 31.296'

From West Union, take OH 41 North less than 2 miles to the entrance of Adams Lake State Park and Adams Lake Prairie State Nature Preserve. The entrance to the park is on the left side of the road. Park your vehicle in the area near the boat ramp.

2 Beaver Creek Wildlife Area:
Siebenthaler Fen

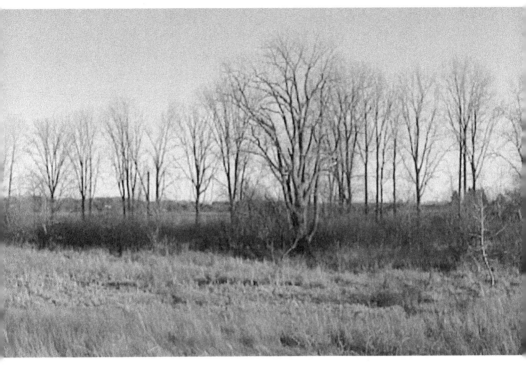

Vista of the wetland complex from the observation tower

In Brief

Beaver Creek Wildlife Area is home to the unique Siebenthaler Fen. The wetland complex serves as a resting spot for migrating waterfowl and Neotropical migrants. The boardwalk allows visitors a chance to explore the wetlands without getting soaked.

Description

The Beaver Creek Wetlands Association's (BCWA) hard work over several years has pulled together different people and organizations to protect vital wetland habitat. By working in partnerships, BCWA helped protect hundreds of acres of wetlands along the Big and Little Beaver Creeks east of Fairborn, Ohio, from development.

LENGTH & CONFIGURATION 1-mile balloon	**MAPS** USGS *Beaver Creek*
DIFFICULTY Easy	**WHEELCHAIR ACCESSIBLE** Boardwalk is accessible, but a gravel/grass area near the kiosk might not be passable for wheelchairs.
SCENERY Woods, wet woods, creek, and floodplain	
EXPOSURE Shaded and full sun	**FACILITIES** None
TRAFFIC Moderate–heavy	**CONTACTS** Ohio Department of Natural Resources Division of Wildlife, 937-372-9261; **wildlife.ohiodnr.gov/beavercreek** or **beavercreekwetlands.org**
TRAIL SURFACE Boardwalk, gravel, and grass	
HIKING TIME 30 minutes	
DRIVING DISTANCE 1.25 hours north of Cincinnati	**COMMENTS** Beaver Creek Wildlife Area is just one part of a wonderful wetland complex supporting an array of waterfowl, songbirds, and butterflies. A shallow water aquifer feeds the Siebenthaler Fen.
SEASON Year-round	
ACCESS Daily, sunrise–sunset; free	

Beaver Creek Wetland Complex locations with trails include Fairborn Marsh, Beaver Creek Wetlands Wildlife Area off New Germany–Trebein Road, Greene County Park Beaver Creek Wetland Nature Preserve, and Siebenthaler Fen in the Beaver Creek Wildlife Area off Fairgrounds Road. We're hiking the Siebenthaler Fen portion of the wetland complex.

Beaver Creek Wildlife Area was purchased by the Ohio Department of Natural Resources (ODNR) Division of Wildlife with the assistance of BCWA and The Nature Conservancy. There are multiple benches throughout this hike to stop and take in the scenery. You can see the evidence of beaver activity along the edge of the creek.

The wetland area includes five of the six wetland types found in Ohio. The most important is the fen portion of the Beaver Creek wetland corridor, which may have been related to the preglacial Teays River.

Siebenthaler Fen is unique in that cool water from a shallow aquifer constantly flows to the surface. This aquifer flows through water-bearing gravel deposited 15,000 years ago when the Wisconsin glacier receded.

The ODNR Division of Wildlife's objective for the 380-acre wetland complex is "to protect, preserve, restore, and enhance wetlands, and improve and protect habitat for nesting and migratory wetland wildlife species."

The accessible boardwalk begins in the northeast corner of the parking lot off of Fairgrounds Road. But before you begin this hike, I highly advise the liberal use of insect repellent. The beginning of the hike is shaded, but the midpoint is in full sun, so you should use sunscreen as well.

Beaver Creek Wildlife Area: Siebenthaler Fen

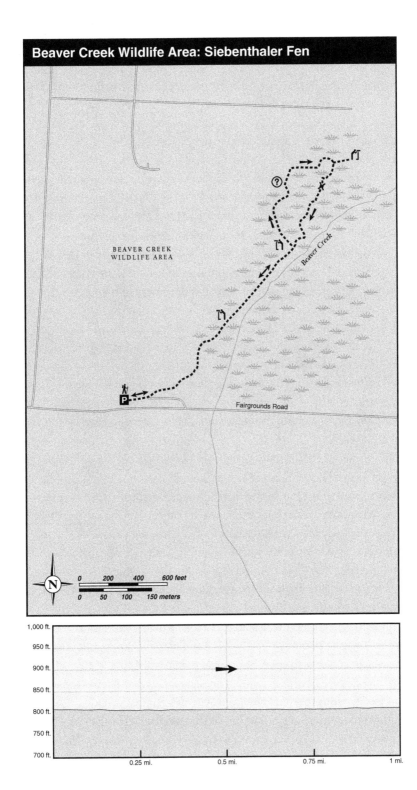

BEAVER CREEK
WILDLIFE AREA

Beaver Creek

Fairgrounds Road

| 0 | 200 | 400 | 600 feet |
| 0 | 50 | 100 | 150 meters |

N

1,000 ft.
950 ft.
900 ft.
850 ft.
800 ft.
750 ft.
700 ft.

0.25 mi.　　　0.5 mi.　　　0.75 mi.　　　1 mi.

Wetlands are the most biologically diverse habitats, both in flora and fauna. Step onto the boardwalk and enter this wet woods. At the junction of the two entrances is an abundance of gray dogwoods. Larger cottonwood, sycamore, and box elder trees act as climbing towers for Virginia creeper and poison ivy.

The sounds of the wetlands dominate urban noise. Expect to see songbirds flitting among the tree branches. Tune into the cacophony of natural sounds and quietly listen for nuthatches, woodpeckers, warblers, and flycatchers, as well as a plethora of frogs. A good spot to stop and call "pssh" to attract birds is at 0.17 mile. More than 470 wetland species have been identified at this incredible wetland complex.

Stay on the raised boardwalk and move silently along so you can view as much wildlife as possible. Don't leave the boardwalk—some of these areas are deeper than they appear. (The water might not be deep, but the mucky bottom is.)

At 0.2 mile is a small side area to step off the main boardwalk. Look for spotted jewelweed, skunk cabbage, and sedges along the sides of the boardwalk.

Continue along the boardwalk, passing the cottonwood trees girdled by beaver at 0.27 mile. Beaver girdle trees by gnawing through the cambium (growing layer) of bark. This prevents nutrients from flowing between the leaves and the roots, killing the tree. Spring, cricket, green, and chorus frogs dominate the natural sounds. Cricket frogs sound like marbles clicking together or a Geiger counter—just depends on your previous experience.

At the intersection at 0.3 mile, take the trail to the left and enter the open wetland area. Sweet flag and common cattail border the trail.

The boardwalk along this side of the hike might be a little squishy at times, especially if there has been a lot of rain. If it has been raining, expect portions of the boardwalk to be partially flooded but still passable—your feet might get a little wet.

My favorite time to visit this wetland is during a rainfall, especially if has rained earlier in the week. Why? Not many people willingly hike when it is raining; wildlife is more active; and the rain dampens (no pun intended) sound, so it is easier to pass quietly along the boardwalk and observe wildlife.

The boardwalk was built with about a 1-inch lip on the sides. During rainy weather the crayfish climb out of the wetland and onto the boardwalk. They cannot, for the most part, manage to escape back over the lip and into the safety of the wetland. This makes them easy prey for hungry raccoons, as I have observed on multiple occasions while getting thoroughly soaked by a springtime shower.

Another observation area at 0.34 mile is surrounded by marsh marigolds and great angelica. In warm weather, expect to see several species of butterflies, skippers, and dragonflies.

You'll reach one of my favorite spots at 0.37 mile. Here you'll see queen of the prairie and elderberry everywhere. Red-winged blackbirds and goldfinches dominate the air and use the cattails as vantage points to defend their territories.

The kiosk is located at 0.42 mile. The identification photos on the kiosk help identify the species of plants, dragonflies, and birds seen in the wetland complex.

After the kiosk, continue on the trail. At the curve at 0.5 mile, be sure to look for frogs and turtles. Immediately after this you'll come upon the observation tower. The tower is tall enough to enable you to view the fen and the wildlife common to this wetland.

The bridge at 0.6 mile passes over a small stream. The water is always cool, but it does not freeze. Look on the stream bottom to the left of the bridge; you'll see white flecks of marl, or calcium carbonate.

The trail loops back on itself at 0.68 mile. Continue on the raised boardwalk until you reach the parking area.

Nearby Activities

To the north, off New Germany–Trebein Road, is the north entrance to the Beaver Creek Wildlife Area. Here, you'll have access via primitive trails to a wet forest and restored seasonal marsh. If you're hungry, there are several restaurants in Xenia and Beavercreek. The National Museum of the United States Air Force is located at nearby Wright–Patterson Air Force Base.

GPS Trailhead Coordinates and Directions

N39° 44.292'   W84° 00.770'

From Cincinnati, take I-75 North to Exit 43/Columbus onto I-675 North. Travel 13 miles to Exit 13A/Xenia. Travel 3.7 miles on US 35 East and turn left onto Factory Road and when it ends turn right onto County Road 142/Dayton–Xenia Road. Turn left onto Beaver Valley Road and travel 1.6 miles to Fairground Road. Turn right onto Fairground Road. The entrance to the wildlife area is on the north side of the road.

3 Buzzardroost Rock Preserve

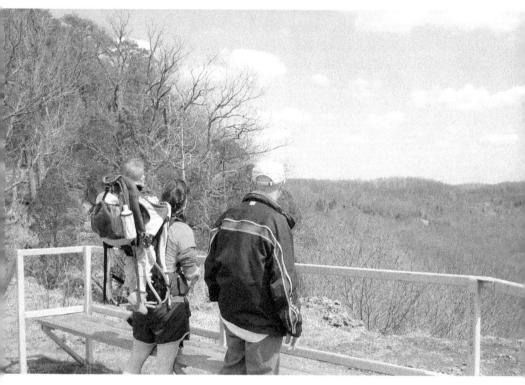

Bird's-eye view at the highest point of Buzzardroost Rock outcrop

In Brief

As you hike from the lowest point in this hike to the highest, you'll pass through several different habitats including old field, prairies, and mature woods. Plan extra time to enjoy the view from the overlook area; you'll have earned it.

Description

Before you start hiking, make sure you have plenty of water, a snack for later, good identification books, and a camera. From the parking lot, look across the drive and to the right for the trail entrance. The singletrack meanders through a meadow before crossing a footbridge and entering the woods at 0.1 mile.

Buzzardroost Rock Preserve is owned and managed by The Nature Conservancy and the Cincinnati Museum of Natural History. The area was opened to the public in

LENGTH & CONFIGURATION 4.63-mile out-and-back	**ACCESS** Daily, sunrise–sunset; free
DIFFICULTY Moderate	**MAPS** USGS *Brush Creek;* Cincinnati Museum of Natural History, Buzzardroost Rock Trail map
SCENERY Woods, cliffs, and overlook	
EXPOSURE Shaded and full sun	**WHEELCHAIR ACCESSIBLE** No
TRAFFIC Moderate–heavy	**FACILITIES** None
TRAIL SURFACE Bare soil, grass, shale, dolomites	**CONTACTS** Cincinnati Museum Center, 513-287-7000; **cincymuseum.org/nature**
HIKING TIME 3–3.5 hours	**COMMENTS** New entrance location. The climb to the overlook is steep. If you are hiking with young children, keep them close to you along the cliff line and overlook.
DRIVING DISTANCE Less than 10 minutes east of West Union	
SEASON Year-round	

1967 and the trail was dedicated in memory of siblings Christian and Emma Goetz, who were instrumental in the creation of nature preserves in Adams County.

Buzzardroost Rock Preserve's trail receives a fair amount of foot traffic. In fact, every time I've visited this unique location, whether it has been snowing or is sweltering hot, I've met plenty of other hikers.

The new trail to Buzzardroost Rock overlook offers plenty of geology, including Lilley–Bisher Dolomite, Peebles Dolomite, and black Ohio Shale. This unique geological area is also home to at least 67 species of land snail. Granted, some of them are so tiny that you could fit several dozen on the head of a penny, but they are there—lurking close to the calcium-rich cliffs.

The land snails lose the race to the diversity and abundance of lichens. Records show 160 species of lichens. You can find lichens growing on the trees and ground as well as on almost any available rock. Look for green shield, speckled shield, ruffle, and reindeer lichens.

Another field that excels in diversity, in Buzzardroost as well as Adams County, is the prairie with 1,170 plant species identified. You'll want to bring a several field guides with you and plan extra time to discover and explore.

Back to the trail, the creek bed to your right is composed of Lilley–Bisher and Peebles Dolomites (Silurian age). The trail follows an old roadbed and to the right is the edge of the Appalachian escarpment. Pass the xeric limestone prairie and borrow pit (an excavated area) at 0.27 mile.

Cross the footbridge over the ephemeral creek and notice the younger forest comprised of red cedar, black locust, Virginia pine, sugar maples, tulip poplar, and

Buzzardroost Rock Preserve

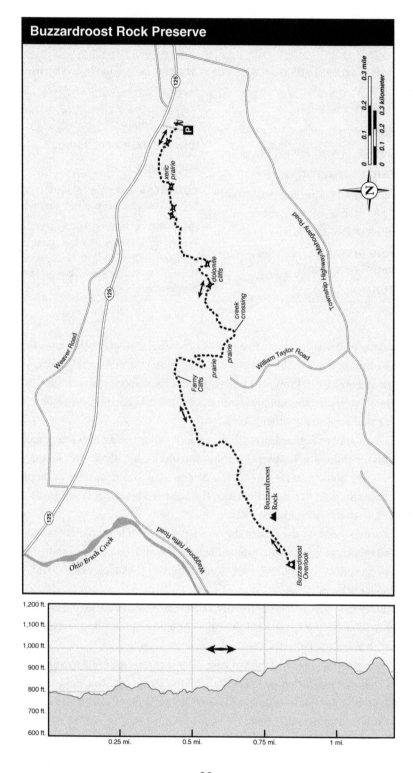

plenty of American beech saplings. Larger trees don't last long in this thin soil as there isn't much earth for the roots to grow into before hitting bedrock. A top-heavy tree, a shallow root structure, and a strong wind are all that is needed to topple some trees.

Cross the footbridge at 0.37 mile and the dynamic of the forest shifts to a slightly older forest with white and chinquapin oaks and shagbark hickories. Before the next footbridge, you can readily see the Lilley–Bisher Dolomite. At 0.5 mile the trail heads uphill and has great views of Brush Creek Valley. This is a good spot to listen for pine warblers.

Right before you cross the footbridge at 0.68 mile, look for the tree with bark that resembles alligator skin. Ta-da! Persimmon tree. The creek flows over where the Peebles and Lilley–Bisher Dolomites meet. Lilley–Bisher is the lower one with rust and yellow tones.

The trail leads into an American beech–dominated woods. After crossing the footbridge at 0.8 mile, peer left uphill and see the dolomite cliffs. Continue following the trail as it slowly leads you uphill and across a stream.

Along this portion of the trail and across the creek to your right, you can see water seeping out of the dolomite. In winter the sides of the cliff are covered with frozen seeps. Farther up the trail and to your right look for the waterfall. It may be hard to see when the leaves are on the trees. The edge of the falls is Lilley–Bisher and the underside is fragile Estill Shale (Silurian age) that the water is carving out.

At 1.06 miles, cross the creek that feeds the falls. Walking down an unfamiliar creek bed is unwise because not only is it is difficult to see where the drop-offs are, but you also could easily walk onto a shelf of rock primed to break away.

The forest opens into a prairie that has several seasonal creeks running through it. As you come up the hill, look for a clump of sycamore trees; nearby are Virginia pines. Watch and listen for song and field sparrows, as well as indigo buntings and prairie warblers. The scrubby area, near 1.24 miles, is perfect for common yellow-throated and blue-winged warblers, as well as yellow-breasted chats.

In the next 0.2 mile you reach Farny Cliffs, named after Adelaide Farny, who donated the money to buy the cliffs. The chestnut oak trees clinging to the edge of the cliff are growing where Peebles Dolomite and Ohio Shale meet. The shale is too acidic for the oaks, so the oak trees are literally clinging to the Peebles Dolomite for dear life. The chestnut oak with the "ripped" side was struck by lightning.

The missing chunk of dolomite is actually far below. Be careful along this edge as it is a long bumpy trip to the bottom.

Through the trees you can see glimpses of the panoramic views of rural Adams County. The trail leads into a forest of white and red oaks, sugar maples, shagbark hickories, and black cherry trees. Follow the trail to the left at 1.73 miles and you'll notice a lot of black cherry trees as the forest transitions to a younger stand of white oaks, sassafras, and tulip poplars. Take a moment at the slight break in the uphill climb at 1.9 miles because more uphill climbing is ahead.

You are now entering the Appalachian Oak Woodland. The black Ohio Shale (Devonian age) provides a foothold for hickories, sour gums, and oak species, including chinquapin and chestnut oaks. This is a good spot to attract birds by calling "pssh." You'll most likely see woodpeckers, nuthatches, vireos, and tanagers.

The trail winds along a ridge of Peebles Dolomite. Be sure to stay on the trail, because although climbing down might appear easy, climbing up won't be.

Continue on this ridge and watch your footing. Cross the boardwalk over the crevasse. The boardwalk and bridge lead to the overlook a few feet ahead at 2.3 miles. The overlook has benches and minimal railing. If you have little ones with you, keep them close for their safety and your sanity. The overlook is a chunk of Peebles Dolomite that juts out some 500 feet above the valley below.

Once you're out on the overlook, take a break and simply enjoy the splendid view of the surrounding hillsides and valleys while you are cooled by the wonderful breeze.

As its name suggests, Buzzardroost Rock provides an ideal vantage point to watch turkey vultures riding the thermal currents from the Ohio Brush Creek Valley. When you're ready, simply retrace your steps to your vehicle.

Nearby Activities

Enjoy shopping at the many Amish stores (don't forget they are closed on Sundays). The best cinnamon rolls ever are found at Miller's Bakery off Wheat Ridge Road near West Union. More hiking is available at Chaparral Prairie State Nature Preserve, Adams Lake State Park and Adams Lake Prairie State Nature Preserve, Lynx Prairie Preserve, Davis Memorial State Nature Preserve, Johnson Ridge State Nature Preserve, and Robert A. Whipple State Nature Preserve.

GPS Trailhead Coordinates and Directions

N38° 46.265'   W83° 25.542'

From West Union, take OH 125 East, almost 7.6 miles to the entrance of Buzzardroost Rock Preserve. The entrance road is easy to miss. On the south side of OH 125 (after you pass County Road 26/Weaver Road the second time on your left), watch for a break in the guardrail on your right. Turn right and follow the lane to the parking area. (If you pass Lynx Road on OH 125, you went a little too far.)

4 Caesar Creek Gorge State Nature Preserve: Gorge Loop Trail

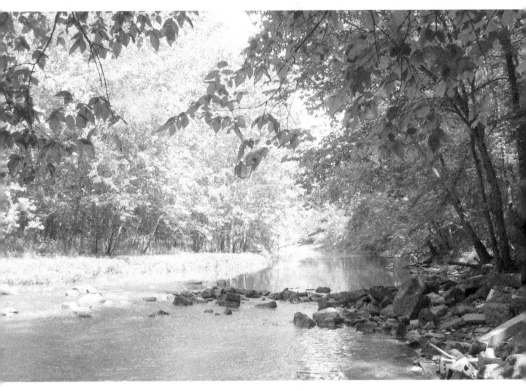

Take one of the many side trails down to Caesar Creek.

In Brief

The Gorge Loop Trail at Caesar Creek Gorge State Nature Preserve offers a pleasant hike through the woods and a nice start or end to your hiking day. It's relatively easy except for portions that lead down a steep hillside.

Description

Caesar Creek Gorge State Nature Preserve is 483 acres of Ordovician bedrock, woods, and Caesar Creek. The meltwater of a glacier carved a path through the area, forming the gorge.

LENGTH & CONFIGURATION 1.53-mile figure eight	**ACCESS** Daily, sunrise–sunset; free
DIFFICULTY Easy–moderate	**MAPS** USGS *Oregonia*
SCENERY Tailwater, forest, and cliffs	**WHEELCHAIR ACCESSIBLE** A portion of the area near the tailwater
EXPOSURE Mostly shaded	**FACILITIES** Restrooms and drinking water at the front of the parking area
TRAFFIC Moderate–heavy	
TRAIL SURFACE Old road, mowed path, gravel, and soil	**CONTACTS** Caesar Creek Gorge State Nature Preserve, 614-265-6453; **tinyurl.com/gorgeloop**
HIKING TIME 1 hour	
DRIVING DISTANCE 1 hour north of Cincinnati	**COMMENTS** Although this trail does not rate as a hard trail, the section that leads downhill has plenty of steps and is a little difficult to navigate in places.
SEASON Year-round	

The nature preserve is located beyond the dam of Caesar Creek Lake. This area is rich in fossils, but you are only allowed to collect them in the nearby emergency spillway. Before doing so, you should obtain a fossil-collecting permit from the U.S. Army Corps of Engineers. You'll most likely find brachiopods, horn coral, and crinoids. Resist the urge to climb up and inspect the rocks of the cut-through because it damages the habitat.

After you've parked your vehicle, walk toward the restroom area. Across the road from the restrooms is a steel bridge spanning the tailwater of Caesar Creek Lake. This bridge is an excellent place to view Caesar Creek.

Continue across the bridge to an intersection of three trails. Follow the Gorge Loop Trail away from the creek. When you reach the woods, follow Gorge Loop Trail to the left and uphill. This trail follows a retired roadbed. It enters a mature forest of American beech, sugar maples, and elms. Butterflies are common here as they take advantage of the small pools of water and salts.

Near 0.13 mile, parts of this trail are marked with blue blazes, as this is also a portion of the Ohio Buckeye Trail. At 0.15 mile a beautiful ravine area begins, with flat stones to the right at 0.28 mile. The trail then transitions from the forest to an open area.

Take a right onto the wide, mulched Gorge Loop Trail. Pass by a small pond to your left and look for the wood duck nesting box. At the next intersection continue straight ahead on the wide, mulched path. The trail enters a young forest and might be muddy if it has rained recently. The forest transitions to a mature woods.

At 0.38 mile, cross a footbridge over a small intermittent stream, then another footbridge shortly thereafter. The trail begins to head uphill over several large steps.

Caesar Creek Gorge State Nature Preserve: Gorge Loop Trail

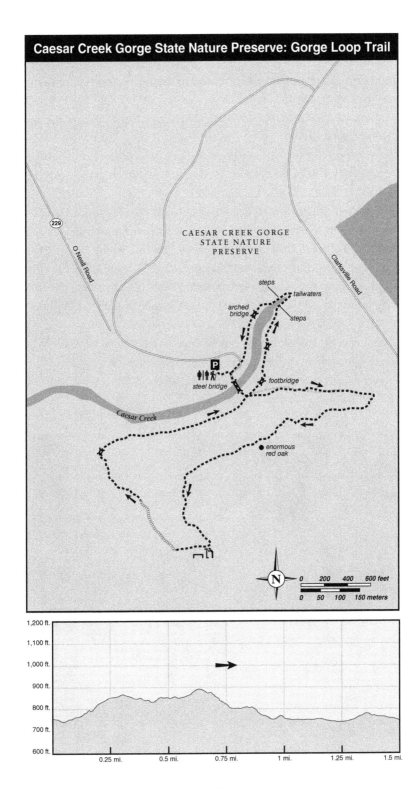

CAESAR CREEK GORGE
STATE NATURE
PRESERVE

steps

tailwaters

arched
bridge

steps

229

O Neall Road

Clarksville Road

P

steel bridge

footbridge

Caesar Creek

enormous
red oak

N

| 0 | 200 | 400 | 600 feet |
| 0 | 50 | 100 | 150 meters |

Beautiful red and white oaks and several shagbark hickory trees fill the forest. The trail winds uphill and passes an enormous red oak tree at 0.47 mile. You can easily identify red oaks by the distinguished dark and light gray bark that, near the top of the tree, looks like ski tracks.

Unlike some gorge trails, this one typically has a good breeze flowing through that makes for a nice, cool hike on a hot summer day. And even though the Gorge Loop Trail is popular, it remains a quiet place to hike.

Near 0.5 mile, trillium covers the hillsides. Dogwoods, basswoods, and elms border the trail along this portion. Pass by the small retention wall and enjoy a break on the bridge at 0.59 mile. Outfitted with benches, this is a wonderful spot to enjoy the view of the gorge. After you cross the bridge, the trail leads uphill for a little bit. It banks and passes by several large trees within 20 feet of each other. The first on the right is a sugar maple, the second one on the right is a red oak, and the next one to the left is a shagbark hickory.

The canopy of the mature woods is now about 60 feet tall. At 0.69 mile, when the trail splits, take the trail to the right and down the steps. It leads downhill and, at 0.71 mile, splits again. The trail to the left leads to the spillway; follow the Gorge Loop Trail to the right and downhill via the steps.

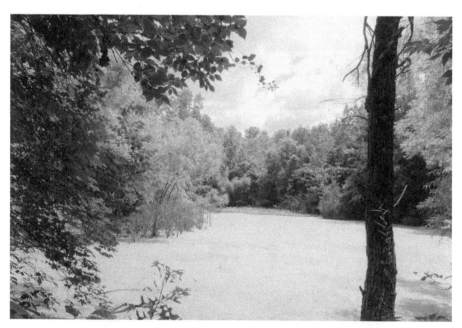

Quiet ponds are full of life. Look for frogs, turtles, and snakes, as well as female ducks followed by ducklings.

Take nearly two dozen steps down to the platform and look to the left at the gorge area. After a dozen more steps, the trail becomes a mulched path. At 0.74 mile, you'll encounter another series of steep steps and a boardwalk. The gorge and stream are to the left.

Decorated by several large, flat stones, the trail winds along a shelf on the hillside. Watch out for the poison ivy on both sides of the trail, especially near 0.86 mile where it overgrows the edges.

Pass through another area with a retaining wall and bench before descending the steps. The steps end at 0.91 mile. The creek bed is just a few feet to the left. Pass over more steps and the mulched path leads to a gravel-covered path. To the left is another bridge.

Take a few moments to enjoy this area and the rock formations.

Follow the gravel road to the right. The creek is to the left. Several spur trails lead to the edge of Caesar Creek. Follow this path to the first intersection and take the concrete path straight ahead.

Cross over the small footbridge and continue along the edge of Caesar Creek. Take the steps up and over the tailwater outlet. At 1.4 miles, cross the bridge with the steep incline. Caesar Creek is to the left and a small stream is to the right.

Follow the concrete path back to the parking lot and your vehicle.

Nearby Activities

Caesar Creek State Park, Spring Valley Wildlife Area, and Fort Ancient offer additional hiking opportunities and are included in this book. Waynesville has several great hometown restaurants as well as plenty of antique stores.

GPS Trailhead Coordinates and Directions

N39° 28.992' W84° 03.904'

From the northeast corner of Cincinnati, take I-71 North (from I-275) 28 miles and turn left onto OH 73. Travel west on OH 73 for 7.7 miles. Turn left, heading south on North Clarksville Road for 2.5 miles. Turn right onto the entrance road to Caesar Creek Gorge State Nature Preserve.

5 Chaparral Prairie State Nature Preserve

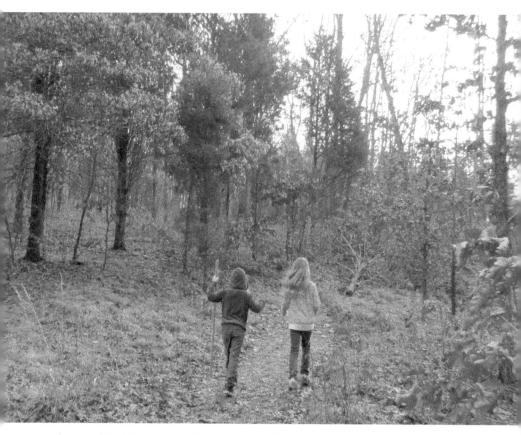

Chaparral Prairie is great to hike any time of the year.

In Brief

More than 14 rare or endangered species are found in this small prairie opening at the remote Chaparral Prairie, located 4 miles northwest of West Union in Adams County.

Description

Chaparral Prairie State Nature Preserve is a playground for any botanist or geology nut. When planning your visit, pack tree, wildflower, prairie, and bird identification books, as well as a camera and binoculars.

LENGTH & CONFIGURATION 1-mile loop plus firebreaks	**ACCESS** Daily, 30 minutes before sunrise–30 minutes after sunset; free
DIFFICULTY Very easy	**MAPS** USGS *West Union;* on-site at kiosk or by calling Ohio Department of Natural Resources Division of Natural Areas and Preserves, 614-265-6561
SCENERY Buffalo beats, prairie, forest, and old field	
EXPOSURE Open except in older wooded areas	**WHEELCHAIR ACCESSIBLE** No
TRAFFIC Light	**FACILITIES** None
TRAIL SURFACE Soil and grass	**CONTACTS** Ohio Division of Natural Resources, 614-265-6561; **tinyurl.com/chapprairie**
HIKING TIME 1 hour	
DRIVING DISTANCE Less than 10 minutes from West Union	**COMMENTS** A botanist's paradise. Follow the rules and regulations of the preserve, which include no pets.
SEASON Year-round	

The 67-acre nature preserve includes prairie, forest, and old-field habitats and is seated on Crab Orchard Shale. This area was once covered by the Illinoian glaciation 200,000 years ago. As the glacier receded, till—the gravel and clay debris from the glacier—covered the area. The area was then covered with loess, a windblown soil.

The loess soil was very susceptible to erosion, and early farming practices hastened the exposure of the Crab Orchard Shale. Common to this region of Adams County are bald spots, or buffalo beats—conical mounds of exposed Crab Orchard Shale on which only hardy, drought-resistant prairie plants are able to grow.

One-third of the Chaparral State Nature Preserve is covered in prairie plants that scientists think migrated to Ohio after the glaciers retreated and the climate was dry and warm. Today the Chaparral is home to diverse plant life, including 15 species of plants rare to Ohio.

Oak species include blackjack and post. Prairie plants such as little bluestem, rattlesnake master, prairie dock, spiked blazing star, and sunflowers flourish in this amazing prairie. It's also home to 11 state-listed species, including spider milkweed, prairie false indigo, pink milkwort, and Carolina buckthorn. Several varieties of butterflies, moths, and songbirds are active in this area during the summer months.

In 1985 the Ohio Department of Natural Resources (ODNR) Division of Natural Areas and Preserves (DNAP) bought Chaparral Prairie State Nature Preserve using funds raised through the voluntary State Tax Checkoff program.

The trailhead is directly behind the large kiosk near the left side of the maintenance building. Take the time to read the interpretive signs scattered throughout the

Chaparral Prairie State Nature Preserve

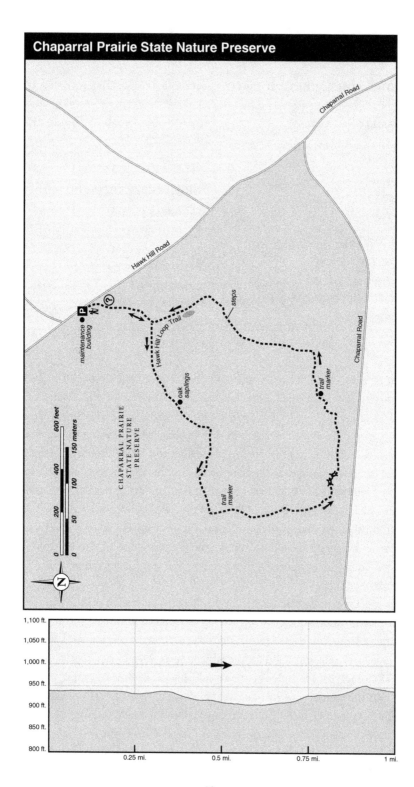

trail. Enter the trail and begin walking into the past. After 100 yards, the entrance trail meets with the Hawk Hill Loop.

Follow the Hawk Hill Loop to the right and up a slight grade. The prairie can survive the constant threat of invasive species thanks to the work of ODNR Division of Natural Areas and Preserves land managers. By using several different eradication methods, including prescribed burns and hand removal, they can keep this moment in time intact for the enjoyment and education of many people. In fact, the Division of Natural Areas and Preserves perfectly describes this area as a "living museum."

Numerous species of oaks border the hiking path. Starting about 400 yards into the Hawk Hill Loop, the diversity of oaks begins to show, including blackjack and post oaks. You'll need patience and a good identification book that uses twig and bud characteristics to determine one oak from another, especially because several of the oaks are not species found in many places in Ohio.

At 0.2 mile, a trail marker notes where the trail joins with a maintenance path. Continue straight ahead on the main trail and enter a stand of red cedar trees. The ground cover is a primitive club moss called ground pine. Please keep in mind that this is a nature preserve; therefore everything is protected. Collecting or removing anything is strictly prohibited. About 100 yards after the trail marker, the ground cover changes to reindeer lichen. As you walk along the trail, blazing stars and other prairie plants show their spectacular blooms during the heat of summer. Cross a series of footbridges near 0.3 mile, under the right-of-way for the power lines, and then the habitat changes to a wooded area with shagbark hickories, red and white oaks, and elms.

The prairie plant rattlesnake master is found over the next 130 yards. According to ODNR Division of Natural Areas and Preserves, this entire prairie area "supports one of the most extensive populations of rattlesnake master in the state."

The trail follows along the right-of-way and heads uphill toward the right at the trail marker. About 70 yards past the marker post is another junction. Remain on the marked trail toward the left.

At 150 yards from the trail junction, five steps lead into a beautiful woodland area. Remain on the trail to the left to return to the open prairie area. Upon exiting the woods, a man-made pond becomes visible. The pond is used by white-tailed deer, as well as a variety of frogs, during the spring and summer months.

Stay on the trail until the junction with the entrance trail, and turn right to return to the parking lot. The firebreak lanes in the old field are also open to exploration. Small prairie openings such as Chaparral Prairie are found throughout the forests in this edge of the Appalachia region, and they are a delightful gateway into Ohio's botanical past. The trails of Adams Lake State Park and Adams Lake Prairie State Nature

Preserve and the Edge of Appalachia Preserve's Lynx Prairie Preserve and Wilderness Trails offer additional opportunities to explore southern Ohio's unique prairies.

Nearby Activities

Located on the edge of the Appalachia Region, West Union offers several Amish and specialty shops, quilt barns, and numerous historic sites, plus additional hikes at Buzzardroost Rock Preserve, Adams Lake State Park and Adams Lake Prairie State Nature Preserve, and Wilderness Trail.

GPS Trailhead Coordinates and Directions

N38° 50.423'   W83° 34.425'

From OH 125 in West Union, turn north onto OH 247 and follow it for 0.7 mile. Turn left onto County Road 22/Chaparral Road and head west for 2.75 miles to Township Road 23/Hawk Hill Road. Continue straight onto Hawk Hill Road for 0.25 mile, where you'll see the maintenance building and parking for the Chaparral on your left. The entrance to the trail is directly behind the kiosk to the left side of the driveway.

6 Chilo Lock 34 Park and Crooked Run Nature Preserve

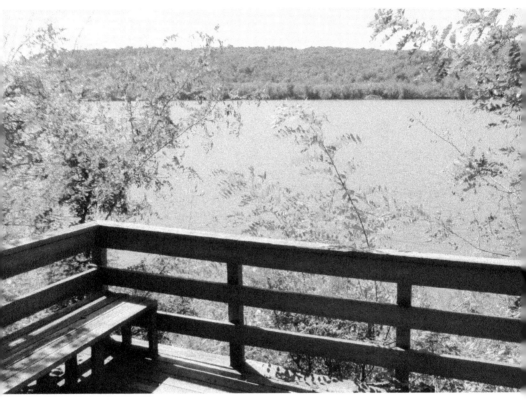

Observation deck along Ohio River in Crooked Run Nature Preserve

In Brief

The Chilo Lock 34 Museum contains interactive displays about the Ohio River and the history of the area, while Crooked Run Nature Preserve is the perfect place to view waterfowl, songbirds, birds of prey, and some wetland-dependent mammals.

Description

Rich in Ohio River history and wildlife diversity, the combination of Chilo Lock 34 Park and Crooked Run Nature Preserve offers a welcome respite from the daily chaos.

LENGTH & CONFIGURATION 2.2-mile series of loops	**MAPS** USGS *Moscow;* **parks.clermont countyohio.gov/ChiloCrookedRunmap.pdf**
DIFFICULTY Easy	**WHEELCHAIR ACCESSIBLE** Some areas are paved or sidewalks.
SCENERY Crooked Run embayment, Ohio River, woods, and wetlands	
EXPOSURE Mostly shaded except for meadow areas	**FACILITIES** Restrooms and water in Chilo Lock 34 Visitor Center and Museum
TRAFFIC Moderate–heavy	**CONTACTS** Clermont County Parks, 513-876-9013; **parks.clermontcountyohio.gov /chilo.aspx** or **clermontparks.org/Crooked .aspx**
TRAIL SURFACE Gravel, soil, mowed paths	
HIKING TIME 1.5 hour	**COMMENTS** In the museum, you can see, hear, and feel Chilo Lock 34 and Ohio River history. Bring your binoculars to explore Crooked Run Nature Preserve, as several blinds offer plenty of places to enjoy watching nature.
DRIVING DISTANCE Less than 1 mile east of Chilo on US 52	
SEASON Year-round	
ACCESS Daily, sunrise–sunset; free	

Crooked Run Robert J. Paul Sanctuary is 78 acres of protected wetlands, estuary, woods, and meadows. The property is owned by the Ohio Department of Natural Resources Division of Natural Areas and Preserves.

Adjacent to the preserve is Clermont County Parks' 39-acre Chilo Lock 34 Park, which includes scenic Ohio River overlooks, a historical river walk, a museum, a playground, picnic areas and shelter, a boat ramp and dock, a basketball court, and horseshoe pits, plus two yurts that are available for rent. Both areas are managed by Clermont County Park District.

Once you turn south off US 52 and enter the park, pass through the 1.5-acre wetland mitigation project and enter the main area of the park. Follow the drive to the parking area to the far west of the large, three-story brick building that houses the Chilo Lock 34 Visitor Center and Museum.

The Chilo Lock 34 building was built in 1925 when a series of wicket dams were installed along the Ohio River to control the average depth of the river and make it navigable. In 1964, Chilo Lock 34 wicket dam was replaced when the Meldahl Lock and Dam, 2 miles downstream, became operational.

The wicket dam's powerhouse was converted into the Chilo Lock 34 Visitor Center and Museum. It is open to the public, but the operating hours vary seasonally. Call for current hours before you visit.

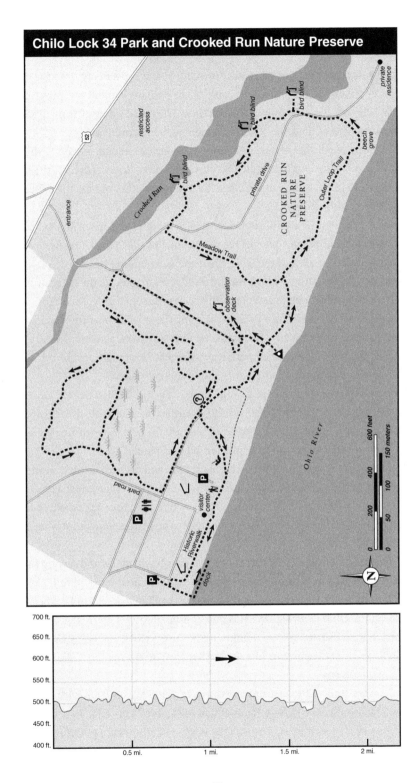

Chilo Lock 34 Park and Crooked Run Nature Preserve

restricted access

entrance

52

Crooked Run

bird blind

bird blind

bird blind

bird blind

private drive

private residence

beech grove

CROOKED RUN NATURE PRESERVE

Outer Loop Trail

Meadow Trail

observation deck

Ohio River

600 feet

150 meters

400

200

100

50

0

0

N

park road

visitor center

Historic Riverwalk

dock

P

P

P

P

700 ft.
650 ft.
600 ft.
550 ft.
500 ft.
450 ft.
400 ft.

0.5 mi.   1 mi.   1.5 mi.   2 mi.

When you get out of your car, walk down the boat ramp and out onto the dock to enjoy up-close views of the Ohio River. Follow the path back uphill and turn right to follow the sidewalk with the railing and benches. The railed sidewalk is the historical walk along the edge of the Ohio River, complete with interpretive signs.

Head to the north side of the large, three-story brick building and enter the Chilo Lock 34 Visitor Center and Museum. The museum's three floors chronicle the history of Chilo Lock 34, the flooding of the Ohio River, and the story of how the people of the region lived and survived.

Inside the museum is a publications area with more information about Clermont County, as well as hands-on activities for young and old alike. The third-floor windows offer a bird's-eye view of the Ohio River and surrounding areas.

Back outside the museum, look for the flood level marker on the exterior of the building before heading northeast, diagonally across the open grass field. The entrance to Crooked Run Nature Preserve is along the treeline near the service road.

The preserve sees a fair number of hikers, bird-watchers, and families, so expect company on the trail. For the most part, a good breeze comes in from the river; however, this area can be hot and humid during the summer months.

Crooked Run Nature Preserve is well known as a great bird-watching location. In fact, during migration you can see a variety of warblers as well as loons and osprey. The latter part of April and the first week of May are the best times during spring migration, while October is the best time for fall migration.

Species you may spot include nesting Baltimore and orchard orioles, prothonotary warblers, yellow-breasted chats, and yellow warblers—to name just a few.

Immediately upon entering Crooked Run is a trail junction. Take the trail leading to the right. In 50 yards, pass the connector trail to the playground and stay on the trail to the left.

At the next junction, 230 feet from the last, pass by the pines and stay on the trail to the right. This trail borders the Ohio River. At the next intersection, pass the trail leading to the observation deck by taking the Outer Loop Trail to the right.

Birds of the Ohio River signage aids in identifying various species that inhabit or frequent the area. Plan to stay a few moments at the overlook and enjoy the serenity of the Ohio River from the comfort of a shaded bench. The river is very relaxing to watch and hear as it rolls past.

Back on the trail and 130 yards from the overlook is the junction with the Meadow Trail. Stay to the right and remain on the Outer Loop Trail. Pass through the stand of American beech trees. The trail turns left and follows the gravel road for 100 yards. (Please respect the privacy of the private residence located at the other end of the gravel road.)

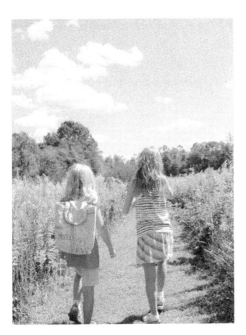

Stroll through the prairie and wetlands.

Throughout Crooked Run are several observation blinds that offer not only a place to rest but also a wonderful glimpse into the wildlife of the backwater estuary system of Crooked Run. The estuary supports many migrating, breeding, and wintering birds. Additionally, great blue herons, green herons, ospreys, and even bald eagles are regularly spotted in the preserve.

The first blind at 0.78 mile and the second blind 200 feet ahead allow you to sit without being noticed by the birds utilizing the Crooked Run embayment. The third observation blind, about 0.1 mile farther down the trail, offers excellent viewing of waterfowl species such as northern pintails and American coots.

The Outer Loop Trail becomes the Meadow Trail 100 yards after the last observation blind. The trail meanders along the road and into a meadow before crossing a small footbridge. The meadow is full of the trill of insects and the calls of red-winged blackbirds. You might also see American woodcock, wild turkey, and white-tailed deer.

Follow the Meadow Trail to the junction of the Meadow and Outer Loop Trails. Take the Outer Loop Trail to the right and follow it until you see the sign for the connector trail to the observation tower. Turn right and follow the trail to the tower. The observation tower is about two stories tall and offers an overview of the meadow below. You can easily spot animal pathways through the meadow from this elevation.

Take the steps back down and stay to your right following the trail along the service road. Continue on the road as it turns left and passes by box elders, hackberries, and maples.

As the trail curves around the pond look for bullfrogs and green frogs hiding in the duckweed. Cross the footbridge. When this trail meets the service road you entered the woods on at the beginning of the hike follow it out of the woods and into the open grassy area.

Continue straight ahead on the road and pass by the yurts and service buildings. At the stop sign turn right on the entrance road (County Park Road) and follow it north. Turn right into the wetland entrance. At the split follow the trail to the left. The trail leads through the meadow and by a wetland.

When the trail reaches the entrance road again follow it back to the parking area and outdoor exhibits. Take some time and look at the various displays before returning to your vehicle.

Nearby Activities

Great Parks of Hamilton County's Woodland Mound and Withrow Nature Preserve, as well as East Fork State Park, offer additional hiking opportunities. The Land of Grant Tours offers a window into the life of Ulysses S. Grant, including his birthplace and schoolhouse.

GPS Trailhead Coordinates and Directions

N38° 47.382'   W84° 07.999'

On the east side of Cincinnati, from the intersection of I-275 and US 52, follow US 52 East approximately 21 miles to the small town of Chilo. Less than 1 mile east of Chilo, off US 52, is the entrance to Chilo Lock 34. Turn right into the park.

7 Clifton Gorge State Nature Preserve

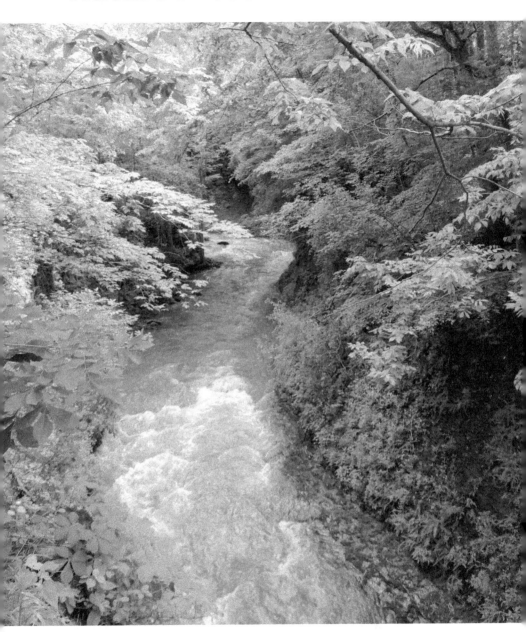

Little Miami River keeps Clifton Gorge moist and cool.

LENGTH & CONFIGURATION 2.7-mile balloon	**ACCESS** Daily, sunrise–sunset; free
DIFFICULTY Moderate–difficult	**MAPS** USGS *Clifton;* Clifton Gorge State Nature Preserve map
SCENERY Gorge, Little Miami River, unique flora	**WHEELCHAIR ACCESSIBLE** A portion of the Narrows Trail
EXPOSURE Mostly shaded	**FACILITIES** Latrine
TRAFFIC Heavy	**CONTACTS** Ohio Department of Natural Resources, Division of Natural Areas and Preserves, 614-265-6561; **dnr.state.oh.us /tabid/882/default.aspx**
TRAIL SURFACE Boulders, loose stone, and soil	
HIKING TIME 1–1.5 hours	
DRIVING DISTANCE 1.5 hours from Cincinnati	**COMMENTS** Everything in the 269 acres of the Clifton Gorge Nature Preserve is protected. Spring is best for bird-watchers and wildflower enthusiasts.
SEASON Year-round, but best in spring, summer, and fall	

In Brief

Step into Ohio's tumultuous geological past and out of the demands of everyday life. This 2.7-mile hike travels through impressive overlooks of the raging Little Miami River, slump-block caves, and a bevy of wildflowers in the spring. The best times to visit are in the spring, summer, and fall.

Description

This 269-acre nature preserve, located a little more than one hour northeast of Cincinnati, is well worth the trip. The nature preserve was created in 1970 to protect this unique geologic area, which was carved out by waters of the melting glaciers. It is also a memorial to geologist and professor John L. Rich, who was instrumental in protecting this area.

If you're hiking the trail with small children, keep them close to you at all times. Never go off-trail on this hike: the trail borders cliff rims, and at the bottom is the powerful Little Miami River.

In Clifton Gorge, you can see plants not found in other parts of the state, including red baneberry and wall rue. In spring the area is a treat for wildflower enthusiasts; expect to see a variety of trilliums, including snow trilliums, as well as hepaticas, jack-in-the-pulpits, and bloodroot. In fact, bring a good wildflower identification book and a camera.

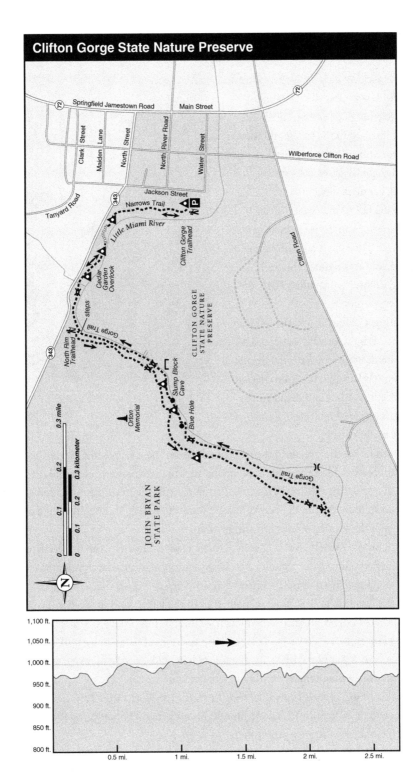

Clifton Gorge State Nature Preserve

Springfield Jamestown Road

Main Street

72

72

Clark Street

Malden Lane

North Street

North River Road

Water Street

Wilberforce Clifton Road

Jackson Street

343

Narrows Trail

Tanyard Road

Little Miami River

Cedar Garden Overlook

Clifton Gorge Trailhead

Clifton Road

steps

Gorge Trail

North Rim Trailhead

343

Slump Block Cave

CLIFTON GORGE STATE NATURE PRESERVE

Blue Hole

Orton Memorial

Gorge Trail

0.3 mile

0.3 kilometer

0.2

0.1

0.2

0.1

0

0

JOHN BRYAN STATE PARK

N

1,100 ft.

1,050 ft.

1,000 ft.

950 ft.

900 ft.

850 ft.

800 ft.

0.5 mi.

1 mi.

1.5 mi.

2 mi.

2.5 mi.

51

The parking area off Jackson and Water Streets is near the trailhead. Before leaving your car, be sure valuables are locked in the trunk and the car is locked. Multiple signs remind visitors that although this area is beautiful and tranquil, crime still occurs.

To the left of the large Clifton Gorge kiosk is the trailhead for the Narrows Trail. The trail is soil- and gravel-covered, and throughout the trail exposed dolomite provides plenty of stumbling points.

Within 122 feet and to the left is an overlook of the river valley gorge. The Little Miami State and National Scenic River funnels through the Silurian dolomite, creating rapids and displaying a perfect example of interglacial and post-glacial canyon cutting.

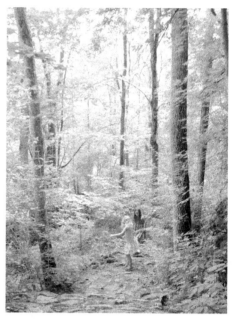

Be careful of your footing over the slick, rocky surfaces.

Continue on the trail until the next overlook on the left at 0.26 mile. In the 1800s several mills were located in this area, including saw, grist, and woolen mills. The mills played an important role in US history: Patterson Mill, for example, provided cloth for American soldiers during the War of 1812. Floods demolished the mills, but a few remnants of the footing stones can still be seen.

Back on the main trail at 0.32 mile, cross a bridge and enjoy the overlook of water cascading down into a deep pool. Here, large chunks of Silurian dolomite have created islands along the corridor of the Little Miami River.

At the junction at 0.47 mile, take the trail to the left to visit the Cedar Garden overlook. From this vantage point you can see uncommon species of plants, including white cedars and Canada yews. Take the loop to connect back to the trail.

This hike is popular with scout groups, college kids, and families. In the open area at 0.62 mile are a maintenance building, latrine, and kiosk.

At this point, several trails intersect. Look for the North Rim Trail trailhead sign and proceed on North Rim Trail. Although this area might be tempting for rock climbers, such climbing is strictly prohibited.

North Rim Trail is a two-person-wide path with exposed dolomite that makes the path uneven and choppy to walk on. The trail passes over many footbridges. The first, at 0.89 mile, is made from recycled plastic. The next footbridge, at 0.94 mile, passes over yet another creek.

One mile into the hike the trail passes a junction with a connector to the lower Gorge Trail. Stay on the trail to the right and head uphill over the exposed stone. Be careful not to follow the access road. If there has been a fair amount of rainfall, the trail near the 1.1-mile point will likely have a stream flowing down the middle of it.

Overlooks at 1.15 and 1.17 miles both offer wonderful views of the gorge below. At the next junction at 1.18 miles, stay to the left on North Rim. Along this trail is a stream and moss-covered trees and rocks. The trail flattens out at 1.39 miles, and at 1.46 miles passes a switchback to the right that leads to the Orton picnic area.

When the trail splits, pass the right side of the trail that leads into John Bryan State Park and take Gorge Trail to the left; this loops back into Clifton Gorge Nature Preserve. This part of the trail is slow and treacherous due to the exposed bedrock.

At 1.54 miles, the trail enters into a valley area adjacent to the Little Miami River. The trestle-style bridge that crosses the waterway leads into John Bryan State Park. Don't cross the bridge. Take a left to continue on J. L. Rich–North Gorge Trail.

This bottomland area is very cool and humid, which allows for a variety of mosses and succulents to grow in the nooks and crannies of the dolomite. American beech, cottonwood, and sycamore trees provide additional shade. In spring look for jack-in-the-pulpits, spring beauties, snow trilliums, bloodroot, and hepaticas.

At several points, Gorge Trail closely parallels the Little Miami River. Another trestle-style bridge at 1.81 miles overlooks a backwater way. At this point the trail meanders through the dolomite cut and it feels as if you stepped into another world.

The vegetation restoration area is at 1.93 miles. The trail leads uphill and past a small waterfall to the left. At 2 miles, cross another footbridge near another waterfall.

The trail soon begins to head back uphill from the bottomland. At 2.09 miles, you'll find another overlook near where the paper mill once stood.

In 1851 the African American artist Robert Duncanson painted a picture of the Blue Hole of the Little Miami River, which you'll see at 2.13 miles. The painting is on display at the Cincinnati Art Museum.

Adventurous hikers can explore a slump-block cave—the only one open to the public—at 2.34 miles. A slump-block cave is formed when water dissolves softer rock and instead of a block of rock falling away from the cliff, the block falls toward the cliff and creates a cave. The cave is several feet deep, wet, a little creepy, and fun with kids.

Another footbridge, at 2.37 miles, is adjacent to a large waterfall. The cliff faces are covered with beautiful light-blue lichens.

At 2.61 miles, take the stairs that lead up to the Narrows Trail. At the top, take a right to return along Narrows Trail to your vehicle about a half-mile away.

Nearby Activities

You'll find several antique shops in the Clifton area. Before setting out on your hike, explore the Clifton Mill area and enjoy a meal. Just north on OH 68 is Young's Dairy— a favorite haunt for ice cream lovers. Shopping in Yellow Springs's many stores is an eclectic adventure.

GPS Trailhead Coordinates and Directions

N39° 47.709'   W83° 49.720'

From Cincinnati, take I-71 North to Exit 65/35A/OH 435 West/Old 35 West. Follow 35 West to OH 72 North for 10.2 miles to Clifton, Ohio. In Clifton, turn left onto Water Street, which at the bend turns into Jackson Street. The parking area is on the west side of the road after the bend.

8 Cox Arboretum MetroPark

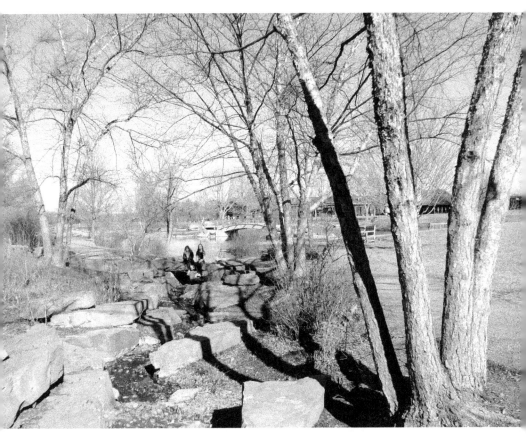

Cox Arboretum gardens during a winter hike

In Brief

Cox Arboretum MetroPark is one of several gems of the Five Rivers MetroParks system. The arboretum includes gardens, display gardens, and water features and holds classes in gardening and nature. The accessible paved trail weaves through many of the planted and watercourse areas.

Description

Located near the intersection of I-75 and I-675 off Springboro Pike, Cox Arboretum offers a beautiful retreat in the 189 acres of formal plantings, forests, and meadows.

LENGTH & CONFIGURATION 3.3-mile loop

DIFFICULTY Easy

SCENERY Formal gardens, ponds, creeks, woods, and wetlands

EXPOSURE Sun and shaded

TRAFFIC Heavy

TRAIL SURFACE Paved, gravel, and soil

HIKING TIME 1.5–2 hours

DRIVING DISTANCE 1 hour north of Cincinnati

SEASON Year-round

ACCESS April 1–October 31: Daily, 8 a.m.–10 p.m.; November 1–March 31: Daily,

8 a.m.–8 p.m.; closed January 1 and December 25; free

MAPS USGS *Dayton South;* Cox Arboretum MetroPark User's Guide and Map

WHEELCHAIR ACCESSIBLE Paved portions

FACILITIES Restrooms and drinking water inside Zorniger Education Center

CONTACTS Cox Arboretum MetroPark, 937-275-PARK (7275) or 937-434-9005; **metroparks.org/parks/coxarboretum**

COMMENTS Plan to spend time wandering through the gardens and at the observation blind.

Arboretum does not adequately define this place. In addition to the enormous variety of tree plantings, several display gardens and watercourses—such as the Woodland Wildflower Garden, Butterfly House, the Bell Children's Maze, and Conservation Corner—provide educational opportunities as well as beautiful landscapes.

The hike begins at the Zorniger Campus. This beautiful glass and stone building houses the office, meeting rooms, restrooms, and a nature shop. Before you start your hike, take a moment to explore the inside of the Zorniger Education Center, including the nature shop. Several brochures on nature and gardening topics are available at the information desk.

Walk around the Zorniger Education Center to the large, open area behind the building and the gardens come into view. The Monet Bridge arches over the water garden, complete with bronze sculptures.

As you continue on the trail, walk to the large, fenced-in garden with a huge pavilion. Step under the archway and enter through the swinging gate.

Follow the pathway to the right and walk around the back of the pavilion, taking in the variety of gardening ideas on display. The pavilion is also used as an outdoor classroom. Check with the naturalist on duty for more information about gardening courses. Exit through the same gate you entered.

Return to the brick path and turn left onto the asphalt trail and continue to lose yourself in the multiple planting areas. All plants are labeled, making it easy for you to identify them and keep track of what you might want to incorporate into your own backyard oasis.

Cox Arboretum MetroPark

- **B** Blue Trail
- **R** Red Trail
- **Y** Yellow Trail

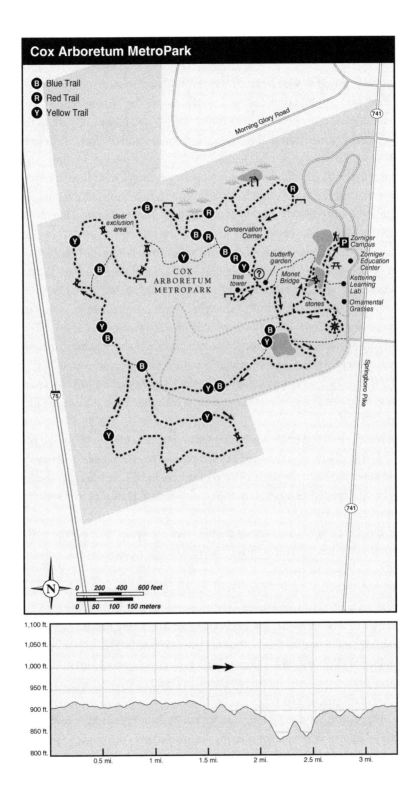

57

Pass the first trail to your right. At the next trail intersection turn right. You'll see a large green butterfly and then the Butterfly House. At the T-intersection follow the trail to your left. At the gazebo take the trail to the left and follow the path to the Tree Tower. The tower created from three Douglas fir trees stands 45 feet tall. Take the 81 steps to the top and enjoy the eerie harmonics the tower makes on a windy day.

Return to the blue/yellow trail near the Butterfly house and follow it to your right. Stay on the blue/yellow trail and when you reach the small lake follow the trail around the lake and enjoy the beauty of the multiple plantings. A bench underneath a shade tree provides a nice place to rest and enjoy the views.

When the trail reconnects with the blue/yellow trail follow the blue/yellow to the left. The color-coded and numbered signposts throughout the area make this an easy trail system to navigate. Another bench is at 1 mile. The trail begins to head downhill.

A service road crosses the trail at 1.2 miles. Continue on the blue/yellow trail. At the next intersection, take the yellow trail to the left. Cross a bridge at 1.4 miles. Red oaks and cottonwoods dominate the forest structure, and you may note that the stream to the right is suffering from a significant amount of bank erosion.

After the bridge, very few saplings cover the forest floor. You will cross a few bridges. At 1.9 miles, the yellow trail reconnects with the blue trail; take the blue/yellow to the left.

You'll find another bench just 170 feet from junction of the yellow and blue trails. The large platform area overlooks a creek ravine at 2.5 miles. Take the blue trail down the steps and over the top of the creek. When you cross the creek, you can turn to the right and explore the creek's exposed bedrock and waterfalls before returning to the hike.

The trail heads uphill, just before the blue trail intersects with the red trail. Take the red trail to the left. Immediately the trail enters into an open prairie wetland area named Conservation Corner.

The goal of Conservation Corner is to educate people about the environment and protecting the land. This area is used to teach people to identify native plants and habitats and how to look for signs of wildlife. Conservation Corner contains tall-grass prairie, shrubs, oaks, and wetlands. Prairie plants include Indian grass, big bluestem, gray-headed coneflower, and bergamot. For a healthy ecosystem, this prairie is burned every three years to destroy the woody plants and nonnative species that would otherwise overtake the prairie plants.

An observation blind at 2.8 miles allows an excellent opportunity to stop and watch the wildlife in the small but thriving prairie wetland. You might see ducks as well as great blue herons. Throughout Conservation Corner are several active bluebird nesting boxes. Goldfinches, sparrows, and red-winged blackbirds are also busily going about their day.

The official trailhead and kiosk appear at 3.1 miles. At the official trailhead, turn left on the blue/yellow trail. You'll soon pass the Butterfly House. Follow the paved pathway to the formal planting areas the Monet Bridge area. Near the Monet Bridge is the stone garden area, which provides plenty of ideas on plants for rock gardens.

To learn more about horticulture and natural history, register for one of the many classes, programs, or seminars that are held here year-round.

Nearby Activities

Need more hiking trails? Germantown and Sugarcreek MetroParks are nearby, and both offer fun hikes for families to enjoy. Dayton Mall, shops, and restaurants are off OH 725. If you like organic food, visit Health Foods Unlimited off OH 725 in the South Towne Shopping Center.

GPS Trailhead Coordinates and Directions

N39° 39.307'   W84° 13.477'

From Cincinnati, take I-75 North toward Dayton and take Exit 44/Miamisburg/Centerville. Turn east (right) onto Miamisburg/Centerville Road and travel for 0.3 miles. Turn north (left) onto Springboro Pike and travel 1 mile to the entrance for Cox Arboretum on the west (left) side of the road.

9 **East Fork State Park:** South Trail

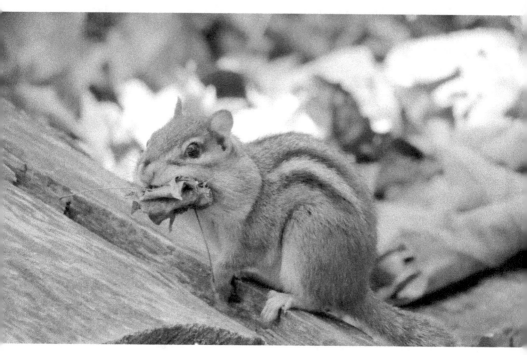

State park chipmunk in the fall

In Brief

East Fork is one of Ohio's largest state parks and is just 25 miles east of Cincinnati. It offers a variety of activities, including fishing, hunting, boating, camping, picnicking, mountain biking, horseback riding, and hiking. South Trail meanders along Clermont County's rolling hillsides.

Description

The East Fork region's rich American Indian history dates back some 3,000 years. Evidence is visible of the Mound Builders, the Adena and Hopewell tribes that once lived in the area. A mound believed to have been built by the Adena is near Elklick Road.

The Erie and Iroquois tribes also lived in the East Fork region. In 1655 the Iroquois devastated the Erie. After that, the region remained relatively uninhabited until

LENGTH & CONFIGURATION 2.91-mile loop	**ACCESS** Daily, 6 a.m.–11 p.m.; free
DIFFICULTY Easy	**MAPS** USGS *Batavia*; East Fork State Park map
SCENERY Forests and ravines	**WHEELCHAIR ACCESSIBLE** No
EXPOSURE Shade	**FACILITIES** Latrine at trailhead; rest-
TRAFFIC Moderate–heavy	room and drinking water at main office
TRAIL SURFACE Soil	**CONTACTS** East Fork State Park, 513-
HIKING TIME 1.5 hours	734-4323; **parks.ohiodnr.gov/eastfork**
DRIVING DISTANCE 45 minutes east of Cincinnati	**COMMENTS** Hikers, mountain bikers, horseback riders, and trail runners all use
SEASON Year-round	the trail, so please be courteous.

the early 19th century. As the new state of Ohio began attracting settlers, commerce grew. Two gold mines once operated near Elklick and Twin Bridges.

The U.S. Army Corps of Engineers, in accordance with the Flood Control Program, created East Fork Reservoir in 1978. The William H. Harsha Lake, East Fork State Park, U.S. Army Corps of Engineers land, and East Fork Wildlife Area comprise southwestern Ohio's largest recreational area.

Turn left into the park entrance and follow Elklick Road to the first intersection after the main office. Turn left, pass by the ponds, and park in the gravel parking area. At the northeast edge of the parking lot is a large kiosk. This display includes hiking and biking information as well as several large overview maps of the area and trails.

Between the kiosk and the latrine is the trailhead. Follow the gravel path to take the South Trail, which is shared with mountain bikers. The trails are also popular with trail runners.

At the trail intersection 400 feet into the hike, take the trail to the extreme left and follow the white blazes. The trail narrows to a single-person-wide path through the open understory of the mature woods. The trail parallels the creek bed as it weaves through young hackberry, red oak, and sycamore trees.

Cross a footbridge at 0.17 mile and a small stream at 0.2 mile. To the right of the trail is the creek ravine about 15 feet below. Shagbark hickory, red oak, and ash trees dominate this portion of the woods.

However, the ash tree population has taken a significant hit from the emerald ash borer and right on that destructive little insects' path is the Asian long-horned beetle. The larvae of both beetles feed on the cambium layer, the part of the tree that carries

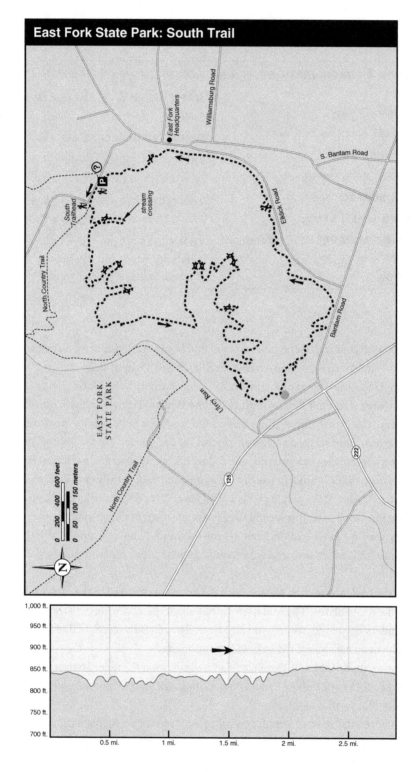

East Fork State Park: South Trail

East Fork Headquarters
Williamsburg Road
S. Bantam Road
Elklick Road
stream crossing
South Trailhead
North Country Trail
Bantam Road
EAST FORK STATE PARK
Ulrey Run
North Country Trail

0   200   400   600 feet
0   50   100   150 meters

125
222

1,000 ft.
950 ft.
900 ft.
850 ft.
800 ft.
750 ft.
700 ft.

0.5 mi.   1 mi.   1.5 mi.   2 mi.   2.5 mi.

water and nutrients between the roots and leaves. This kills the tree. To help protect all forests do not remove anything from any forest.

At roughly eye level and attached to trees are yellow medallions with the icon of a mountain biker or painted white blazes on the trees to mark the trail's path through the woods. In the fall with the abundance of leaves on the forest floor, the trail might be a little difficult to follow. If at any time you are confused about whether or not you're on the trail, simply look for the bright yellow medallions or white blazes.

A beautiful valley area is visible at 0.39 mile. Walking through this valley's open understory, tall canopy, and moss-covered trees seems like stepping into a children's storybook tale, minus the dragons. But, if you walk slowly and quietly, you may see wild turkeys and white-tailed deer.

In the bend of the trail is a large shagbark hickory, and at 0.47 mile, you'll cross a footbridge. Less than 100 feet ahead, you'll come upon another footbridge. The path curves into an area with larger red oak, sycamore, and American beech trees.

At 0.58 mile, lovely black cherry trees flourish to the left of the trail. One of my favorite trees is the sycamore, and at 0.6 mile, near another footbridge, is a stunning group of sycamores complete with platy yellow, gray, and tan bark and ghostly white trunks.

Eastern screech owls seem to prefer sycamore trees. The diminutive owls sound similar to a child's baby-doll cry. In southern Ohio, the red color morph is more common than the gray, which is more common farther north. Maybe that is why the small owls are often overlooked when perched along the tawny branches of sycamore trees.

Within 250 feet of the sycamores, three ridges become visible through the open woods. Higher along the ridge at 0.68 mile is a great view of the valley to the right. Continue along the ridgeline and enjoy the valley views.

Be careful of your footing crossing over the series of 2-foot-high bumps at 1.13 miles. Cross two more footbridges within 100 feet of the bumps.

The forest at 1.2 miles is a young and dense grouping of sugar maple, black cherry, hackberry, American beech, and elm trees. Grapevine and multiflora rose are plentiful in this area.

The trail crosses a series of bridges for the next 0.1 mile. Another footbridge at 1.4 miles is surrounded by red oak and sugar maple saplings. You'll see an exposed streambed and surrounding bedrock in the valley area at 1.74 miles.

The sycamore- and oak-dominated forest transitions to brambles at 1.88 miles and into a successional field at 1.94 miles. Stop and listen for the chorusing of frogs at a small pond at 2.04 miles. Along the forest edge at 2.09 miles, several flat stones line the trail where it parallels the road, passing several storm water manhole access points.

A footbridge crosses the creek at 2.46 miles. The trail passes in front of the park office (across the road) at 2.73 miles. The trail curves and a stone path leads through the brambles and honeysuckle.

The footbridge at 2.76 miles passes by a pond area with wood duck nesting boxes and leads back to the parking lot. Return to the parking lot, opposite from the kiosk.

Nearby Activities

Stonelick State Park, Cincinnati Nature Center, and Chilo Lock 34 Park and Crooked Run Nature Preserve provide additional hiking opportunities. East Fork State Park also is home to portions of the Buckeye Trail, the North Country National Scenic Trail, and the American Discovery Trail, as well as the Steve Newman Worldwalker Perimeter Trail—it's just 31.5 miles long.

GPS Trailhead Coordinates and Directions

N39° 00.411'   W84° 08.528'

From I-275 on Cincinnati's east side, take Exit 65/Beechmont/Amelia. Travel east on OH 125 for 9.5 miles. Turn northeast onto Bantam Road and travel 0.3 mile. Turn north onto Elklick Road to enter the park.

10 Edge of Appalachia Preserve:
The Wilderness Trail

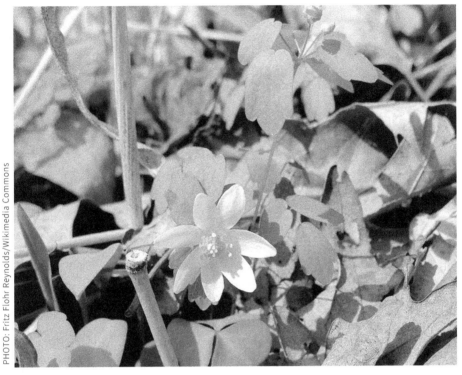

Rue anemone along the trail

In Brief

This wonderful trail is part of The Nature Conservancy's Edge of Appalachia Nature Preserve System and is a National Natural Landmark. The area offers a variety of habitats as well as a fantastic "all alonely" hike. Throughout the hike are beautiful dolomite cliffs, waterfalls, and a diversity of wildlife. Be aware of the multiple cliff edges—stay on the trail and pay attention.

Description

The Wilderness Trail's small parking area is at the end of Shivener Road. This preserve honors Charlie A. Eulett, an Adams County teacher who during the 1960s and 1970s

PHOTO: Fritz Flohr Reynolds/Wikimedia Commons

LENGTH & CONFIGURATION 2.45-mile loop	Museum of Natural History's The Wilderness Trail Map
DIFFICULTY Moderate	**WHEELCHAIR ACCESSIBLE** No
SCENERY Woods, cliffs, waterfalls	**FACILITIES** None
EXPOSURE Shade and some sun	**CONTACTS** The Nature Conservancy, 614-717-2770; **tinyurl.com/wildernesstrl;** Appalachian Discovery, **appalachiandiscovery .com**
TRAFFIC Light	
TRAIL SURFACE Gravel and dolomite	
HIKING TIME 1.5–2 hours	**COMMENTS** Multiple cliffs and ravines offer incredible views. If hiking with young children, keep them close at all times. This trail is rugged and travels along the leading edge of several cliffs. Includes Appalachian Discovery Birding and Heritage Trail.
DRIVING DISTANCE 20 minutes east of West Union	
SEASON Year-round	
ACCESS Daily, sunrise–sunset; free	
MAPS USGS *Brush Creek;* Cincinnati	

taught people about the county's prairies and woodlands. From the gravel parking area, the entrance to the trail is near the corner of the fence along the south corner of the parking lot.

To find the entrance, look for the bright yellow markings to the Appalachian Discovery Birding and Heritage Trail. Enter the trail through a narrow passageway along the fence. To stay on the trail, follow the yellow blazes.

The Cincinnati Museum of Natural History manages the Wilderness Trail area for educational and scientific use, and the trail is a National Natural Landmark. Please stay on the trail and refrain from climbing the cliffs.

The trail heads downhill through a forest dominated by sycamore and red and white oak trees. Just 422 feet after you begin the hike, you'll cross a small footbridge in the valley. The waterway flowing into the valley under the bridge is Saw Mill Branch. American beech, tulip poplar, chestnut oak, sugar maple, and black gum trees cover the hillsides.

Take a moment to register at the Charles A. Eulett sign-in box. Odds are pretty good that you won't see another person while you're on this hike. Add in the remote location and you end up with an extremely serene hike.

The wooded area is a great example of a balanced forest, one with a good mixture of understory, saplings, and canopy trees. Watch for the small grove of American beech saplings that bracket the trail. Also notice the absence of invasive honeysuckle

Edge of Appalachia Preserve: The Wilderness Trail

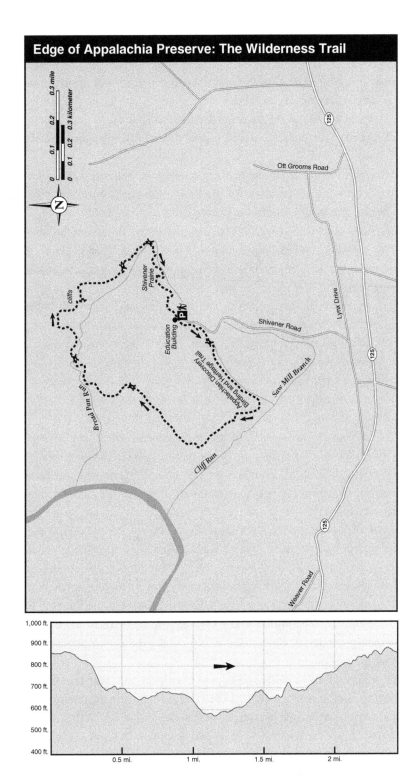

67

in this area. This is important for the natural succession of the woodland to take place and for wildflowers to survive and thrive.

In spring, at 0.2 mile you'll be rewarded with an abundance of wildflowers. The trail meanders through the woods, up and down hills, and runs parallel to the stream below.

At 0.25 mile, the trail heads uphill to rocky outcrops. The trail at this point is one person wide. Cross a small stream at 0.47 mile and enter into an eastern red cedar stand. The dolomite under your feet is also the stone of the cliffs.

Along this stretch of the hike, look left and peer down the edge of the cliff into the valley 60 to 80 feet below. Head downhill at 0.53 mile. Be careful on the loose, gravelly surface of the dolomite. The path is especially slippery when leaves cover it and when it's been raining.

As you walk through the forest of sugar maple, white oak, dogwood, and redbud trees, you might be fortunate enough to startle a deer or see a wild turkey. The trail rounds a bend at 0.65 mile. At 0.82 mile, lichen-covered cliffs come into view.

At 1 mile the hike crosses another footbridge. You are warned—this footbridge has a lot of wiggle to it. Take a left and pass between the American beech trees. You'll cross a few more streams near 1.08 miles. Look for the tracks of raccoons and skunks, as well as those of deer.

At 1.23 miles, you'll see a waterfall and small ravine stream. Bread Pan Run Creek passes through the valley. Look for the yellow marks on the trees to stay on the trail. Cross a bridge 100 feet ahead. The narrow trail leads uphill through red cedar and tulip trees. Use the stepping-stones to cross the small stream cascading through the dolomite at 1.5 miles.

As the trail goes up the hill, cliffs border the trail to the left and right. You'll see several large chunks of dolomite covered in lichens and moss near 1.55 miles. Sugar maples and chinquapin oaks dominate the forest. During spring migration, scarlet tanagers, warblers, and flycatchers bring color and lively songs to the quiet woods.

During the next 100 feet, cross several streams as the path continues to head uphill. After crossing the footbridge at 1.87 miles, the trail is relatively flat. To the right are multiple waterfalls. The trail at this point is parallel to the stream some 30 feet below.

At 2 miles you'll reach what appears to be a trail junction. Take the trail to the right downhill and cross a footbridge. As you continue on the trail, the stream to your left cascades over a series of block-shaped limestone.

The trail takes a hard right at 2.1 miles and heads uphill. Again, if you're unsure exactly where the trail is, look for the yellow marks on the trees. This portion of the trail suffers from a fair amount of erosion.

At 2.2 miles the path enters into an open area named Shivener Prairie, once known as Floyd Shivener's corn patch. Now it's a prairie, complete with blazing star, rue anemone, and western sunflower.

Squeeze through the entrance/exit at 2.31 miles, leaving the woods and entering into an open, grassy area. To the right is a latrine and to the left is the education building. Take the gravel road uphill to your vehicle.

Nearby Activities

Adams County is home to a multitude of hiking opportunities, including Chaparral Prairie State Nature Preserve, Adams Lake State Park and Adams Lake Prairie State Nature Preserve, Buzzardroost Rock Trail, and several other shorter hikes. Adams County is also home to the Audubon automobile birding trail as well as Quilt Barn Squares. Donna Sue Groves began the Quilt Sampler project to honor her mother, who is a master quilter. The Quilt Barns each have one large quilt square painted on them. The artwork and patterns are truly beautiful.

GPS Trailhead Coordinates and Directions

N38° 46.813'   W83° 25.030'

From West Union, drive 7 miles east on OH 125. Turn northeast (left) on Lynx Drive and in 0.2 mile, turn north (left) onto Shivener Road. The preserve is located at the end of Shivener Road.

11 Fernald Preserve

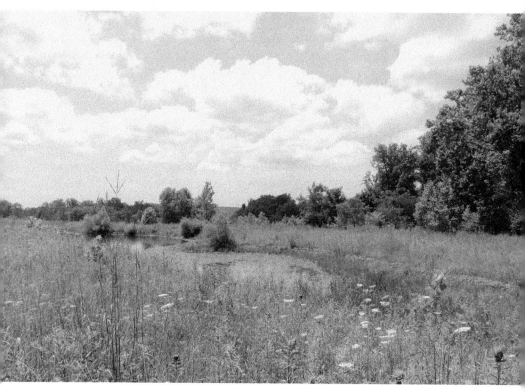

Meadow views and pocket wetlands make this the perfect spot for a variety of birds.

In Brief

Fernald Preserve was a uranium-processing facility. In 2006 remedial actions were completed to address the long-term groundwater safety, and environmental restoration projects were underway. In 2008 the preserve opened to the public and offers more than 7 miles of hiking trails through woods, prairies, meadows, and wetlands, and a sustainably designed visitor center.

Description

Fernald Preserve is a site where uranium production used to occur. The land was bought in 1951 by the U.S. Department of Energy (DOE), and its predecessor agency, the Atomic Energy Commission. Uranium processing began in 1952 and in 1986 the state of Ohio initiated a claim against the DOE for violations of multiple environmental

LENGTH & CONFIGURATION 5.8-mile loops

DIFFICULTY Easy–moderate

SCENERY Prairie, wetlands, ponds, and forests

EXPOSURE Sun and shade

TRAFFIC Moderate

TRAIL SURFACE Gravel, earth, and mowed grass

HIKING TIME 2–3 hours

DRIVING DISTANCE Less than 30 minutes from Cincinnati

SEASON Year-round

ACCESS Daily, 7 a.m.–sunset. Visitor center: Wednesday–Saturday, 9 a.m.–5 p.m.; free

MAPS USGS *Shandon;* Fernald Preserve Trails Map

WHEELCHAIR ACCESSIBLE The trails around the visitor center are compacted gravel.

FACILITIES Water fountains, restrooms, and benches inside the visitor center

CONTACTS Fernald Preserve Administrative Office, 513-648-6000; **www.lm.doe .gov/Fernald/sites.aspx**

COMMENTS This site is a former uranium-production facility, and after uranium-contaminated groundwater was discovered and much controversy, the facility was closed. The site has undergone remedial actions and restoration.

regulations. This resulted in the site being listed on the Environmental Protection Agency's national priority list in 1989, and in that same year, uranium production was ceased at the site.

In 1991 remediation efforts began and in 2006 remedial actions such as the long-term groundwater remedy were in place and nature restoration projects had begun. The site officially opened to the public in 2008.

Follow the main entrance road to the visitor center. Take a few minutes to explore the visitor center to gain a clearer picture of what occurred at this site and the changes that have been made to improve it. If you have children, be sure to grab a copy of the scavenger hunt before starting on the trails. Back outside, walk to the far back corner of the large parking lot and look for the trail entrance.

The Shingle Oak Trail takes you through diverse habitats including wetlands, prairies, and woodlands. This trail has a variety of milkweed plants along the borders and plenty of butterflies. Songbirds zip overhead and take much-needed breaks on the overhanging branches near the water. You might even get lucky and startle a wild turkey dusting on the wide gravel trail.

A few hundred feet after the trailhead is the old site of the Fernald silo which is now a wetland area. Expect to see dragonflies and red-winged blackbirds flitting through the willows. At the trail intersection, turn right and follow it to Paddy's Run Overlook and take in the scenery of the cottonwoods and sycamore trees from the bench.

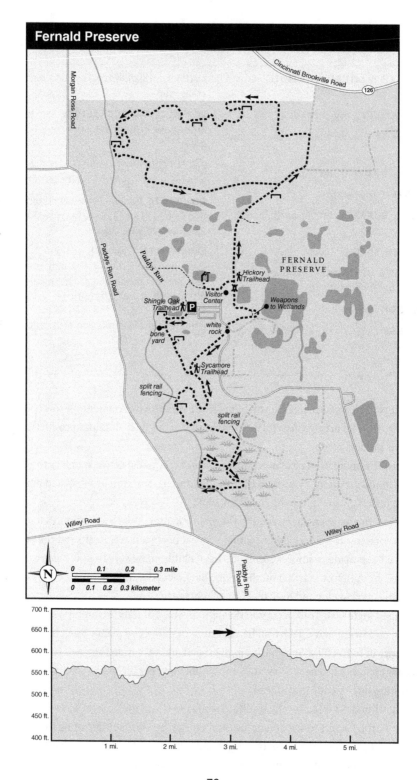

Fernald Preserve

FERNALD
PRESERVE

Cincinnati Brookville Road
126

Morgan Ross Road

Paddys Run Road

Paddys Run

Hickory
Trailhead

Visitor
Center

Shingle Oak
Trailhead

P

Weapons
to Wetlands

bone
yard

white
rock

Sycamore
Trailhead

split rail
fencing

split rail
fencing

Willey Road

Willey Road

Paddys Run Road

N

| 0 | 0.1 | 0.2 | 0.3 mile |

| 0 | 0.1 | 0.2 | 0.3 kilometer |

700 ft.
650 ft.
600 ft.
550 ft.
500 ft.
450 ft.
400 ft.

1 mi.   2 mi.   3 mi.   4 mi.   5 mi.

Retrace your steps to the intersection and continue to the right. On the right side of the trail, immediately before you reach the intersection with the short trail to the Bone Yard, is a walnut tree and just a few feet away is a great example of a sycamore tree. Take the short trail to the Bone Yard and then continue on the Shingle Oak Trail through the riparian habitat.

At the next intersection turn left. Pass by the area where thousands of saplings and shrubs were planted as part of the ecological restoration before reaching the wildlife-viewing area 0.27 mile into the hike. Return to the main trail and continue to the left.

When you reach the junction with the Sycamore Trail at 0.44 mile into the hike, follow the Sycamore Trail to the right. The surface of the trail changes to a mowed grass path. Stay on the trail as you pass by grasses, bee balms, and thistles before entering a wooded area.

The small pond at 0.59 mile is filled with a plethora of frogs chorusing during the summer months. The trail meanders through a meadow becoming gravel again. While it may look as through the trail ends, travel on the gravel path until you reach the wooded area. Look to the right for the sycamore trees and the small footpath leading into the woods comprised of hackberries, walnuts, and hickories. At 0.72 mile is an enormous sycamore tree on the right side as the trail curves.

Pass by the split rail fencing at 0.76 mile into the hike. Watch for the lichen-covered trees along this section of the trail. This portion of the hike is a peaceful retreat from the chaos of daily life. At 0.83 mile take a break at the bench while you enjoy the views of the valley.

In 300 feet, the trail exits the cool shade of the woods and enters a meadow skirting by the other side of the pond passed earlier. When you reach the split rail fence at 1.06 miles, continue to the right. At the next trail intersection follow the trail to the left and enter a wet meadow area filled with willows, bee balms, cattails, and coneflowers. Take a break on the bench before continuing on the trail.

When you reach the trail intersection retrace your steps on the Sycamore Trail to the Shingle Oak Trail junction. Turn right and follow the Shingle Oak Trail. Pass by the pine plantations. At the next trail split is a large white rock. The visitor center is visible to the left.

Take the trail across the road 2.56 miles into the hike and continue on the gravel path through the open meadow filled with songbirds. Pass the Weapons to Wetlands Grove and walk down to the boardwalk overlooking of the pond. This was once the site of the uranium-production area.

As you continue on the trial the visitor center is off to the right. Follow the trail around the backside of the visitor center at 2.85 miles. Watch for the solstice marker and the restoration garden.

Look for the trailhead for the Hickory Trail as you cross the trestle-style bridge. Don't accidently take the side trail to the left—you'll take this later. Continue straight ahead on the Hickory Trail. At the split, take the trail to the right. The trail takes a hard left and follows along an access road before taking another hard left at the green shed.

When the trail rounds the bend to the right you are treated with a woodland of hickory trees before the trail turns left and is surrounded by red oaks and elms. Sit at the bench and look straight ahead at the snags. Hummingbirds use the tiny limbs as resting spots.

Continue on the trail and stop to examine the chew marks on the bench located 4.18 miles into the hike. The trail ducks in and out of the woods before reaching the bench at 4.73 miles that overlooks a steep valley. Take a few moments at this spot to see how many birds you can identify by their calls. The tree at the right end of the bench is a white oak.

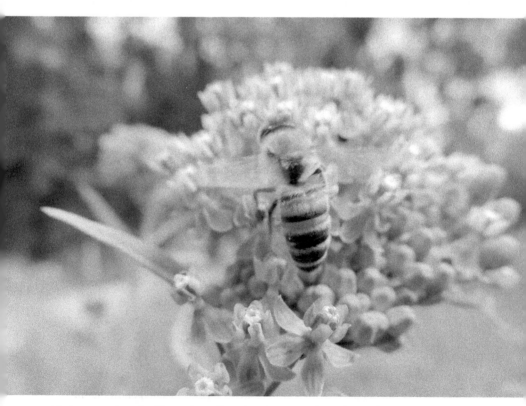

Various species of milkweed grow in abundance and are the perfect place to capture photos of bees and butterflies.

At 4.75 miles the trial skirts along a split rail fence protecting you from the steep hillside leading to Paddy's Run. The forest is comprised of white oaks, hackberries, and sugar maples. The trail enters an open area with a pond that is home to plenty of green frogs and bullfrogs. Watch for butterflies on the coneflowers and blazing stars.

At 5 miles the trail comes out onto a service road; continue straight on the service road. The wetlands are closely monitored and part of the remediation of the land. When you reach the trail split turn right and retrace your steps back to side trail you passed earlier. Turn right and follow the side trail to the observation platform. Return to the trail and follow it back to the visitor center and then to your vehicle.

Nearby Activities

More trails are nearby at Miami Whitewater Forest, Hueston Woods State Park, Miami University's Bachelor Preserve, and Governor Bebb MetroPark. If you are hungry or need supplies there are plenty of options in Ross as well as the Northgate area.

GPS Trailhead Coordinates and Directions

N39° 17.871'   W84° 41.740'

From I-275 near Northgate take Exit 33 for US 27/OH 126 North. Travel north on US 27 for 5 miles to the Hamilton–Ross exit. Turn left (south) onto OH 128/Hamilton–Cleves Highway and travel 4 miles, passing through Ross. Turn right onto Willey Road. The entrance is 0.25 mile ahead.

12 Fort Ancient State Memorial

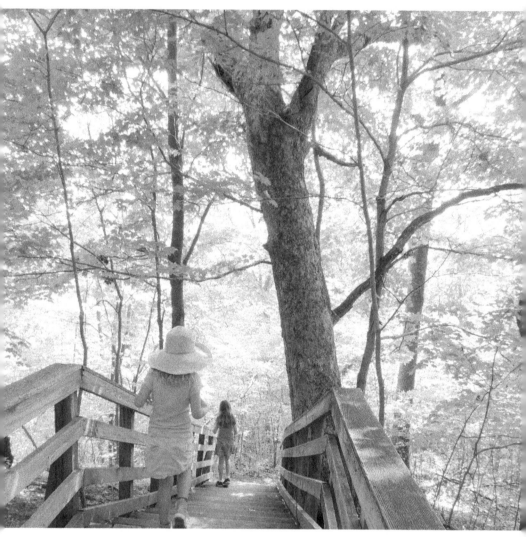

The boardwalk snakes above the fragile forest floor.

In Brief

Expect the unexpected along the trail at Fort Ancient. An elaborate array of earthworks and a stone serpent grace the trail through the woods. Enjoy the many displays in the museum and visitor center. The children's discovery area is full of opportunities for hands-on learning.

76

LENGTH & CONFIGURATION 3.9-mile out-and-back

DIFFICULTY Easy–moderate

SCENERY American Indian earthworks, mounds, serpent mounds (only one is visible from the hike), woods, and the Little Miami River

EXPOSURE Shade and full sun

TRAFFIC Moderate–heavy

TRAIL SURFACE Soil, wooden stairs, asphalt, and mowed meadow

HIKING TIME 2.5–3 hours

DRIVING DISTANCE 1 hour north of Cincinnati

SEASON Year-round

ACCESS April–November: Tuesday–Saturday, 10 a.m.–5 p.m.; Sunday, noon–5 p.m. Closed Mondays. December–March: Saturday, 10 a.m.–5 p.m.; Sunday, noon–5 p.m. Adults, $6; students ages 6–16 and seniors age 60 and older, $5; children age 5 and younger and members, free

MAPS USGS *Oregonia*

WHEELCHAIR ACCESSIBLE No

FACILITIES Restrooms and water at visitor center and museum

CONTACTS Fort Ancient, 513-932-4421; fortancient.org

COMMENTS A stone serpent? Yes, that's right. You'll find that and more at this National Historic Landmark.

Description

After entering the grounds, park in the lot near the visitor center and museum. Inside you'll find information on Fort Ancient's current events as well as a detailed series of displays about its history. Hands-on interactive learning displays in the children's room keep young and old intrigued. Outside the center is a prehistoric garden Fort Ancient staff and volunteers create each year.

Archaeological evidence shows that the Hopewell American Indians built the earthworks and mounds at Fort Ancient as well as throughout the Ohio River Valley. Evidence also shows that the Hopewell relied on hunting and gathering for their food supplies, but they were also part of a trade network encompassing parts of North America. In fact, copper from the upper peninsula of Michigan, alligator teeth from Louisiana, and mica from the southern Appalachian Mountains have been discovered on this site.

The museum's 9,000 square feet of interpretive displays and exhibits show visitors the history of American Indians in Ohio. Many artifacts found at the site are exhibited, including everyday tools such as the ones the Hopewell used to create the earthworks.

Earthmoving tools were made from available resources. To create a shovel, the Hopewell bound the shoulder-blade bones of large mammals, such as deer or elk, to a long piece of wood. They split elk antlers to create rakes, and to create hoes they used sinew and rope to fasten clamshells and stones to pole-sized saplings or branches.

Fort Ancient State Memorial

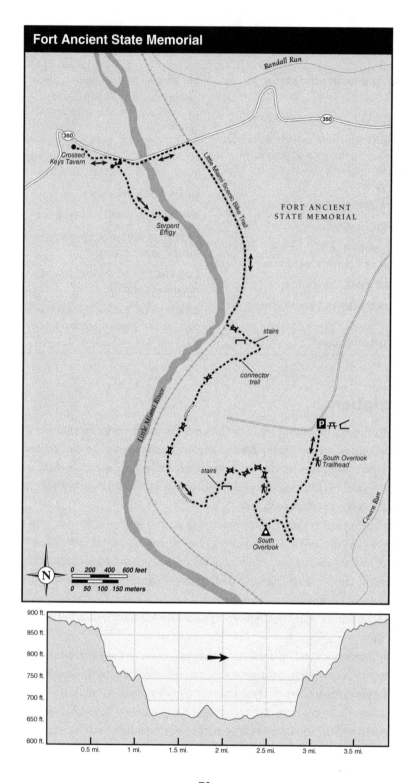

78

After digging, they collected soil into baskets and transferred it to the earthworks site. Archaeologists estimate the soil-laden baskets weighed 35–45 pounds. Radiocarbon dating shows that it took the Hopewell nearly 200 years to create the elaborate earthworks and mounds.

The height of the walls varies 4–23 feet. They enclose 100 acres and stretch an astonishing 3.5 miles. In several places, the walls form regular geometric patterns. The noncontinuous walls are marked by 70 openings. Archaeologists theorize that the alignment of the mound and the walls' openings served as a type of calendar for the tribe. They could use the sun to track annual events and the moon to track events a decade apart.

To begin the hike, return to your vehicle after exploring the visitor center and drive to the shelter houses and picnic area near the South Fort. Park your vehicle in the large parking lot to the south of the main road. A small sign points the way to the South Overlook and Earthworks Trails. Cross the mowed grass to the South Overlook trailhead. Interpretive maps are inside the mailbox near the trailhead.

The earthworks enclosure was built in three main parts: the North, Middle, and South Forts. Interpretive signs throughout the hike explain the history of the earthworks. At the trail split at 0.2 mile, stay to the left. The trail is a narrow path through the woods dominated by sugar maple trees.

At the bench at 0.26 mile, follow the trail to the right, passing in front of a large wooden sign. You'll see multiple spur trails in this area and it's easy to take one by accident. The approved trails do not impact the earthworks and are relatively flat. If you find yourself hiking up a small hill, backtrack until you are in the flat area again and look for the approved trail.

The hills in front of you are the earthworks. Continue following this trail as it leads you back near the trail split. Turn left and continue on the trail among the hickory and tulip poplar trees.

The Hopewell constructed and used the earthworks between 100 B C and A D 300. The Hopewell culture consisted of several American Indian tribes and encompassed a wide range of economic, political, and spiritual beliefs and practices. The common thread was the construction of earthen walls built in geometric patterns and mounds. The Hopewell were also known for their diverse network of contacts extending from the Atlantic coast to the Rocky Mountains. This vast trading network brought mica, sharks' teeth, obsidian, copper, and seashells to Ohio.

Before the Hopewell culture, the Adena lived in this area from 700 BC to 0. Long after the Hopewell culture at this site disappeared, the Fort Ancient culture, believed to be descendants of the Hopewell, lived and farmed here from A D 890 until 1650.

Walk to the benches under the large hickory and oak trees. Follow the boardwalk to the South Overlook of the Little Miami River Gorge, which is some 270 feet deep. This gorge was created during the Wisconsin Ice Age 18,000 years ago. Glacial meltwaters created new watercourses throughout this region.

Return to the trail along the edge of the woods and grassy area. Along the wood line at 0.44 mile, follow the trail to the left and into the woods. The path leads downhill, with a fair amount of poison ivy on both sides of the trail. The forest is composed of sugar maples, oaks, and basswoods. Cross the bridge at 0.49 mile. This area is full of periwinkle, planted in the 1930s by the Civilian Conservation Corps in an effort to stabilize the easily eroded hillsides. Cross two more bridges over the next 200 feet.

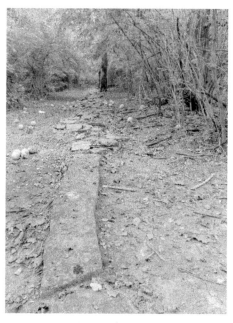

Kern Effigy 2

Here you'll find plenty of redbuds and dogwoods, which in spring burst with lavender redbud blooms and pinkish-white dogwood blooms. Cross several more footbridges over the next 0.2 mile as the trail winds along a hillside through a forest of hickory, box elder, spicebush, sugar maple, and sassafras trees. You might even be surprised by a person zip-lining above your head.

At 1 mile you'll reach a junction with a connector trail to the Little Miami River, which you will take. Follow the switchback and descend the staircase. When this trail connects with a bike path, turn right and follow the asphalt path 0.4 mile to the canoe livery. Turn left onto State Route 350. Carefully cross the bridge on the left side of the road.

Turn left immediately after the bridge, slip around the cattle fence (don't worry—no cattle), and into an open field. Walk toward the Little Miami River and follow the treeline for 760 feet until you reach the opening marked with a white blaze. Follow the mowed path to the stone serpent, Kern Effigy 2. (Kern Effigy 1 is farther to the east and not included in this hike.)

Kern Effigy 2 is a prehistoric stone serpent created with carefully positioned slabs of limestone. Don't remove stones or walk on this historic landmark. It was discovered in 1983 and fully uncovered by team effort in 1985. The stone serpent's sinuous body stretches nearly 154 feet and is more than 4.5 feet wide. Carbon dating places the construction of the effigy during the time of the Hopewell culture.

By standing outside at 8:40 a.m., in the middle of winter, scientists proved their hypothesis. The stone serpent was used as an astronomical marker to pinpoint the winter solstice. The Kern Effigies are on the National Register of Historic Places.

Return to OH 350, turn left and walk uphill, through the grassy opening, and to the stone house that was the Crossed Keys Tavern, which operated from 1809 until 1820. This building is on the National Register of Historic Places because of its architectural and engineering significance.

Retrace your steps along OH 350, turn right on the bike path, follow it to the Fort Ancient Trail entrance, and retrace your steps to your vehicle.

Nearby Activities

Caesar Creek State Park and Caesar Creek Gorge State Nature Preserve are just minutes away to the north and offer additional hiking trails. Waynesville is known for its antiques shops as well as down-home-cooking restaurants.

GPS Trailhead Coordinates and Directions

N39° 23.977'   W84° 05.651'

From Cincinnati, take I-71 North to Exit 36 and turn right on Wilmington Road. In about 300 feet turn right on Middleboro Road. Travel less than 2 miles and turn right on OH 350. The entrance is 0.7 mile on the left.

13 Germantown MetroPark

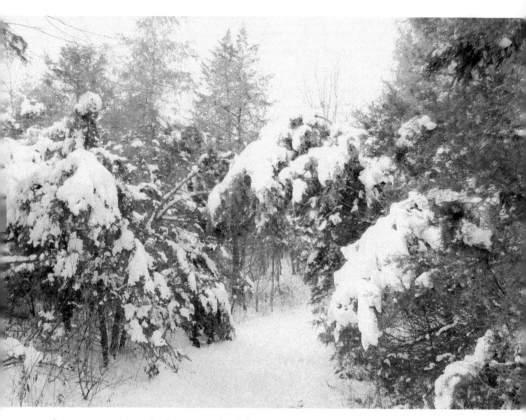

Germantown MetroPark is a popular hike even in winter.

In Brief

Germantown MetroPark is a beautiful area to hike. As with other Five Rivers MetroParks, the trails are well marked and maintained. The eco-friendly and hands-on nature center is a fun place to learn more about this area and green practices.

Description

Germantown MetroPark came into being in the 1930s during the Great Depression, when 1,665 acres of diverse habitat was reserved for public use and enjoyment by the Miami Conservancy District. Several small tributaries throughout the park drain into Twin Creek, which flows through the heart of park. In fact, the varying topography and watersheds create a mosaic of forests, prairies, cedar stands, and ponds.

LENGTH & CONFIGURATION 7.36-mile loop

DIFFICULTY Moderate–difficult

SCENERY Woods and waterways

EXPOSURE Shade and some sun

TRAFFIC Moderate

TRAIL SURFACE Boardwalk, soil, and exposed rock

HIKING TIME 4–5 hours

DRIVING DISTANCE 1 hour north of Cincinnati

SEASON Year-round

ACCESS April 1–October 31: Daily, 8 a.m.–10 p.m.; November 1–March 31: Daily, 8 a.m.–8 p.m.; closed January 1 and December 25; free

MAPS USGS *Farmersville;* Germantown MetroPark map

WHEELCHAIR ACCESSIBLE Boardwalk area

FACILITIES Restrooms and drinking water in nature center

CONTACTS Five Rivers MetroParks, 937-275-PARK (7275); **metroparks.org/Parks /Germantown/Home.aspx**

COMMENTS This hike gives you time to think as it weaves through the forest along Twin Creek.

The combination of habitats works well for bobcats, as sightings of this elusive animal have been confirmed by biologists. You have little to fear from bobcats. The nocturnal animals are extremely reclusive and rarely, if ever, seen.

After turning off Boomershine Road, follow the signs to the nature center. Park in the lot and walk to the kiosk, then follow the sidewalk path downhill to the nature center. This ecologically friendly feature is almost completely underground.

Sit and watch squirrels and songbirds through the large plate-glass windows in the "Window on Wildlife" area inside. Be sure to poke around the nature center and explore the multiple exhibits. When you return outside to the wooden deck, examine the totem pole–style trail-marker post. It is marked with different-colored circles, each specific to a looped trail that will return you to the trail's point of origin.

Turn left and follow the red/orange/green trail. The boardwalk is about 15 feet above ground, which provides a unique perspective through the canopy of deciduous trees.

Below the right side of the trail is a streambed, complete with a waterfall. Stop and enjoy the view, and try to identify the assortment of birds by their songs. At the end of the boardwalk, take the stone stairs to the gravel path. At 0.4 mile, turn left onto the red/orange/green trail (post 1).

The trail leads into an eastern red cedar forest. Hardwood trees are selectively removed from this area to prevent the cedar trees from being shaded out. Five Rivers MetroParks does an excellent job of actively managing their land for diverse habitats.

Germantown MetroPark

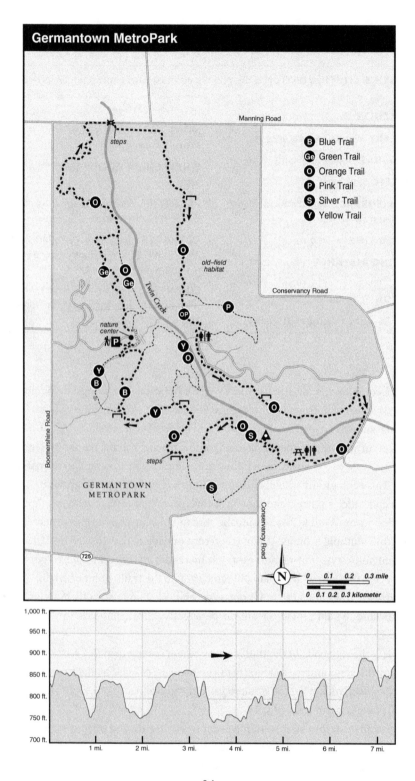

B Blue Trail
Ge Green Trail
O Orange Trail
P Pink Trail
S Silver Trail
Y Yellow Trail

Manning Road

steps

old–field
habitat

Conservancy Road

Twin Creek

nature
center

GERMANTOWN
METROPARK

steps

Boomershine Road

Conservancy Road

725

N

| 0 | 0.1 | 0.2 | 0.3 mile |
| 0 | 0.1 | 0.2 | 0.3 kilometer |

1,000 ft.
950 ft.
900 ft.
850 ft.
800 ft.
750 ft.
700 ft.

1 mi. 2 mi. 3 mi. 4 mi. 5 mi. 6 mi. 7 mi.

The trail passes a small pond, and you might be fortunate enough to scare up a great blue heron. Continue on the main trail past the spur trail at 0.5 mile. In 200 feet, the green trail splits from the red/orange trail (post 3). Continue on the green trail to the left.

The forest transitions from a cedar forest to mixed hardwoods. Pass another pond. At 0.9 mile (post 4), the green trail intersects with another portion of the green trail and the orange trail. Follow the orange trail to the left. The orange trail meanders through an upland forest and switchbacks over the hillsides to decrease the amount of trail erosion.

The trail leads uphill and out of the woods and into a large open field. If you are here in winter and there is snow on the ground, you'll likely see sled riders racing down the hill or trudging back up.

Continue on this trail as it ducks back into the woods and then crosses an open field. Turn right and follow the trail down the embankment to Manning Road at 1.9 miles. Turn right and continue along the edge of the road for 0.2 mile while keeping a watchful eye for fast-moving traffic.

Immediately after the guardrail, take the steps and follow the trail as it parallels Manning Road. If it has rained, this portion may be flooded. If that is the case, continue on Manning Road and immediately after Farmersville Road on the left, look for the orange trail's entrance on the right side of the road. The orange trail continues into the woods. The first portion of the trail is lined with wild ginger, Ohio buckeyes, and a multitude of wildflowers.

You'll enter into an open, grassy area at 3.1 miles. This old-field habitat is slowly being taken over by red cedar trees. Continue watching for the orange markers to make sure you stay on the main trail. At 3.36 miles, the pink trail intersects and merges with the orange trail (post 5). Continue on the pink/orange trail, which is the trail on the right. (The pink trail is to the left.)

At 3.59 miles, continue on the orange trail at the pink and orange trail intersection (post 6). Cross the dam at 4.5 miles. When the silver trail joins the orange trail (post 16) continue on the orange/silver trail. At 5.87 miles is an excellent view of Twin Creek. Follow the orange trail to the right (post 8) when the orange and silver trails diverge.

At 6.25 miles, rest a while on the bench. In spring, take a few moments to enjoy the trillium-covered hillsides. In some areas the blooms are so dense that the hillsides appear covered in a blanket of snow. At 6.44 miles, enjoy a pleasant spot on yet another bench. At the trail junction (post 9), continue on the yellow trail to the left.

At the intersection of the yellow and blue trails at 7 miles (post 12), turn to the right and take the blue trail. Continue following this trail through the woods.

When the blue and the white trails connect (post 11), follow the white/blue trail straight ahead. The forest floor is relatively open with a just few saplings under the tall shagbark hickory, beech, and white oak trees.

The orange/yellow trail and blue/white trail connect with each other at 7.3 miles (post 10). Turn left and continue on the orange/blue/yellow/white trail. Give yourself the freedom to enjoy the multitude of shelf waterfalls along the right side of the trail.

This trail crosses a small stream and returns to the nature center. From the nature center, retrace your steps back to your vehicle in the parking area.

Nearby Activities

Hueston Woods State Park, Cox Arboretum MetroPark, and Sugarcreek MetroPark provide more hiking and nature-viewing opportunities. The Dayton Mall shopping area is just minutes to the east.

GPS Trailhead Coordinates and Directions

N39° 38.578'   W84° 25.512'

From Cincinnati, take I-75 North. Exit onto OH 725 West. Follow OH 725 for 11 miles to Boomershine Road and turn north (right). Take Boomershine Road 1 mile and turn east (right) into Germantown MetroPark. Follow the signs to the nature center.

14 Gilmore MetroPark

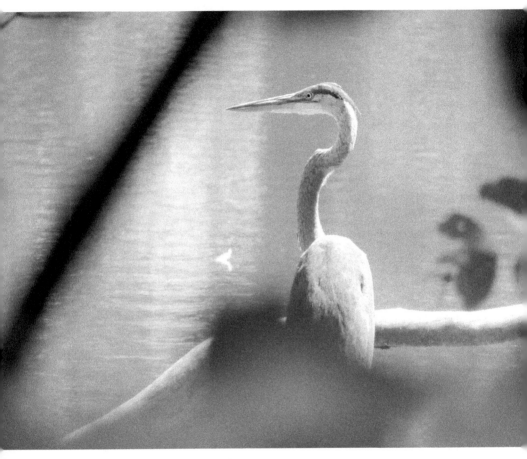

Great blue heron at Kingfisher Pond

In Brief

A gem in the middle of suburbia, Gilmore MetroPark offers wetland-dependent creatures a safe haven and wildlife watchers opportunities to view songbirds, turtles, kingfishers, butterflies, and waterfowl.

Description

It's hard to believe that in the middle of suburbia flourishes a 200-acre park composed primarily of wetlands. The complex provides important habitat for waterfowl,

LENGTH & CONFIGURATION 2.4-mile loop

DIFFICULTY Easy

SCENERY Wetlands, ponds, marshes, and meadows

EXPOSURE Sun and shade

TRAFFIC Moderate

TRAIL SURFACE Soil, access road, mowed path, and decking

HIKING TIME 2 hours (includes time at the observation blind and decks)

DRIVING DISTANCE 30 minutes northwest of Cincinnati

SEASON Year-round, though spring rains may flood portions of the trails

ACCESS Daily, sunrise–sunset; Butler County residents, free vehicle permit; nonresidents, $10 annual vehicle permit or $5 daily vehicle permit

MAPS USGS *Greenhills;* Butler County Parks Gilmore MetroPark map

WHEELCHAIR ACCESSIBLE No

FACILITIES None

CONTACTS MetroParks of Butler County, 513-867-5835; **butlercountymetroparks .org/gilmore.asp**

COMMENTS This low-lying wetland complex accumulates water from the surrounding parking lots and roadways. As a result, the trails might be flooded—after all, it *is* a wetland.

songbirds, and shorebirds. Other species such as frogs, salamanders, turtles, white-tailed deer, and raccoons also thrive here.

Gilmore MetroPark has a unique history. In the early 1800s, this area was part of a large wetland complex dubbed the Big Pond. The Miami–Erie Canal flowed through Mill Creek Valley to the Gilmore MetroPark and on to the Great Miami River Valley. The Miami–Erie Canal system was abandoned in 1929 due to the growing popularity of the railroad system.

Park in the lot and walk north to the wet woods. The trailhead for the Conservancy Loop is also the start of the floating dock. Step onto the dock—well, it will be floating if there's water, and if not it will be on the ground. If it's floating don't step too quickly across the dock, as the up-and-down motions of your footfalls will cause water to squirt out of the small holes in the dock boards and right up the inside of your pant leg.

Keep moving along the dock; if you don't, the section you're standing on will begin to sink. Red, silver, and sugar maples and cottonwoods provide ample shade. If you enter quietly and move slowly along the dock, you may glimpse some of the waterfowl that utilize this area.

Continue on the dock to the slight hill leading to the access road at 300 feet, and turn right. This trail follows along the old Miami–Erie Canal on the left. It's also an access road that receives traffic from heavy utility vehicles, and as a result, portions of the trail have deep ruts. In the spring and summer, look for tadpoles here.

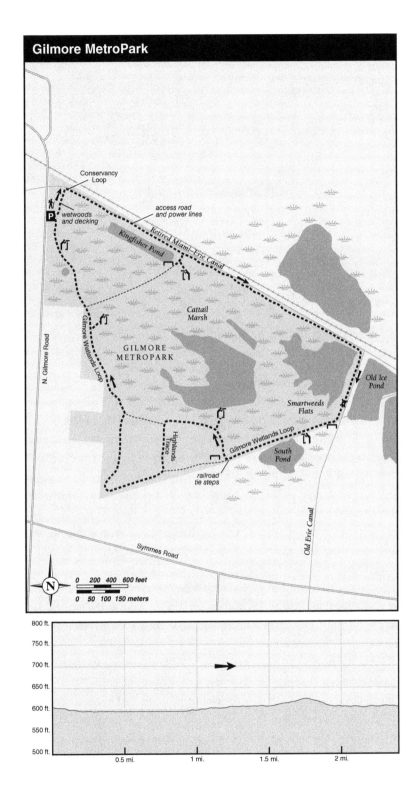

Gilmore MetroPark

Conservancy Loop

access road and power lines

wetwoods and decking

P

Kingfisher Pond

Retired Miami–Erie Canal

N. Gilmore Road

Gilmore Wetlands Loop

Cattail Marsh

GILMORE METROPARK

Old Ice Pond

Smartweeds Flats

Highlands Trace

Gilmore Wetlands Loop

South Pond

railroad tie steps

Old Erie Canal

Symmes Road

N

0   200   400   600 feet
0   50   100   150 meters

800 ft.
750 ft.
700 ft.
650 ft.
600 ft.
550 ft.
500 ft.

0.5 mi.   1 mi.   1.5 mi.   2 mi.

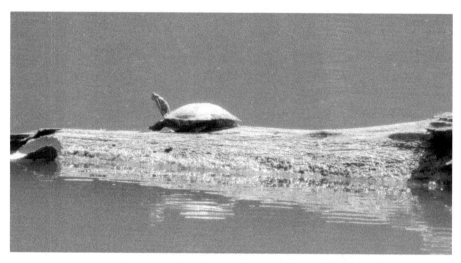

Painted turtle sunning on log in Kingfisher Pond

You'll have a minimal amount of shade along this portion of the trail. Keep watch in the wet woods to the right for waterfowl species, including pintails and grebes. Also, listen for the distinctive calls of the great blue heron and the kingfisher.

On the right at 0.26 mile, you'll pass a large body of water with several snags (dead trees). Continue on the Conservancy Loop Trail until you see the hiker medallion that leads to the right at 0.38 mile. Take this trail up a small hill and into the wetland area. The trail proceeds straight ahead, but I have yet to hike this portion due to flooding.

To the left of the trail is a two-story blind that looks over the marsh and provides a spot for quietly viewing the wildlife activity. To the right is an opening that overlooks Kingfisher Pond. Approach the opening slowly because turtles often sun themselves in this open area.

When you return to the access road turn right. This trail is Gilmore Wetland Loop. At 1 mile the trail takes a right and passes Old Ice Pond to the left and Smartweed Flats to the right. Old Ice Pond provided ice to the Cincinnati area during the late 19th and early 20th centuries.

At the trail junction at 1.12 miles is a bench. Follow Gilmore Wetland Loop to the right. At 1.22 miles you'll reach an observation deck over the South Pond. The deck offers a pleasant spot to look out over the wetlands dominated by smartweed, willows, cottonwoods, and silver maples.

The trail passes through a tunnel of bush honeysuckle so dense that you can't see the wetlands to either side of the trail. At the intersection at 1.39 miles, take a right, staying on Gilmore Wetlands Loop. Follow the trail down the railroad-tie steps to the boardwalk and through the open prairie and marsh. Take a moment and enjoy sitting on the bench and watching the wetlands and prairie for activity.

The trail borders the marsh. At 1.46 miles take the side trail to the edge of the marsh and then return to Gilmore Wetlands Loop. At 1.5 miles at the intersection with Highlands Trace Trail (red medallions), turn left and follow it through the prairie. At 1.6 miles turn right, staying on Highlands Trace as it winds through prairie plants and briefly through a woodland area. Follow it until it reconnects with Gilmore Wetlands Loop (blue medallions) at 2 miles.

Another observation platform at 2.2 miles looks out over Cattail Marsh. Sit down, get comfortable, and watch for waterfowl species, especially during the early morning and late afternoon hours.

Continue on Gilmore Wetlands Loop. Pass the spur trail and look for the bluebird nesting boxes throughout this area. Red-winged blackbirds are common throughout this portion of the hike.

Pass the Conservancy Loop connector trail to the observation tower blind at 2.33 miles. Continue on the left side of the Conservancy Loop. Pass another spur trail that leads to the left. The Conservancy Loop passes through a prairie busy with songbirds and butterflies and then a small pond at 2.45 miles before opening into the manicured lawn area.

Continue to the outdoor classroom platform and onto the boardwalk on the other side. The boardwalk leads back to the parking lot and your vehicle.

Nearby Activities

Winton Woods, Caldwell Preserve, and Spring Grove Cemetery offer additional hiking trails. Stop by Jungle Jim's for pretty much any kind of food or beverage you can imagine and Bass Pro Shops for outdoor supplies.

GPS Trailhead Coordinates and Directions

N39° 21.382'   W84° 31.137'

From Cincinnati, take I-75 North to I-275 West. Take Exit 41 to OH 4 North. Travel 2.5 miles and turn north onto OH 4 Bypass. In 1.4 miles, turn left onto Symmes Road. Travel less than a mile and turn right onto North Gilmore Road. The park entrance is less than 0.7 mile ahead on the right.

15 Governor Bebb MetroPark and Pioneer Village

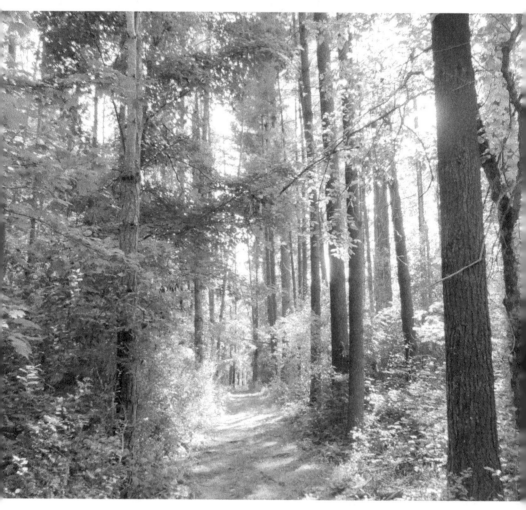

Look and listen for songbirds along the edges of the woodland trail.

In Brief

Complete with log cabins and a covered bridge, Governor Bebb MetroPark and Pioneer Village provides a trip back into Ohio's pioneering past. Enjoy a peaceful retreat by hiking through the upland woods, pine stand, and meadow area.

LENGTH & CONFIGURATION 1.6-mile loop	30 minutes after sunset; Pioneer Village Memorial Day weekend–Labor Day weekend: Saturday and Sunday, 1 p.m.– 5 p.m.; Butler County residents, free vehicle permit; nonresidents, $10 annual vehicle permit or $5 daily vehicle permit
DIFFICULTY Easy	
SCENERY Woods, prairie, pine stand, and re-created pioneer village	
EXPOSURE Sun and shaded	**MAPS** USGS *Harrison* and *Riley*; Governor Bebb MetroPark map
TRAFFIC Light–moderate	
TRAIL SURFACE Soil, exposed rock, and grass	**WHEELCHAIR ACCESSIBLE** No
	FACILITIES Restrooms
HIKING TIME 1 hour	**CONTACTS** MetroParks of Butler County, 513-867-5835; **butlercountymetroparks .org/governor-bebb.asp**
DRIVING DISTANCE 1 hour northwest of Cincinnati	
SEASON Year-round	**COMMENTS** Be sure to enjoy the Pioneer Village and covered bridge.
ACCESS MetroPark: Daily, 8 a.m.–	

Description

Take a glimpse into pioneer times in Butler County, at the Governor Bebb MetroPark and Pioneer Village. The 264-acre nature preserve is named after William Bebb, the 19th governor of Ohio who served from 1846 to 1849. Authentic log cabins include Bebb's birthplace and boyhood home. Pioneer Village hosts educational programs and events throughout the year.

When you enter the park, take a few moments on foot to explore the covered bridge. Originally located near Oxford and built in 1850, the bridge was moved and reassembled at the park entrance in 1970.

Immediately beyond the covered bridge on the right of the entrance road is the Pioneer Village and a small parking area. If you come on summer weekends, you'll have the chance to explore the village.

Continue following the entrance road downhill. Pass the manager's office and residence on the right and continue on the road as it parallels Dry Fork Creek on the left. The road ends at a turnaround and small parking area near the W. Murstein Youth Hostel.

Park in the small parking area. The Pelewa Trailhead is to the right. This trail is a 0.45-mile loop, but we'll be joining it with Meadow Loop Trail.

Within 50 feet of the trail's start, it passes over a bridge built in 2001 by Jim Montgomery as an Eagle Scout project, with the assistance of Troop 967. After the bridge, continue uphill via the large steps thanks to Eagle Scout Ray J. Koch. Watch

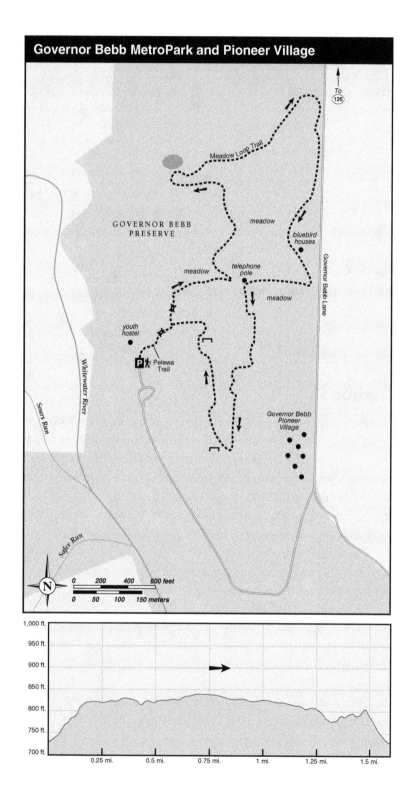

Governor Bebb MetroPark and Pioneer Village

To 126

Meadow Loop Trail

GOVERNOR BEBB PRESERVE

meadow

bluebird houses

meadow

telephone pole

meadow

Governor Bebb Lane

youth hostel

P Pelewa Trail

Governor Bebb Pioneer Village

Whitewater River

Sours Run

Safer Run

N

0   200   400   600 feet

0   50   100   150 meters

1,000 ft.
950 ft.
900 ft.
850 ft.
800 ft.
750 ft.
700 ft.

0.25 mi.   0.5 mi.   0.75 mi.   1 mi.   1.25 mi.   1.5 mi.

your footing over the pathway; a significant amount of erosion has left several large rocks and roots exposed. The upland forest includes sycamore, white oak, Ohio buckeye, and box elder trees. In the woods expect to see wild turkeys, fox squirrels, white-tailed deer, and pileated woodpeckers.

The trail intersects with the Meadow Trail 265 feet into the hike. Follow the Meadow Trail to the left, slightly downhill, and cross another footbridge built in 2005 by Aaron Tharp for his Eagle Scout project, with the assistance of Troop 433. The bridge passes over a small stream. Along the stream corridor you can readily see the exposed bedrock.

Along the trail, landscaping ties are used to decrease erosion. This area has red, white, and chinquapin oaks, as well as sugar maples. At the apex of the hill, turn and look over the ridges and the waterway. The forest has little understory but plenty of wildflowers in early spring.

At 0.1 mile enter the open meadow area and follow the Grenadier Squaw Meadow Trail markers along the mowed path. At the split, follow the trail to the left and continue on this 1-mile loop through the open meadow.

The mowed trail meanders through the meadow, including several wet spots and drainage areas. Look for deer tracks in the wet soil. In a small pond to the left at 0.4 mile, frogs call during the spring mating season. The trees bordering this area include white oak, cottonwood, and Ohio buckeye.

Several bluebird houses pepper the meadow area. Find a dry spot along the edge of the trail and settle in. Sit quietly and soon the birds will resume their normal activities, such as feeding and coming and going from birdhouses.

Also look for a variety of butterflies and other insects. Continue on the trail, turn to the right at 0.6 mile, and follow the wide, mowed path.

Ahead at the telephone pole is a sign for the trail. One mile into the hike, turn left and take the trail that passes through the fence line. On the other side of the fence line, the trail leads to the left and enters a white and red pine forest.

A pine stand is a truly unique forest to experience. The forest floor is open and quiet due to the thick accumulation of pine needles. The sound of the wind moving through the pine needles high above you is reminiscent of a waterfall. Despite this white noise, pine stands are eerily quiet. I highly recommend taking advantage of one of the many stumps to sit down and relax in this quiet forest.

Be careful of the multiple spur trails after you reach the 1.1-mile point. To remain on the trail, stay to the right at each junction. You'll have a little bit of help from trees marked with the blue medallion hiker symbol. A bench at 1.3 miles allows you to sit and possibly observe deer going about their day.

A good example of a honey locust tree presents itself at 1.4 miles. The honey locust produces plenty of thorns, used throughout history as sewing and fishing implements. Just ahead the trail corners and on the right is a small pond. The forest is composed of cottonwood, white pine, and sycamore trees.

At the pond at 1.5 miles is a bench that encourages you to sit and enjoy the view. Continue on the trail and in 50 feet is another trail junction. Here, stop and listen for towhees, chickadees, and juncos.

Follow the trail to the left down a very steep grade as it parallels a power line right-of-way. The forest is composed of sugar maples, Ohio buckeyes, red oaks, and hackberries.

The combination of this steep incline, exposed rocks, and wet conditions make this section a test of your balance and agility. Continue down this trail until it rejoins itself. Take the trail to the left to return to your vehicle.

Nearby Activities

Within 30 minutes of this park, Hueston Woods State Park and Nature Preserve, Miami University, Mounds State Recreation Area (in Indiana), and Miami Whitewater Forest offer additional hiking opportunities. You'll find plenty of restaurants along High Street/US 27 in Oxford, Ohio.

GPS Trailhead Coordinates and Directions

N39° 22.304'   W84° 48.522'

From Cincinnati, take US 27 North toward Millville. Turn left on High Street and continue on Hamilton–Scipio Road/OH 129 for 8.6 miles. Take a sharp left onto Cincinnati–Brookville Road/OH 126, go 1 mile, then turn right onto Bebb Lane.

16 Hueston Woods State Park

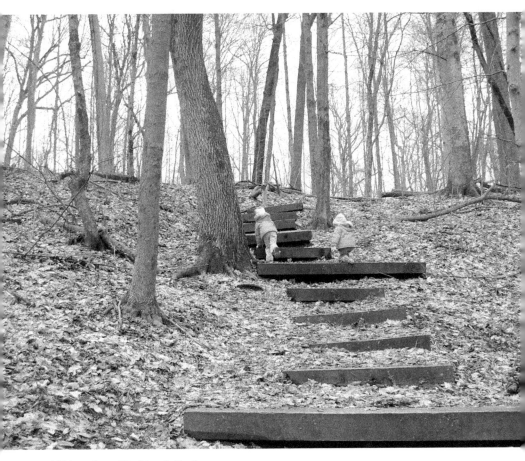

Hiking along Big Woods Trail

In Brief

Hueston Woods State Park has camping, a rustic lodge, nature center, wildlife rehabilitation center, archery range, and marina. The grounds also include the Hueston Woods State Nature Preserve, which is home to an old-growth, nearly virgin, forest.

Description

To get to the starting point of this hike, turn right onto Loop Road from Butler–Israel Road. Stay on Loop Road until you reach the fifth turn on the left. Turn left and into a

LENGTH 5.8 miles	**ACCESS** Daily, 30 minutes before sunrise–30 minutes after sunset; free
CONFIGURATION Series of loops and out-and-back	**MAPS** USGS *College Corner;* Hueston Woods State Park map
DIFFICULTY Moderate–difficult	
SCENERY Woods, old-growth forest, and lake	**WHEELCHAIR ACCESSIBLE** No
EXPOSURE Shaded	**FACILITIES** Restrooms and water at main office near nature center and at the lodge
TRAFFIC Moderate	
TRAIL SURFACE Soil and exposed rocks	**CONTACTS** Hueston Woods State Park office, 513-523-6347; **parks.ohiodnr.gov /huestonwoods**
HIKING TIME 3–3.5 hours	
DRIVING DISTANCE 1 hour from Cincinnati	**COMMENTS** The American Discovery portion of this trail will be impassable if there has been rainfall or flooding. Wipe your shoes to prevent the spread of weed seeds before entering the preserve.
SEASON Year-round	

small parking area at Hueston Woods State Nature Preserve. Once you're in the parking area, look to the south to find the kiosk and trailhead for Big Woods Trail.

Hueston Woods State Nature Preserve is designated as a National Natural Landmark by the U.S. Department of the Interior. The path is a one-person-wide trail through the forest. In spring this old-growth and nearly virgin forest is filled with a multitude of spring wildflowers, including Dutchman's breeches, squirrel corn, trilliums, mayapples, and bloodroot.

In addition to the bevy of spring wildflowers, this 200-acre nature preserve is also home to old-growth woods with beech, sugar maple, white ash, and red and white oak trees. A forest like this is extremely rare in western Ohio because this area was once heavily farmed.

Expect a fair amount of traffic on the trail, but all of it will be bipedal, as bicycles and pets are not permitted on state nature preserve trails. Cross a trestle-style bridge over the small creek nearly 500 feet into the hike. After the bridge, the trail descends a decent grade. It's slippery in wet weather because of the leaf-litter covering.

Cross another bridge over a creek bed at 0.1 mile. After this bridge the trail goes back uphill. Watch your step over exposed roots. Several steps lead up the hill. A blanket of wildflowers covers the edges of the trail in the spring, and the rolling hills are especially beautiful during the spring bloom.

Cross the creek at 0.25 mile. This creek is a good example of how water flows and creates oxbows. Cross the bridge over the dry creek bed at 0.49 mile. This part of the

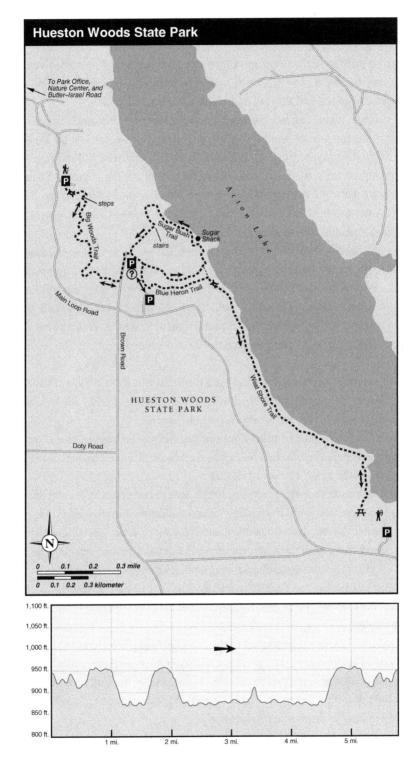

Hueston Woods State Park

To Park Office,
Nature Center, and
Butler–Israel Road

steps

Big Woods Trail

Sugar Bush Trail

Sugar Shack

stairs

Blue Heron Trail

Main Loop Road

Brown Road

Acton Lake

West Shore Trail

HUESTON WOODS
STATE PARK

Doty Road

N

| 0 | 0.1 | 0.2 | 0.3 mile |
| 0 | 0.1 | 0.2 | 0.3 kilometer |

1,100 ft.					
1,050 ft.					
1,000 ft.					
950 ft.					
900 ft.					
850 ft.					
800 ft.	1 mi.	2 mi.	3 mi.	4 mi.	5 mi.

trail is also a portion of the American Discovery Trail, and you'll notice icon medallions on structures and trees. Cross the bridge and enter the bottom woodland area with the stream to the left. Rainfall makes this area wet and muddy.

Remember, if you sink into the mud, pull your foot out while pushing your toes up and into the top of your boot. If you just yank your foot out of the mud, then that is exactly what will happen. Your foot will come out, but your boot will stay buried.

Continue on the trail, crossing the creek along the stepping-stones at 0.6 mile. Take a deep breath and stop to enjoy the scenery of this beautiful forest. You'll see plenty of American beeches along this trail. The beech tree has smooth, gray bark and an excellent branching structure.

The trail heads uphill before entering an open, flat area. Turn left on the road and walk to the turnaround and parking area. On the left side of the parking area is a kiosk. Walk down the road heading toward the lake and look for hiker medallions on the right. Follow the American Discovery Trail, which connects to the Sugar Bush Trail.

The entrance to Sugar Bush Trail is to the right at 0.92 mile. This trail has a nice, wide path through a forest composed primarily of dogwood, redbud, beech, and sugar maple trees.

At the marker for Sugar Bush and Blue Heron Trails, stay on Sugar Bush Trail straight ahead. This forest is very well maintained, as evidenced by the lack of invasive species such as garlic mustard and honeysuckle.

The forest is changing from an older stand of trees to younger trees and more saplings, especially near the lake 1.13 miles into the hike. Continue on the trail to the left until you reach the Sugar House at 1.28 miles.

You'll find outhouse-style restrooms here. Close to the Acton Lake shoreline are several picnic benches. Cross the parking lot and walk along the lake's edge to the woods. Reenter the woods on Sugar Bush and West Shore Trails 1.35 miles into the hike. If it has rained, this part of the trail is very muddy as it borders the edge of the lake.

At 1.5 miles the trail switchbacks near a small backwater area. It is easy to get confused here because there are so many user-made trails. Look uphill and parallel to the service road for the large sycamore tree to find the base of the stairs. Follow the stairs uphill.

At the trail junction near the top of the hill, take Sugar Bush Trail to the right. It'll cross the road again and eventually retrace the short portion of the trail where Sugar Bush and Blue Heron Trails overlap. However, this time at the split take Blue Heron Trail to the right. Blue Heron Trail exits into another turnaround and parking lot. A seasonal drinking fountain is at this location.

Enter the cul-de-sac area and veer slightly left to reenter the woods at 1.9 miles. Use the stepping-stones at 2.07 miles to cross the stream. Sugar Bush Trail parallels

Blue Heron Trail. At the junction at 2.22 miles, take the trail to the right immediately before the footbridge. You are now on the West Shore and American Discovery Trails.

Over the next 0.1 mile, you'll cross several streams. This trail meanders along the edge of the lake. Watch your step in several spots—one wrong step and you'll be going for an unexpected swim.

If there has been a significant amount of rain, odds are that parts of West Shore and American Discovery Trails will not be passable due to high water. Cross the streambed at 2.71 miles. The stepping-stones across this have several fossils embedded in them.

Here, the trail enters an open area with an access road and a power station at the edge of the lake. The trail enters into a red pine stand at 2.9 miles. Follow the orange-tape (on trees) trail along the edge of the lake. West Shore Trail exits at the Archery Range with restrooms available.

Take a few moments to enjoy a break and one of the many benches or explore closer to the dam before retracing your steps and following West Shore and American Discovery Trails back to the access road turnaround. Turn left and follow the road to the entrance to Big Woods Trail and retrace your steps to your vehicle.

Nearby Activities

Mounds State Recreation Area and Whitewater Memorial State Park in Indiana, as well as Miami University and Governor Bebb MetroPark in Ohio, offer additional hiking opportunities. You'll find plenty of shopping and dining opportunities in Oxford, Ohio.

GPS Trailhead Coordinates and Directions

N39° 34.466'   W84° 45.687'

From Cincinnati, take US 27 North to Oxford. As you leave Oxford, you'll see a large shopping center on the right. Look for Todd Road and turn right. When this road intersects with Butler–Israel Road, turn right and follow the road as it immediately jogs to the left. Continue on this road and follow the signs to Hueston Woods State Park office and nature center.

17 John Bryan State Park

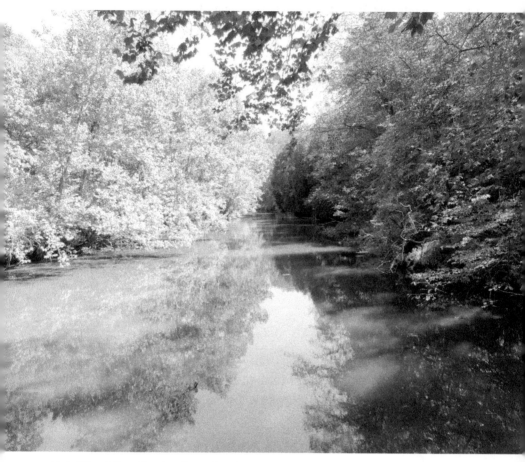

Little Miami River flowing through John Bryan State Park

In Brief

Step out of southwestern Ohio and into the scenic views of John Bryan State Park. Pittsburgh–Cincinnati Stage Coach and South Gorge Trails offer incredible views of the gorge and Little Miami River, plenty of songbirds, and an array of wildflowers.

Description

John Bryan purchased 335 acres along the gorge in 1896 and named it Riverside Farm. Out of respect for nature, John Bryan bequeathed Riverside Farm to the state of Ohio

LENGTH & CONFIGURATION 2.9-mile loop	**ACCESS** Daily, 30 minutes before sunrise–30 minutes after sunset; free
DIFFICULTY Moderate	**MAPS** USGS *Clifton;* John Bryan State Park map
SCENERY Gorge, river, waterfalls, and wildflowers	**WHEELCHAIR ACCESSIBLE** No
EXPOSURE Mostly shaded	**FACILITIES** Latrines, drinking water, and camping
TRAFFIC Moderate–heavy	**CONTACTS** Ohio Department of Natural Resources, Division of Ohio State Parks, 937-767-1274; **parks.ohiodnr.gov /johnbryan**
TRAIL SURFACE Boulders, loose stone, and soil	
HIKING TIME 1–1.5 hours	
DRIVING DISTANCE 1.5 hours north of Cincinnati	**COMMENTS** Spring is best for bird-watchers and wildflower enthusiasts. John Bryan State Park is a hidden gem. This park has great trails and incredible views.
SEASON Year-round; best in spring, summer, and fall	

in 1918, "to be cultivated by the state as a forestry, botanic and wildlife reserve park and experiment station."

John Bryan State Park is a continuation of the dolomite gorge carved first by glacial meltwaters and now by the Little Miami River. The Little Miami River became Ohio's first designated State Scenic River in 1969. With every dip, bend, and riffle, it also earned the designation as a National Wild and Scenic River in 1973. Additionally, a portion of the gorge is designated as a National Natural Landmark.

Glaciers deposited flora from the colder Canadian climate that are able to survive in the cool, moist recesses of the gorge. Species include Canada yew, redberry elder, arborvitae, mountain maple, and even a few hemlocks.

Definitely bring tree, wildflower, and bird identification books for this hike. More than 100 species of trees and shrubs and more than 340 species of wildflowers call this area home! In spring, snow trillium, Virginia bluebell, bellwort, wild ginger, Dutchman's breeches, jack-in-the-pulpit, and wild columbine decorate the dolomite outcrops.

Also along this river corridor are more than 87 species of fish and 36 species of mussels, including five state-endangered species. Wildlife such as salamanders, songbirds, Neotropical migrants, and white-tailed deer are also abundant in the park.

Before hiking John Bryan, brush up on your birdsong identification skills. More than 90 species of birds reside in or visit the park during the year and not all of them

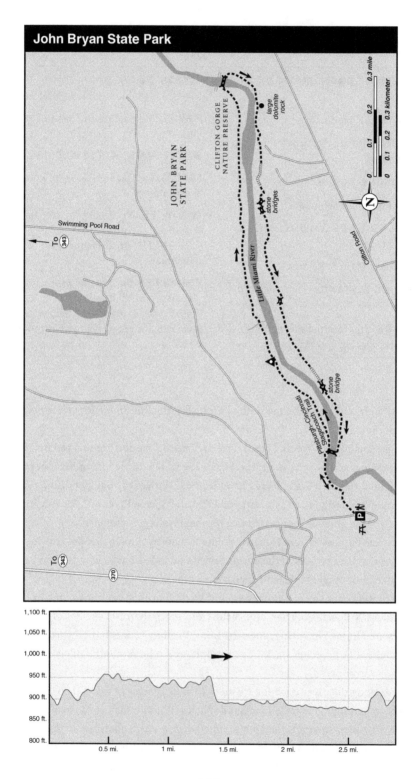

will slow down long enough for you to see them, but you can hear their songs. And you can always try calling "pssh" to see which birds will come to investigate.

After entering John Bryan State Park, follow the drive all the way down to the lower picnic area and park. Look to the left of the pavilion for the trailhead, marked by a sign that reads RIVER GORGE. Take the large, irregular stone steps downhill to the open area with cedar, white oak, and black cherry trees. Just 0.1 mile into the hike, a sign on a large rock identifies the Little Miami River's status as a National Wild and Scenic River.

Take the trail to the left over the craggy dolomite, which has pockets of mud during the wet season. Along the edge of the Little Miami River, the trail weaves through white oak, sugar maple, and sycamore trees that shade the path.

At 0.25 mile, a sign marks the Pittsburgh–Cincinnati Stagecoach Trail, which is named after the stagecoach route that once served this area. Do not cross the river on the footbridge; stay on the trail and continue to follow it as it parallels the Little Miami River. At this point, the trail is a two-person-wide path. When the trail splits at 0.3 mile, stay on the main trail by taking the trail to the left and uphill.

The trail passes through the woods and receives heavy use by day hikers, as well as people out for a stroll. Don't be surprised to see Miami University classes practicing their rock-climbing skills along the cliff face. Although this trail sees a fair amount of use, it is still extremely peaceful and quiet, and other hikers are extraordinarily polite.

Use the stepping-stones to cross a small stream at 0.7 mile. To the left are large chunks of dolomite that broke off the cliff. In springtime, spring beauties bloom over the top of the dolomite rocks and look like a light covering of snow.

The trail enters Clifton Gorge Nature Preserve at 1.47 miles and intersects with its Gorge and Rim Trails. Follow the trail to the right and cross the fast-moving Little Miami River on the trestle-style bridge connecting to South Gorge Trail.

After crossing the bridge, follow South Gorge Trail to the right. The area to the left is closed to the public to help protect the fragile ecosystem.

Many cold-climate plants were deposited in the gorge when glaciers passed through. Today these plants are able to survive only in the unique microclimate created by the combination of the gorge and the flowing waterway. At 1.5 miles, you'll pass an intersection with a trail to the left that leads to 4-H Camp Clifton. Continue on South Gorge Trail.

Within 500 feet of the intersection, a waterfall cascades between the chunks of dolomite. After this point, cross a series of footbridges that keep travelers out of the streams as well as reduce damage to the soil structure. At this point, moss completely covers the stones, and the water flowing downhill is trickling over the top.

South Gorge Trail is comprised of exposed dolomite, mud, footbridges, and plenty of roots. To the left, ocean blue–colored lichens that appear to be dappled sunlight completely cover the cliff faces.

Several large chunks of dolomite near 1.7 miles look as if they're cleaved in half and have sprouted trees. At this point, slow down and enjoy the unique flora of this area, especially in spring.

The trail levels out at 1.8 miles as it weaves through a forest dominated by white oak, sycamore, and elm trees. Roughly 2 miles into the hike, cross a series of stone bridges over the tops of several spectacular waterfalls. In this area is a 6-acre parcel donated by Martin and Mary Cook in 1982. Stay on the main trail by avoiding the spur trails to your right.

Enjoy crossing on the stepping-stones over the tops of two waterfalls that cascade across the path at 2.7 miles. Near 2.8 miles is the first bridge (you passed this earlier from the other side) over the Little Miami River. As you approach the bridge, watch your step over the exposed roots of the sycamore trees.

Cross the bridge over the Little Miami River and return to the Pittsburgh–Cincinnati Stagecoach Trail. Turn left and retrace your steps to the parking area.

Nearby Activities

Additional hikes in this area include Clifton Gorge State Nature Preserve and Glen Helen Nature Preserve. The shops in Yellow Springs offer a little bit of everything. If you are craving something sweet, head for Young's Dairy, which is off of US 68 north of Yellow Springs. Another nearby attraction is Wright–Patterson Air Force Base in Fairborn, which is home to historic Huffman Prairie, where Wilbur and Orville Wright took their first flight, as well as the National Museum of the United States Air Force.

GPS Trailhead Coordinates and Directions

N39° 47.105'   W83° 51.833'

Take I-71 north to US 68 North to Yellow Springs. Turn right onto Yellow Springs Pike/OH 343 East. In 1 mile turn right onto OH 370 South. The entrance to the park is 1.1 miles ahead on the left.

18 Miami University Natural Areas

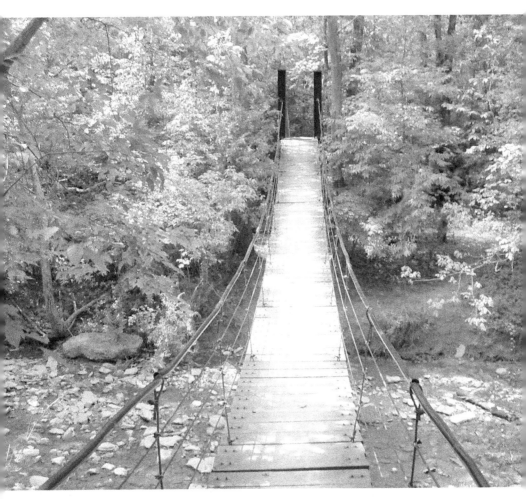

Minimize bouncing and swaying by stepping slowly on this bridge at Bachelor Woods.

In Brief

Miami University Natural Areas and hiking trails just might give you the opportunity to be a kid again. Imagine living in an enormous crevice of one of the sycamore trees; skip across the concrete stepping-stones over the creek; or test the sway limits of the swinging bridge.

LENGTH & CONFIGURATION 4.3-mile loop	**ACCESS** Daily, sunrise–sunset; free
DIFFICULTY Easy–moderate	**MAPS** USGS *Oxford;* Miami University Natural Areas Hiking Trail map
SCENERY Forest, stream, and swinging bridge	**WHEELCHAIR ACCESSIBLE** No
EXPOSURE Mostly shaded	**FACILITIES** None
TRAFFIC Moderate	**CONTACTS** Miami University Natural Areas, 513-524-2197; **www.units.muohio .edu/naturalareas/Miami_University_ Natural_Areas/Trails.html**
TRAIL SURFACE Soil and exposed roots and rocks	
HIKING TIME 3 hours	**COMMENTS** Bachelor Pond and the swinging bridge make for a fun and interesting hike through second-growth and old-growth woods. The trails are well marked with a map of the area and a "you are here" notation at each trail junction.
DRIVING DISTANCE 1 hour north of Cincinnati	
SEASON Year-round	

Description

From the parking area, walk north (toward the bridge) along the gravel road. Cross over the bridge and turn right to go down the set of stairs. This is a narrow path that leads down to the stream. Continue along the edge of Harkers Run, where hackberry trees and wild ginger surround the trail. Grapevine is also prevalent throughout this lowland area.

Enormous sycamore trees bracket Harkers Run. Many have decayed heartwood, which leads to the tree becoming hollowed out and looking much like a home for hobbits. Throughout this portion of the trail, several small spur trails lead down to the stream's edge.

Continue on the main trail and pass by a massive dead tree at 0.47 mile. The soil in this area is sandy as the path winds underneath an arching sycamore. At the trail intersection, follow the trail to the right and use the concrete posts to cross Harkers Run. The concrete posts have gravel embedded on the top, are about 20 inches wide, and are spaced about 12–18 inches apart. This is a fun path to cross, especially with young children.

After crossing the creek, continue on the trail to the left, uphill over several telephone pole–style steps, and enter the upland woods of white and red oak, sugar maple, American beech, ash, black cherry, and shagbark hickory trees at 0.62 mile. Be careful of your footing over exposed roots.

You are entering an outdoor classroom and are likely to see markers, laundry baskets to collect leaf litter, or deer exclusion areas.

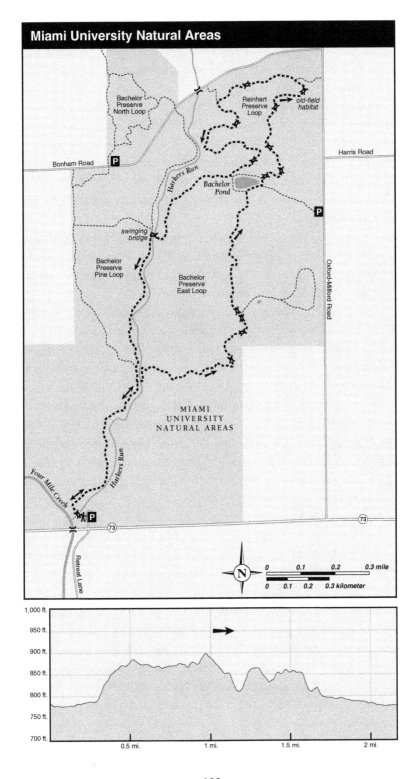

Miami University Natural Areas

Bachelor Preserve North Loop

Reinhart Preserve Loop

old-field habitat

Harris Road

Bonham Road

P

Bachelor Pond

Harker's Run

swinging bridge

P

Oxford-Milford Road

Bachelor Preserve Pine Loop

Bachelor Preserve East Loop

MIAMI UNIVERSITY NATURAL AREAS

Harker's Run

Four Mile Creek

Harker's Run

P

73

73

Retreat Lane

N

| 0 | 0.1 | 0.2 | 0.3 mile |
| 0 | 0.1 | 0.2 | 0.3 kilometer |

1,000 ft.
950 ft.
900 ft.
850 ft.
800 ft.
750 ft.
700 ft.

0.5 mi.   1 mi.   1.5 mi.   2 mi.

This forest is quiet, and the only noise other than the sounds of nature would be of your own making. Pass by several large red oak trees at 0.78 mile. The trail curves at 0.9 mile and then passes near black cherry and white oak trees. The bark of a black cherry tree looks as if someone glued burned potato chips onto the dark, blackish-gray bark. White oaks typically have flat patches of bark along the light gray trunks.

Cross the footbridge at 0.94 mile as the habitat transitions to red cedars and honeysuckle with a few elm trees. Cross another footbridge at 1.04 miles and immediately spot a honey locust tree complete with thorns. Pioneers used the thorns for fishing and sewing implements.

After crossing a footbridge at 1.08 miles, the trail intersects with another one. Follow the trail to the left and into an area dominated by red cedar trees. The trail crosses another footbridge at 1.12 miles and passes through a stand of beautiful redbud trees. In early spring, delicate lavender blossoms cover these trees.

At Bachelor Pond, follow the trail on the right to the end of the pond. At the trail junction at 1.53 miles follow the trail to the left and around Bachelor Pond. Here you can watch for kingfishers, great blue herons, songbirds, and of course waterfowl. At the trail junction at 1.55 miles, follow the trail to the right and enter a stand of white pine and red cedar trees, which smells wonderful. Follow the trail downhill to yet another footbridge near 1.63 miles, surrounded by dogwood and locust trees.

The eroded trail continues downhill, crosses a footbridge at 1.72 miles, and then crosses an extremely bouncy footbridge at 1.83 miles. The habitat transitions again into one with not much canopy; in fact, it's going through succession. Cross another footbridge at 1.95 miles and pass through the old-field habitat with Russian and autumn olive, red cedars, and plenty of poison ivy.

At 2.05 miles return to the upland woods of oaks, tulips, redbuds, dogwoods, and sugar maples. Cross the footbridge over the top of the creek and continue along the trail, heading uphill over the exposed roots. At the trail junction at 2.25 miles follow the trail to the left and enter a stand of sugar maple, red oak, birch, redbud, and dogwood trees.

Cross two more footbridges, and at the trail intersection at 2.9 miles follow the flat trail straight ahead through pawpaw, sweet gum, and pine trees. You may well spot deer here during the late summer months. Look for tulip, sycamore, and dogwood trees.

The trail leads to the steps for the swinging bridge over the top of Harkers Run. This is fun, especially with obnoxious friends who bounce the bridge while you are trying to cross. On the other side, follow the trail to the left that parallels Harkers Run.

Look into the streambed for the large, green-tinted rock with several smaller rocks embedded in it. This unique boulder is tillite. Tillite boulders were created when the rocks and boulders of glacial till were compressed under the weight of the glacier. Often made up of granite, basalt, and feldspar, tillites have a greenish-black tint.

The valley along the edge of Harkers Run is full of hackberry, sycamore, and paw-paw trees. Continue following this path, and at the trail junction at 3.6 miles follow the trail to the left. Note the large sycamore trees throughout this area. The trail will soon start to look familiar. Continue on this trail until you reach the steps next to the bridge. Walk up the steps, turn left onto the gravel road, cross the bridge, and walk back to the parking lot and your car.

Nearby Activities

You'll find additional hiking trails at Miami University Natural Areas, as well as at Hueston Woods State Park and State Nature Preserve. Downtown Oxford offers plenty of shopping and dining opportunities.

GPS Trailhead Coordinates and Directions

N39° 30.504'   W84° 42.967'

From I-275 and US 27 on the west side of Cincinnati, follow US 27 North for 20 miles to Oxford. In Oxford, look for the Pulley Tower at the corner of Oxford–Trenton Road, turn right and in less than 1 mile turn left into the parking area with the kiosk.

19 Miami Whitewater Forest:
Shaker Trace Outer Loop

In Brief

Several trails, including the Shaker Trace Outer Loop, are found inside the expansive Miami Whitewater Forest Park. The paved Outer Loop trail meanders through several different habitats, including the Shaker Trace Wetlands. A variety of users take advantage of the serenity of this lengthy, yet easily accessible, trail.

Description

Miami Whitewater Forest began in 1949, when Great Parks of Hamilton County acquired 709 acres of land. Today, the park encompasses 4,345 acres, making it the largest park in the Great Parks of Hamilton County district.

The visitor center's interactive displays and Nature Niche Store are fun to explore. At the center of the park is the 85-acre Miami Whitewater Forest Lake, created in 1969 when the dam was completed. The marina rents pontoons and paddle-, row-, and motorboats. Pirate Parky's Cove is a unique water-play area on the lake.

The park has multiple picnic areas and playgrounds, a dog park, a marina, a campground with electricity, a 9-hole disc golf course, an 18-hole golf course, a driving range, and a wet playground. Bicycle rentals are also available.

Miami Whitewater Forest is home to more than 150 acres of restored wetlands, including the Shaker Trace Wetland Restoration Project on the north side of the property.

Once you enter the park, follow the signs to the visitor center, Nature Niche Store, and Parky's Pirate Cove. Park in the parking area, face the visitor center, and look to the right to find the footpath.

Follow the footpath down the stone steps and around the back side of the visitor center to see the lake. Continue along the edge of the lake, following the path to the north to the other side of the visitor center and the boardwalk.

Walk along the boardwalk until you reach the gazebo that serves as the trailhead. Follow the paved trail to Shaker Trace Outer Loop to the northwest and away from the visitor center and Miami Whitewater Forest Lake. The trail crosses several roads. Each approach is clearly marked.

LENGTH & CONFIGURATION 7.7-mile loop	**ACCESS** Daily, sunrise–sunset; annual vehicle permit, $10; daily vehicle permit, $5
DIFFICULTY Moderate	**MAPS** USGS *Shandon* and *Harrison;* Miami Whitewater Forest map
SCENERY Prairie, farm field, river corridor, and restored wetlands	**WHEELCHAIR ACCESSIBLE** Yes
EXPOSURE Mostly sun, some shade	**FACILITIES** Restroom and water at visitor center
TRAFFIC Heavy	
TRAIL SURFACE Paved	**CONTACTS** Great Parks of Hamilton County, 513-367-4774; **greatparks.org/parks/miami-whitewater-forest**
HIKING TIME 3.5–4 hours	
DRIVING DISTANCE 45 minutes west of Cincinnati	
SEASON Year-round	**COMMENTS** This hike meanders through beautiful farmland and restored wetlands.

This trail passes the disc golf course at 0.54 mile. Disc golf is a fun, easy game in which you toss a disc from a tee and try to make it into a goal. It's also a relatively inexpensive sport—a disc costs between $8 and $12 at most sporting goods stores. The first time or two that you play you'll need a lot of patience. Discs tend to go exactly where you didn't throw to, such as tree branches. *Hint:* If your disc does get stuck in a tree, use a full water bottle to knock it out. If you use another disc, odds are you'll need to retrieve two discs from the branches.

At the trail split at 0.6 mile, take the trail to the right. This two-lane paved trail is shared with hikers, in-line skaters, bicyclists, and stroller-pushing parents. When someone faster than you is trying to get by, step aside and let them pass. Stop at the bench at 2.1 miles to enjoy the scenery before continuing on the trail.

The trail meanders along the Dry Fork Whitewater River corridor. The river corridor area to the right of the trail is abundant with sycamore, hackberry, and locust trees. The trail splits and the right goes under the New Haven Road bridge. At 2.5 miles the trail splits and the left crosses Willey Road while the right passes under the bridge before rejoining.

At 2.8 miles the trail crosses Atherton Road, then takes you through an open prairie and crop field near 3.2 miles. Near 3.5 miles take a break and observe the wildlife activities in the brushy fencerow.

Brushy fencerows are important habitat for cottontail rabbits, pheasants, red foxes, and many other small mammals and birds. With modern farming practices removing fencerows, many of these wildlife populations have decreased in numbers.

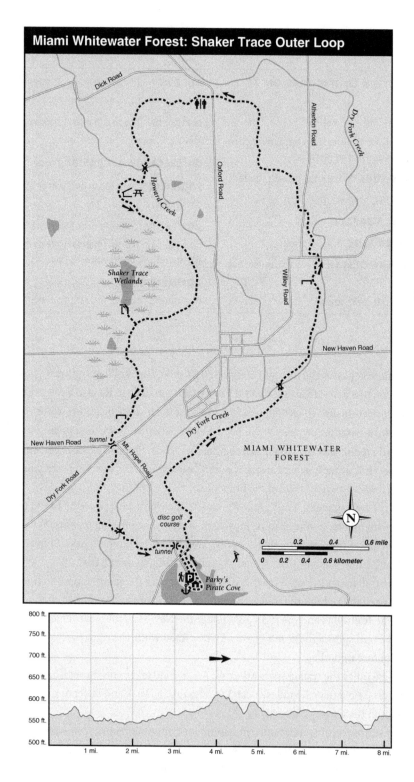

Miami Whitewater Forest: Shaker Trace Outer Loop

Dick Road

Atherton Road

Dry Fork Creek

Oxford Road

Howard Creek

Shaker Trace Wetlands

Willey Road

New Haven Road

New Haven Road   tunnel

Dry Fork Creek

Mt. Hope Road

MIAMI WHITEWATER FOREST

Dry Fork Road

N

disc golf course

tunnel

0   0.2   0.4   0.6 mile

0   0.2   0.4   0.6 kilometer

Parky's Pirate Cove

800 ft.
750 ft.
700 ft.
650 ft.
600 ft.
550 ft.
500 ft.

1 mi.   2 mi.   3 mi.   4 mi.   5 mi.   6 mi.   7 mi.   8 mi.

The trail crosses Oxford Road at 3.8 miles. If you need a restroom break, look for the latrines shortly after crossing Oxford Road. The road crossing is well marked on the trail. The prairie and fencerow near the crossing provide good habitat for red foxes, meadow voles, and white-tailed deer.

Cross a bridge shaded by sycamore trees at 4.6 miles and pass a large shingle oak tree to the right side before taking a break at another shelter house at 4.9 miles. The Wilz family, in honor of Peggy Frey Wilz, made this shelter possible. From this vantage point, Shaker Trace Wetlands is visible.

Shaker Trace Wetlands is a restoration project that began in 1991 via partnerships between Great Parks of Hamilton County, the Ohio Department of Natural Resources, Hamilton County Soil and Water Conservation District, and the U.S. Fish and Wildlife Service. Numerous Ducks Unlimited wood duck nesting boxes pepper the terrain of the wetland complex.

And what would a wetland be if it didn't have plenty of frogs? The wetlands are managed to keep the fish population low to protect the amphibian populations. This wetland is a perfect habitat where frogs can thrive, and in spring and summer their chorusing can be intense (if not a bit deafening).

Several benches bracket the side trail that leads down to the observation area for Shaker Trace Wetlands. Quietly take the side trail to the right and enjoy a glimpse of this beautiful wetland complex. Return to the main trail and turn right to continue.

The trail crosses Baughman Road at 6.4 miles. Prior to being settled 200 years ago, this area supported prairies and wetlands before being destroyed to create farmland. The 96 acres of wetlands and 390 acres of prairie have been beautifully restored and give a peek into how Ohio's landscape must have appeared to early settlers.

Look for kestrels hunting the open field area. The slate-gray to blue, reddish brown, and white birds are nearly the size of a robin. They hunt by hovering over a grassy area to search for meadow voles and field mice. When kestrels find prey, they fold in their wings, plunging down to capture it. This area also is prime habitat for northern harriers, which use drainage corridors and open fields as hunting grounds. While on the hunt these large birds of prey slowly and gently glide a few feet above the ground.

Another bench at 6.8 miles is a nice place to stop, rest, and watch wildlife. Pass through a tunnel at 6.9 miles. The trail crosses a bridge at 7.5 miles, and at the trail intersection near the bridge, take the trail to the right. Continue on this trail, passing through another tunnel at 7.8 miles.

This area opens up into a well-manicured area where the parking lot and visitor center soon come into view. Now all you need to do is recall where you parked your car.

Nearby Activities

Nearby hikes include Shawnee Lookout, Fernbank Park, and Mitchell Memorial Forest in Ohio, and Whitewater Memorial State Park and Mounds State Recreation Area in Indiana. In Cincinnati, the Cincinnati Museum Center and Cincinnati Zoo and Botanical Garden offer plenty of activities to enjoy.

GPS Trailhead Coordinates and Directions

N39° 15.497'   W84° 44.640'

From Cincinnati, take I-74 West to Exit 3/Dry Fork Road. Turn north (right) onto Dry Fork Road. Take Dry Fork Road north 2.4 miles and turn right onto Mt. Hope Road. Follow the signs to the visitor center.

20 Pyramid Hill Sculpture Park & Museum

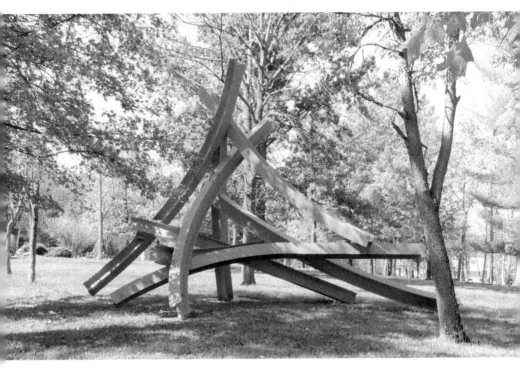

#51 The Web *by Brian Monaghan at Pyramid Hill*

In Brief

The 265-acre Pyramid Hill Sculpture Park & Museum is a unique hiking experience. Take a day to explore all that this wonderful celebration of the arts has to offer. Massive sculptures are on display with nature as the backdrop. Plus, you can explore the Ancient Sculpture Museum's Egyptian, Greek, Roman, and Etruscan sculptures. The entrance fee is well worth the price.

Description

Pyramid Hill is an outdoor sculpture park covering 265 acres of rolling hillsides and forests. Whereas you typically see one sculpture at a university or business, here you can take in the beauty and artistry of more than 60 sculptures in wood, metal, and

LENGTH & CONFIGURATION 3.3-mile loops	7:30 p.m. Adults, $8; children ages 6–12, $3; children age 5 and younger, free
DIFFICULTY Easy–moderate	**MAPS** USGS *Hamilton* and *Greenhills*; Pyramid Hill Sculpture Park map (most current is available at museum office)
SCENERY Sculptures, ponds, forests	
EXPOSURE Mostly shaded	
TRAFFIC Moderate–heavy	**WHEELCHAIR ACCESSIBLE** Paved portions
TRAIL SURFACE Mowed path, gravel, soil, golf cart paths, and roads	**FACILITIES** Restrooms and drinking water in museum
HIKING TIME 2–2.5+ hours	
DRIVING DISTANCE 30 minutes north of Cincinnati	**CONTACTS** Pyramid Hill Sculpture Park & Museum, 513-868-8336 or 513-868-1234; **pyramidhill.org**
SEASON Year-round (winter weather permitting)	**COMMENTS** Enjoy beautiful sculptures while you hike. You can rent an Art Cart— a fun and different way to explore.
ACCESS 8 a.m.–5 p.m. Exit gate closes at	

stone. Pyramid Hill's mission is "the eventual establishment of a collection which will demonstrate the complete history of sculpture by mankind, making Pyramid Hill the only art park in the world working on the accomplishment." Special events are held throughout the year, as well as educational programs in art, horticulture, geology, and the environment.

Once you enter Pyramid Hill follow the road to the Ancient Sculpture Museum and park your vehicle. From the Ancient Sculpture Museum's parking area, look down the road to the right of the museum, and in a small clearing you'll see the sign for the gold and red trails. Immediately after stepping off the road and onto trail you'll encounter the first sculpture, *Gyro Chair II* by Jim Killy.

At the next intersection, follow the gold/red trail to the left. At 0.1 mile the trail crosses a road and transitions from paved to gravel. Pass by a few shagbark hickory trees before crossing another road at 0.19 mile. When you reach the road turn right and walk uphill. At the first intersection, you'll see signs for one-way, amphitheater, and post 24. Turn left at the post and continue on the gold/red trail.

When you reach the traffic circle, look for *The General,* artist unknown, to your right. The trail continues on the other side of the traffic circle. Look for post 23 and follow the red/gold trail through the grassy area to *Melinda at the Beach* by Bill Barrett. Look straight ahead along the woodland edge for the next trail marker post 15 and turn left onto the small golf cart road.

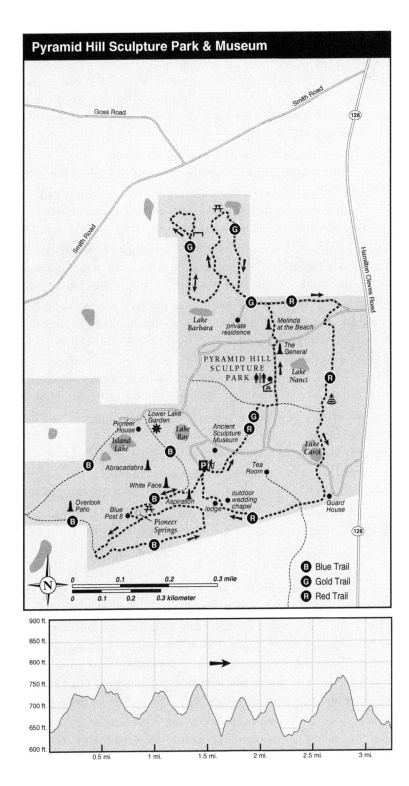

Pyramid Hill Sculpture Park & Museum

Goss Road

Smith Road

128

Smith Road

Hamilton Cleves Road

Lake Barbara

private residence

Melinda at the Beach

The General

PYRAMID HILL
SCULPTURE
PARK

Lake Nanci

Lower Lake Garden

Pioneer House

Island Lake

Lake Ray

Ancient Sculpture Museum

Lake Carol

Abracadabra

White Face

Overlook Patio

Aspiration

Blue Post 8

Tea Room

outdoor wedding chapel

lodge

Guard House

Pioneer Springs

128

B	Blue Trail
G	Gold Trail
R	Red Trail

N

0   0.1   0.2   0.3 mile

0   0.1   0.2   0.3 kilometer

900 ft.
850 ft.
800 ft.
750 ft.
700 ft.
650 ft.
600 ft.

0.5 mi.   1 mi.   1.5 mi.   2 mi.   2.5 mi.   3 mi.

119

At post 16 turn right and follow the footpath into the woods. Watch your step as there are a lot of walnuts. Like many forests with ash trees this one has also been damaged by emerald ash borers killing the white ash trees. Many of the trees in this area are identified, making this a great spot to test your identification skills. When you reach the split in the trail at 0.56 mile, take the trail to your left.

At post 20 is the intersection of three trails, follow the trail to your left. At the next trail intersection go to your right and follow the trail through the woods. Take a left at the next intersection and follow the loop trail through a sugar maple forest. At the bend in the trail is a large white oak tree to the left.

Take in the scenery from the bench before reconnecting with the trail you followed in; follow the trail all the way back to the three-trail intersection and at post 20 turn left and head downhill. Go to the right at post 19. At 1.47 miles take a break at the picnic table near the pond. Sit quietly and you may just get serenaded by the plethora of frogs calling this small body of water home. While this is remote, you occasionally will have a plane fly overhead.

Continue on the trail and when you reach the paved road you came in on take the road left and downhill. When you reach the Y intersection and can see the barn down the hill, take a sharp right and continue on the cart path. Cross the next road (cars use this road so be careful). Walk to the left side of the pond at 1.7 miles and into the woods following the red trail markers.

Watch your footing over the exposed roots and don't take any side trails. Continue on this trail straight ahead and uphill. To your right you'll pass by *The Web* by Brian Monaghan, *Paul* by Martin Gantman, and *Untitled Bench* by Jon Isherwood before the trail crosses the cart path. At this point the trail tracks along the cart path, but you can walk through the woods paralleling the cart path to reach *A Smile from Bayon* by Joseph Mannino and Lake Carol, surrounded by river birch and weeping willow trees.

Walk along the cart path, follow it uphill, and cross the entrance road. Continue following the cart path until you reach the smaller asphalt trail. Take this trail around the lodge at 2.3 miles. Follow the path around the lodge, keeping the building to your left. Soon you'll see a pretty bridge as well as a field wagon. Enjoy walking under the stunning wisteria-covered arbor. Any of these focal points are great for photos.

When you reach the road turn left (the museum will be to your back) and go up hill to follow the blue trail. Immediately after the curve in the road and to the left, you'll see one of my favorite sculptures, *Aspiration* by Ann Melanie, tucked neatly into the corner of an open grassy area surrounded by woods. Behind this sculpture is a large sycamore tree.

Look for the Stone Wall Trail/blue trail (which parallels the road on the downhill side). This trail is aptly named because of the stone wall that was built in the 1830s to prevent the cleared hillside from sliding into the creek. Originally cleared to grow grapes, the hillside is now home to magnificent sculptures.

You can see the large white marble sculpture *White Face* and the enormous red sculpture *Abracadabra,* both by Jon Isherwood, from this lower trail, or before you leave take your time and examine the sculptures up close. Take a break at the picnic table at 2.5 miles.

A tenth of a mile later, turn left and follow the trail away from the road. Walk up the hill passing by the stone wall and pond (Pioneer Springs) to your left. At the next intersection take the trail to your right and walk uphill. Pass side trails and continue straight ahead. The next trail intersection is a Y; head to the right and you'll see a blue post 40.

Bush honeysuckle as well as white oaks, elms, and locusts make up much of the flora. The trail leads up a really steep hill and loops to the left. At the next intersection continue on the trail to your right and uphill. Pass two connector trails and continue on the trail straight ahead. When the trail begins heading downhill, watch for large walnuts along the path. It is all too easy and painful to roll an ankle on one of those bright green orbs.

At blue post 36 the trail enters an open area and 3.0 miles into the hike the trail splits. Take the trail downhill and to your right. When the trail splits again stay to your right. Several ash trees have been felled along this area. Avoid taking side trails, and when you reach the Pioneer Springs site, retrace your earlier steps to the museum and your vehicle. Or, you can cross the road and take a closer look at the sculptures before heading back to your vehicle. Just saying . . . .

Nearby Activities

If you like migratory birds, wetlands, and forests, head to Gilmore MetroPark, Fernald Preserve, or Miami Whitewater Forest. Need new boots? Bass Pro Shops is located in nearby Forest Park. If you are hungry, there are plenty of restaurants around the area.

GPS Trailhead Coordinates and Directions
N39° 22.350'   W84° 34.902'

From I-275 turn north onto US 27/OH 126. In 5.2 miles take OH 128 North and travel almost 5 miles to the entrance to Pyramid Hill on the left.

21 Spring Valley Wildlife Area

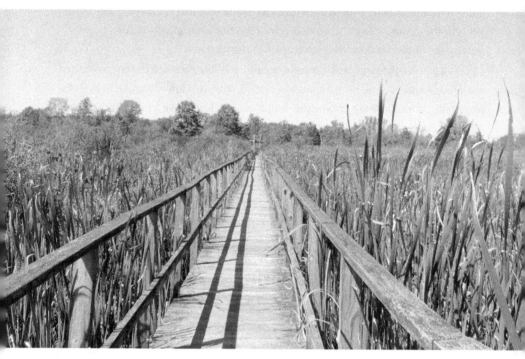

Spring Valley Wildlife Area's boardwalk to observation deck

In Brief

Spring Valley Wildlife Area's wetland is a diverse habitat that is home to a variety of shorebirds, waterfowl, songbirds, snakes, turtles, fish, and mammals. From the boardwalk, you can sit and enjoy views of the wetland.

Description

Located 8 miles southeast of Xenia, off US 42, this 842-acre wildlife area has a variety of habitats to explore, including upland and bottomland hardwoods and wetlands. In the early 1900s the area was a commercial fur farm. In 1953–1954, Spring Valley Wildlife Area was created when the fur farm, marsh, and 80-acre lake were purchased by the Ohio Department of Natural Resources Division of Wildlife.

Today, nearly 90% of Ohio's wetlands have been drained, and Spring Valley Wildlife Area is recognized by the Ohio Historical Marker program because of its wetland features.

122

LENGTH & CONFIGURATION 2.75-mile loop	**SEASON** Year-round
DIFFICULTY Easy	**ACCESS** Daily, sunrise–sunset; free
SCENERY Woods, wetlands, and lake	**MAPS** USGS *Waynesville;* Spring Valley Wildlife Area map
EXPOSURE Shade and sun	**WHEELCHAIR ACCESSIBLE** No
TRAFFIC Moderate	**FACILITIES** No
TRAIL SURFACE Soil, grass, and access roads	**CONTACTS** Wildlife District Five, 937-372-9261; **wildlife.ohiodnr.gov/springvalley**
HIKING TIME 1.5 hours	**COMMENTS** An excellent destination for bird-watching. Wear shoes that can get wet, as some parts of the trail might be under more than 6 inches of water.
DRIVING DISTANCE 1 hour north of Cincinnati	

Spring Valley Wildlife Area is very popular with bird-watchers, which is no surprise because more than 230 species of birds—including the occasional greater white-fronted goose, long-tailed duck, sandhill crane, bald eagle, and worm-eating warbler—use the wetland complex at some point during their life cycle. The wetland complex is also well known for attracting migrating birds such as flycatchers, vireos, and warblers. Definitely brush up on your birdsong identification skills prior to this hike.

This area was also selected as one of several locations throughout the state for the osprey reintroduction project that began in 1996. The project has been a success, and visitors frequently can see ospreys hunting the marsh. Ospreys hover high over the water. When prey is spotted, they fold their wings and dive to hit the water talons first. Often osprey go completely underwater; after emerging, they shake off the water much like a dog.

Note that the area is open to hunting. If you are unfamiliar with the hunting seasons, call 937-372-9261 or stop by the wildlife area headquarters for detailed information. Archery, shotgun, and firearms ranges are located on the property, off Houston Road. Additional information about the wildlife area and range is available at the headquarters off Roxanna–New Burlington Road.

The trail is located off Pence Jones Road. After turning right onto Pence Jones Road, turn right onto the paved driveway and follow it to a small parking area. The trail circles the 150-acre marsh and lake wetland complex.

The wetland is an excellent breeding ground for deerflies, horseflies, mosquitoes, and ticks. Unless you're hiking in the dead of winter, you'll absolutely, positively need insect repellent. I cannot stress this enough—bring it along with you in case you

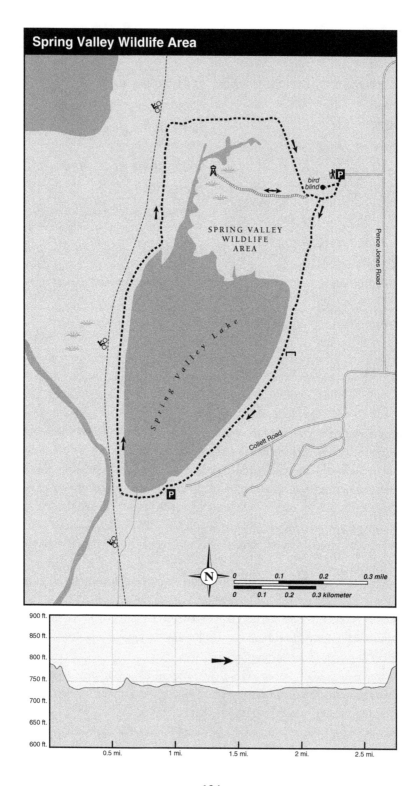

Spring Valley Wildlife Area

SPRING VALLEY
WILDLIFE
AREA

Spring Valley Lake

bird blind

Pence Jones Road

Collett Road

0   0.1   0.2   0.3 mile
0   0.1   0.2   0.3 kilometer

N

900 ft.
850 ft.
800 ft.
750 ft.
700 ft.
650 ft.
600 ft.

0.5 mi.   1 mi.   1.5 mi.   2 mi.   2.5 mi.

need to reapply. I also highly recommend a hat, because a portion of this hike is in the direct sun, and it also helps to keep the bugs out of your hair.

From the parking lot, walk west to the edge of the woods. The very nice and well-built bird blind faces into the woods at several feeding stations. Inside the blind is a sturdy bench and desk-like shelf that works well for holding binoculars and notebooks. In summer the area around the bird blind is a good place to watch for dragonflies and damselflies.

After you leave the bird blind, you'll see along the woodland edge a chained-off access road. This is the trailhead. The trail leads downhill over exposed stones. At 0.1 mile, when the trail splits, take the trail to the right, following it downhill.

Pass the access road at 0.14 mile and continue straight ahead. Cattails grow along the edge of the trail in the lower areas, and water is visible on both sides of the trail.

The Spring Valley Wildlife Area is home to the eastern massasauga rattlesnake, also known as the swamp rattlesnake. Count yourself lucky if you're fortunate enough to see one of these beautiful snakes, as they are very reclusive and timid.

The single footpath trail to the boardwalk is very narrow and in the midst of summer might be hard to find due to the overgrown vegetation. You'll come upon a boardwalk area at 0.23 mile. On either side of the boardwalk is an array of wetland plants, from cattails to water lilies to the diminutive duckweed. Along the boardwalk are benches to stop and enjoy the cacophony of wetland sounds. The boardwalk extends into the wetland for more than 600 feet. At the end is a 13-foot observation tower.

From the observation tower, take a break on the Leopold benches while enjoying the panoramic view of the wetland complex. It's easy from this vantage point to watch several species of birds, including red-winged blackbirds and waterfowl, as well as to see the passageways large mammals have made through the cattails. To the north are several old snags, and throughout the wetland complex are a multitude of wood duck nesting boxes.

Retrace your steps along the boardwalk. At the trail junction at 0.62 mile, take the trail to the right and into the woods. The benches at 0.96 and 1.05 miles overlook the wetland area and a few wood duck nesting boxes.

The trail enters another parking area at 1.2 miles. Continue across the parking lot with the wetland complex on the right and walk to another chained access road. Cross this barrier and proceed on the trail along the edge of the wetland complex.

If it has rained, this portion of the trail might not be passable unless you don't mind wading through water and mud. This is where the shoes that you don't care about getting wet and muddy come into play.

At 1.43 miles, the trail borders the edge of the wetlands. To the right is a large wetland complex and to the left is a ditch between the trail and the railroad bed that is now a bike trail. At 1.61 miles, the hiking trail enters an open area.

If there has been a lot of rain (as there often is in springtime), be prepared to walk through standing water as deep as 12–18 inches near the 2-mile mark. At the intersection at 2.3 miles, take the trail to the right. Continue on the trail to the right at the next intersection at 2.52 miles. Take the trail to the left at 2.7 miles to return to the parking area and your vehicle.

Nearby Activities

Waynesville has several antiques shops and plenty of hometown places to grab a bite to eat. Additional hiking opportunities in the area are Caesar Creek State Park, Caesar Creek Gorge State Nature Preserve, Fort Ancient State Memorial, and Beaver Creek Wildlife Area.

GPS Trailhead Coordinates and Directions

N39° 34.366'   W84° 000.644'

In Waynesville, from the intersection of US 42 and OH 73, take US 42 North 5.6 miles. Turn right onto Roxanna–New Burlington Road and follow it 1.5 miles. Turn right onto Pence Jones Road and travel 0.3 mile. Turn west (right) onto the paved lane leading to a parking area.

22 Stonelick State Park

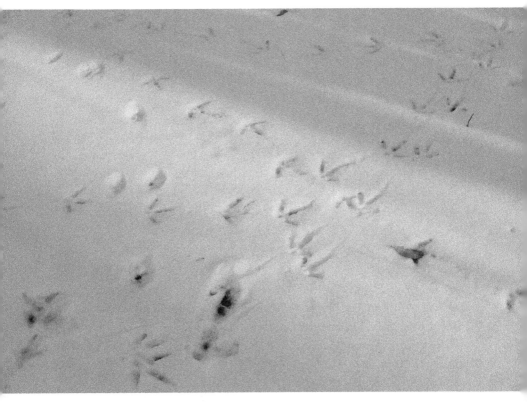

Wild turkey tracks in the snow on Red Fox Trail

In Brief

Stonelick State Park rests atop a portion of the Cincinnati Arch and is rich in fossil history. Activities include camping, boating, fishing, hunting, swimming, picnicking, and several hiking trails.

Description

The Stonelick State Park area is one of the best spots in the state to see some amazing fossils. Erosion has exposed some of the oldest rocks in the arch, ranging in age from 350 million to 500 million years old. The fossils in the Cincinnati Arch include trilobites, brachiopods, and cephalopods, which have attracted fossil hunters since the early 1800s. You can look, but keeping the fossils is forbidden. If you want to collect

LENGTH & CONFIGURATION 6.7-mile balloon and out-and-back	**SEASON** Year-round
DIFFICULTY Easy–moderate	**ACCESS** Daily, 6 a.m.–11 p.m.; free
SCENERY Woods, wetlands, and lake	**MAPS** USGS *Newtonsville;* Stonelick State Park map
EXPOSURE Mostly shaded	**WHEELCHAIR ACCESSIBLE** No
TRAFFIC Light–moderate	**FACILITIES** Restrooms and water
TRAIL SURFACE Soil, exposed rocks and roots	**CONTACTS** Stonelick State Park office, 513-734-4323; **parks.ohiodnr.gov/stonelick**
HIKING TIME 2.5–3 hours	**COMMENTS** Enjoy panoramic views of the lake from any of the many benches along Lakeview Trail. Portions of the Beechtree Trail might be flooded.
DRIVING DISTANCE 25 minutes northeast of Cincinnati	

them, the U.S. Army Corps of Engineers allows fossil collecting via permit in designated areas of Hueston Woods, East Fork, and Caesar Creek State Parks.

In 1948 the state of Ohio began purchasing land to create Stonelick State Park. In 1950 the dam across Stonelick Creek was finished, creating 200-acre Stonelick Lake.

Enter Stonelick State Park from OH 727 and park in the small parking area across the road from the maintenance service center. Walk to the right of the service center to find the trailhead for Beechtree Trail, which parallels the fence.

This trail meanders through the forest. Large low spots are scattered along the trail. During winter, the low spots are full of water, offering exciting mini ice-skating rinks when temperatures are low enough for the water to freeze. In spring the same low spots are great areas to look for tadpoles, frogs, and salamanders.

At 0.93 mile, you'll see a water tower. The trail continues on the other side of the water tower and into the woods, then turns left at 1.12 miles. Portions of this trail are marked with blue blaze marks. The forest at 1.2 miles is codominated by sweet gum, American beech, and maple trees. This is unusual because sweet gums are usually a subordinate tree.

When the trail intersects with private property at 1.44 miles, continue on Beechtree Trail to the left. Cross the road at 1.48 miles, look for the Lakeview sign, and reenter the woods. Immediately ahead of you are the entrances for Lakeview and Southwoods Trails.

Take Southwoods Trail to the right over a short, steep hill and into a small stand of red cedars. The trail on this portion of the hike is extremely eroded, with roots that crisscross the trail, making it treacherous for your ankles.

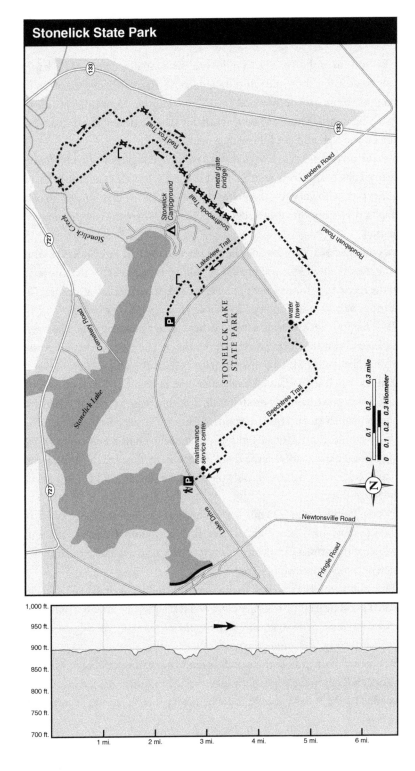

Stonelick State Park

At the bottom of the hill at 1.55 miles is a small stream. Stop and look for tracks of animals, such as raccoon and white-tailed deer. Cross the bridge over the small stream and continue on Southwoods Trail. Cross another footbridge at 1.63 miles before heading uphill. There are no markers for this portion of the trail, so be alert to staying on the trail and not following a deer path.

Cross the metal bridge at 1.66 miles and enter a younger forest with plenty of white and red oak trees. Cross another footbridge at 1.76 miles and notice that the forest is more open, with very few understory plants under the high canopy of oaks and sugar maples. Cross another footbridge at 1.79 miles, where the campground is visible from the trail.

Cross the road at 1.88 miles and the entrance to the Red Fox Trail is to your right. At the split near the Red Fox Trailhead sign, follow the trail to the left. The terrain is flat, and the forest transitions from open hardwoods to red cedars at 2 miles. Cross the footbridge at 2.19 miles, and at 2.23 miles enjoy a break on a bench.

Follow the trail left and walk a little farther to the wetland area at 2.35 miles and listen for frogs chorusing during spring and summer. The trail curves and crosses a footbridge at 2.59 miles. This narrow footpath borders the edge of the lake for more than 0.2 miles. You'll see a pleasant backwater cove at about 2.77 miles before the trail heads uphill along an extremely eroded trail. Stop and watch for herons, waterfowl, and other wetland critters. This is a wonderful escape, especially in the winter.

Pass the connector trail at 2.84 miles and continue on Red Fox Trail to the left, following the red blaze marks on the trees. Walk quietly through the older forest of sugar maple, oak, and beech trees, and you might encounter a wild turkey scratching along the forest floor.

Cross the footbridge at 3.23 miles, and continue through the forest of sugar maple, beech, shagbark hickory, and white oak trees. Ignore the user-made trails. Continue following the primary trail, and when it connects to itself take the trail to the left, which becomes Southwoods Trail.

Follow Southwoods Trail back to the steep hill and the entrance to Lakeview Trail. Take Lakeview Trail to the right, and you'll see the lake after 0.2 mile. Elm trees border the trail close to the road. The trail briefly passes along the edge of the road, crosses the waterway, and enters the woods on the other side.

This portion of the trail in the woods is muddy in wet weather. Spur trails radiate along Lakeview Trail to the edge of the lake. At 0.39 mile into the Lakeview Trail, you're shaded by red cedar trees. Multiple benches provide excellent vantage points to view the lake.

Cross the creek at 4.5 miles, turn around in the parking area, and retrace your steps to the junction of Lakeview, Southwoods, and Beechtree Trails. Turn right and follow Beechtree Trail back to your vehicle.

Nearby Activities

East Fork State Park, Cincinnati Nature Center, and Sharon Woods offer additional hiking opportunities. Cowan Lake State Park and Indian Creek Wildlife Area are also nearby. Loveland has a variety of shops and dining. Roads Rivers and Trails in Milford is the nearest outfitter.

GPS Trailhead Coordinates and Directions

N39° 12.977'   W84° 04.647'

From I-275 on the east side of Cincinnati, take OH 28 North 2.6 miles. Turn east (right) onto Woodville Pike and travel 7.7 miles. Turn right onto Newtonsville Road and immediately turn right onto OH 727/Newtonsville Road. Travel 0.8 miles and turn left onto Lake Drive.

23 Sugarcreek MetroPark

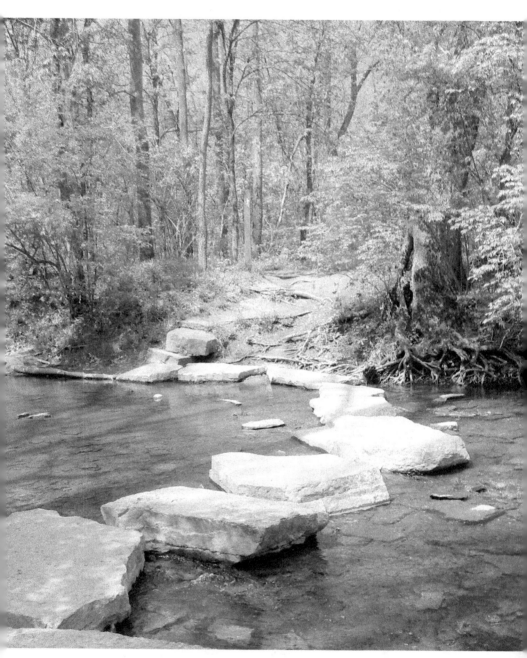

Enjoy hopping from stone to stone as you cross Sugar Creek.

LENGTH & CONFIGURATION 5.21-mile loop	8 a.m.–10 p.m.; November 1–March 31 8 a.m.–8 p.m.; closed January 1 and December 25; free
DIFFICULTY Easy–moderate	
SCENERY Woodlands, tallgrass prairie, and creeks	**MAPS** USGS *Waynesville;* Sugarcreek MetroPark User's Guide & Map
EXPOSURE Sun and shade	**WHEELCHAIR ACCESSIBLE** Some portions are paved. There is an additional 0.25-mile paved accessible trail through the prairie.
TRAFFIC Heavy	
TRAIL SURFACE Paved, soil, and gravel	
HIKING TIME 3.5–4 hours	**FACILITIES** Latrine and drinking water
DRIVING DISTANCE 1 hour from Cincinnati	**CONTACTS** Sugarcreek MetroPark, 937-275-PARK (7275); **metroparks.org/Parks /Sugarcreek/Home.aspx**
SEASON Year-round	**COMMENTS** Great hike for the navigationally impaired
ACCESS April 1–October 31: Daily,	

In Brief

Located on Dayton's lower east side, Sugarcreek MetroPark is part of the Five Rivers MetroParks system. With 618 acres, complete with 550-year-old oak trees, creek crossings, a fossil-collecting area, tallgrass prairie, woodlands, and an Osage orange–tree tunnel, you'll find several places to lose yourself.

Description

Five Rivers MetroParks actively manages Sugarcreek MetroPark for a variety of habitats that support an array of wildlife, including white-tailed deer, red fox, waterfowl, and a multitude of delightful songbirds. Most of the trails, as with other Five Rivers MetroParks, are clearly marked and color coded with numbered intersections. All color-coded trails are also loop trails that will return to the beginning of the loop.

The Sugarcreek MetroPark trail system is peppered with signposts, which benefits anyone who is navigationally impaired. Many different users visit Sugarcreek MetroPark, so expect to encounter joggers, dog walkers, and families out for a woodland adventure. In fact, for most of the hike you'll encounter plenty of people. If you are looking for a little solitude, cross the creek and take the more primitive Big Woods Trail loop. Not many people venture onto it because of its primitive qualities—it's a one-person-wide earthen path.

Sugarcreek MetroPark

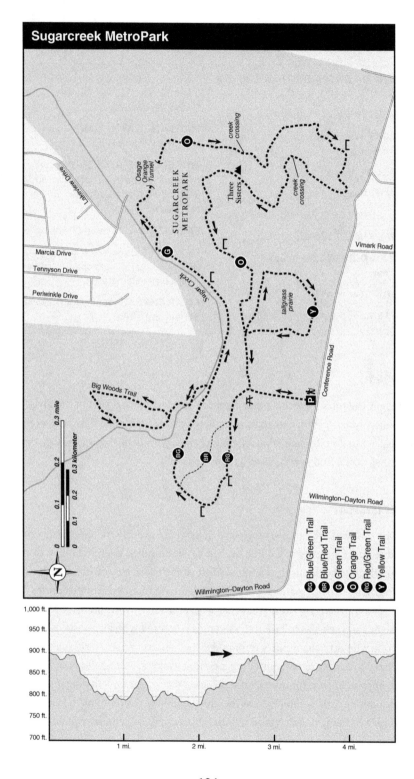

On the north side of the Sugarcreek MetroPark parking area is a kiosk. At the far side of it, take a moment to look for and investigate the geocache. At this location are water fountains for humans and dogs as well as a latrine facility. Proceed down the paved path that connects directly to the water fountain and latrine area. Along the edges of the paved entrance trail are informational signs about the emerald ash borer.

At 0.13 mile the trail intersects with the other trailheads at a spot that includes a pavilion and picnic tables. Follow the signpost marked with blue, green, and red circles. The trail leads straight ahead from the trail you came in on, then left into the woods.

After 0.25 mile you'll see an intersection labeled number 18. Take the red/green trail to the left and uphill along Sycamore Ridge. Stop at the bench at 0.3 mile to enjoy the view of the woods and listen to the birds singing.

When you reach intersection number 17 at 0.5 mile, take the blue/green trail to the left. In a few feet, Sugar Creek becomes visible in the valley to the left of the trail. In spring trout lilies line this area.

The trail begins to parallel Sugar Creek at 0.75 mile. The bench and kiosk for the fossil area are at 0.81 mile. The kiosk explains the fossil collecting rules and regulations and notes the access point to the area where fossil collecting is allowed. Some of the basic rules: no tools, no more than three fossils per day per person, and no fossils larger than your hand. Please read the regulations posted at the kiosk prior to collecting fossils. Fossils of interest include horn coral, brachiopods, crinoids, trilobites, and gastropods.

This area is also intersection number 16. Look down the hillside to the left and follow the enormous stone steps to the creek and then across Sugar Creek. Take a few steps up a small hill and follow the trail to the left to go on the Big Woods Trail loop.

This trail is dense with vegetation and is a single-person-wide footpath through the undergrowth. At 0.85 mile plenty of wild ginger and spring wildflowers border the trail. Enormous sycamore trees also bracket the trail, so be careful of your footing as you step over exposed roots.

Be wary of the multiple spurs that radiate to the left from this trail, especially near the 0.92-mile mark. But, don't stress out too much. If you take a spur by accident you'll just wind up at the edge of the creek and need to retrace your steps back to the trail.

Big Woods Trail follows along the creek corridor. Take a little time to sit and watch the water in the creek. In the elbows, the water is deep and clear, and you can watch the fish swimming. Just be careful to not stand on an overhang, or you might take an abrupt trip into one of those pools.

The trail begins to diverge from Sugar Creek, and at 0.96 mile you'll encounter an older signpost with a yellow hiker symbol. Follow the trail to the right as it curves up the steep hill. As the trail leads downhill and passes through the low-lying area check out the large beech trees and trillium (in spring).

When the trail rejoins itself, retrace your steps to Sugar Creek, across and up the stone steps to the bench at intersection number 16. Continue on the blue/green trail to the left.

The hike continues to parallel Sugar Creek. The ambient sounds of the flowing water readily cancel out the ruckus of surrounding suburbia. Continue following this trail along the edge of the creek, and at 2.16 miles you'll reach intersection number 10. Take the connector trail to the right.

The connector trail meets intersection number 11 at the start of the Osage Orange Tunnel at 2.23 miles. Depending on the time of day, the tunnel under the curved branches of the Osage orange trees would either be the perfect spot for wedding photos or a reenactment of Sleepy Hollow. Follow the path through the archway of the tunnel to intersection number 8.

At intersection number 8, take the orange/green trail to the right. At intersection number 7 continue on the green trail.

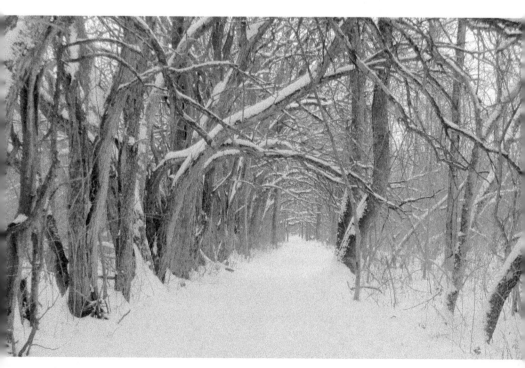

Osage Orange Tunnel at Sugarcreek

After the stream crossing at 2.56 miles, the trail enters Beech Woods. The trail leads downhill and runs parallel to a small creek. At 3.2 miles the trail crosses the creek and heads up a steep hill for the next 400 feet.

Intersection number 4 is 3.27 miles into the journey. The trail to the right connects to the Three Sisters, three impressive and massive 550-year-old white oak trees. At intersection number 5, take the trail to the right to view the Three Sisters. One of the Three Sisters died in 2005, but it still is an integral part of the forest ecosystem. Take a break on the nice swing and enjoy the view of the woods. The medallion is part of Five Rivers MetroParks' Venture Quest adventures—think geocaching meets letterboxing with a twist.

Return to the orange trail and continue to intersection number 6 at 3.5 miles, then take the connector trail to the left to intersection number 12, where it joins the other side of the orange trail. Take a left onto the orange trail and follow it through intersection number 13 (3.88 miles) by taking a right.

The orange trail leads to intersection number 14, which connects with the blue trail. Continue to the left on the blue/orange trail. At 4 miles at intersection number 2, turn left and follow the yellow trail as it meanders through the tallgrass prairie. Watch and listen for the variety of songbirds that call it home.

When the looped yellow trail reconnects with intersection number 2, take a left onto the yellow/blue/green/orange trail. Follow this path to the open area with the pavilion and picnic tables. At the paved path you came in on, turn left and return to the trailhead.

Nearby Activities

Stock up on delicious treats for the trail and home at Dorothy Lane Market near the corner of OH 48 and Whipp Road, or at Health Foods Unlimited off OH 725 near the Dayton Mall. To work off those treats, head over to Germantown MetroPark.

GPS Trailhead Coordinates and Directions
N39° 37.054'   W84° 05.794'

From Cincinnati, take I-75 North to Exit 43/I-675 North. Continue on I-675 and take Exit 7/Wilmington Pike. Turn right and follow Wilmington Pike south. Take Wilmington Pike south for 2.8 miles. At the bend the road changes to Wilmington Dayton Road. At the next turn, continue straight onto Conference Road and follow it to the main parking area on the north side of the road.

24 Withrow Nature Preserve

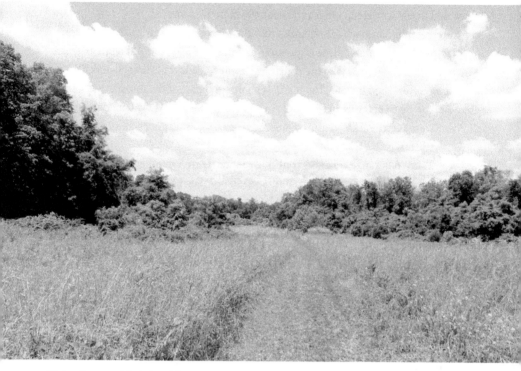

Listen for songbirds in Withrow Nature Preserve's meadow.

In Brief

At Withrow Nature Preserve, a Great Parks of Hamilton County park, hikers can spy on the Ohio River, enjoy a cool trek through upland woods, and meander along the grass path through the open field to watch butterflies and several types of songbirds during the summer months.

Description

Nestled into the Greater Cincinnati area, this nature preserve serves as an easily accessible destination to get away from it all. The Highwood Lodge sits at the end of the parking area and often hosts small outdoor celebrations such as weddings.

The rest of the 270-acre nature preserve is home to many upland animals, including white-tailed deer, gray squirrels, and red-eyed vireos, in addition to an abundance of

LENGTH & CONFIGURATION 2.1-mile loops and out-and-back	SEASON Year-round
DIFFICULTY Easy	ACCESS Daily, sunrise–sunset; annual vehicle permit, $10; daily vehicle permit, $5
SCENERY Ohio River overlook, woods, and open field	MAPS USGS *Newport* and *Withamsville;* signage at Trout Lily Trailhead
EXPOSURE Mostly shade except open field	WHEELCHAIR ACCESSIBLE No
TRAFFIC Light	FACILITIES Semipermanent latrines at edge of parking lot
TRAIL SURFACE Mostly gravel and grass	CONTACTS Great Parks of Hamilton County, 513-521-7275; **greatparks.org /parks/withrow-nature-preserve**
HIKING TIME 1.5–2 hours (depends on how much time you spend at the bench at the overlook)	
DRIVING DISTANCE Less than 10 minutes from I-275's Five Mile Road exit	COMMENTS The open field is a perfect place to see plenty of butterflies, goldfinches, and bluebirds.

butterflies and skippers. The jaunt is relatively easy and an ideal place to introduce your children to hiking. A fair amount of the winding trail is wide enough to walk side by side.

You'll pass through mature uplands with an abundance of sugar maples, white and red oaks, slippery elms, and hickories along paths lined with a spectacular variety of spring wildflowers. Along the way, look for a large, open field area that serves as a butterfly paradise and nesting home for eastern bluebirds. But the gem of the property is the scenic overlook of the Ohio River.

From the parking area, head toward the Highwood Lodge, being careful not to crash any weddings in progress. With the lodge to the right, look to the left for the Trout Lily trailhead sign with general information about the hike and an overview map of the area. Just beyond the sign is the entrance to the trail and the woods.

Descending the steps into the cool air of the mature forest, you'll find the first section of woods to be a canopy of hefty white oaks and sugar maples. Aromatic spicebush lines both sides of the path, as does the occasional bunch of poison ivy. The steps in this area are steep and require your attention, lest you catch a toe and trip (not that I would know).

At the base of the hill, ignore the closed trail and continue on the Trout Lily Trail to your left. A small footbridge transports you into a wonderful second-growth forest.

You'll notice several portions of the hike are very open and there are several trees that have been cut down. The trees are ash and land managers decided to remove the trees due to the damage caused by the small but devastating emerald ash borer. Emerald ash borer larvae eat the cambium, or growth layer, of the tree. The cambium is the

Withrow Nature Preserve

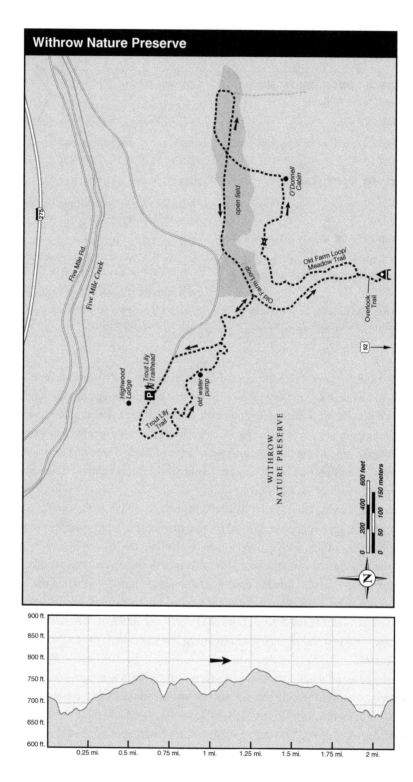

part of the tree that transfers nutrients and water between the leaves and the roots. If you look closely at the tree remains you can see the tunnels left behind from the insects eating the cambium.

Land managers cut down infected trees to reduce the spread of the emerald ash borer as well as to improve safety along the trail. Please help keep the forest healthy by not removing firewood or any wood (walking sticks you find included) from the woods. You could inadvertently give an invasive insect a free ride to a new delectable forest.

Along this portion go the trail you'll pass a small grove of pawpaws. The pawpaw tree grows wide, ovate-shaped leaves that, when pinched, smell of diesel fuel and lemons. In the late fall pawpaws also produce an edible fruit that tastes similar to banana pudding. But you'll need to restrain yourself, as the rules of the nature preserve prohibit taking or damaging plants, minerals, and animals.

The path then climbs slowly uphill to a small clump of black cherry trees and an old water pump at 0.28 mile. The path winds downhill into a nice, open woods and another footbridge. Soon after the footbridge, the trail meets up with another trail that leads back to the parking area. At the intersection of these trails, follow the arrow signage and continue straight ahead. At 0.48 mile when you reach the next intersection, turn right and head to the Overlook Trail. On the left you'll pass the intersection with Old Farm Loop/Meadow Trail at 0.68 mile and continue on the trail to the Overlook. The Overlook Trail ascends a few steps before winding uphill and downhill through a younger upland forest.

Keep heading straight, and in another 80 yards, you'll reach the overlook, which ends at a park bench situated perfectly to gaze through a window in the trees to the Ohio River below. Relax on the bench and take a few minutes to watch the river traffic from far above.

Once you have had your fill of the Ohio River, retrace your steps and turn right to follow Old Farm Loop/Meadow Trail. The irregular rise and tread of steps on the sloped portions of the trail, meant to control trail erosion, are a bit tricky to navigate.

After 0.2 mile from the turn, a forest clearing appears. Look for the footprint left by the cabin built by the O'Donnell family in the grassy opening. Two benches allow reflection on what it must have been like to build and live in a cabin here.

To preserve the wildlife and habitat of the area, the Nellie R. and James B. O'Donnell Jr. family and The Nature Conservancy led the acquisition of Withrow Nature Preserve and the surrounding land. In 1980 Adelaide Withrow donated the lodge and surrounding property to Great Parks of Hamilton County.

The path leads back into a wooded area with an ample supply of both sugar maples and rambunctious gray squirrels; soon it widens into a lane that enters an incredible butterfly paradise. For approximately 0.4 mile, the path loops through milkweeds, grasses, daisies, ironweed, purple coneflowers, black-eyed Susans, thistle, and clover. During the late spring and summer months, butterflies such as fritillaries, monarchs, and swallowtails flit from flower to flower.

At the trail signpost, take the mowed grassy path to the right that cuts through the middle of the field. Several bluebird nesting boxes are located in the open field beneath a sky alive with eastern bluebirds, barn swallows, and goldfinches. Stay on the path until you reach another gravel access road. Follow the arrow and head left, staying on this path as it meanders along the edge of the open field and woods.

When the trails through the field converge, stay on the trail to the right and head back into the woods. (The connector trail on the right leads to the parking area.) Retrace your steps back to the trailhead and parking area.

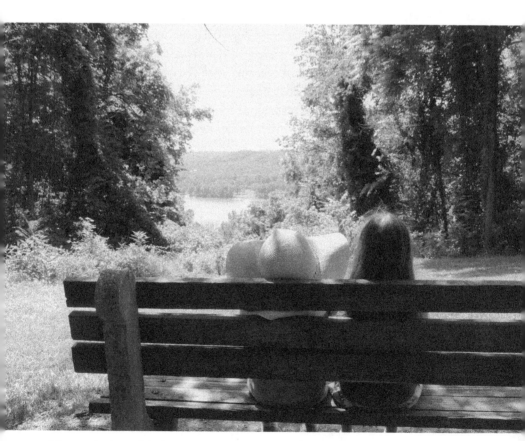

The overlook is a fabulous spot to sit and watch the Ohio River.

Nearby Attractions

Incredible ice cream is just minutes away at Graeter's off Beechmont Avenue/OH 125. At the intersection of Beechmont Avenue and Five Mile is an open-air mall, plenty of restaurants, a pharmacy, and a grocery store. Take Five Mile south to US 52 East and follow the signs for another Great Parks of Hamilton County gem, Woodland Mound, which offers a great disc golf course, nature center, plenty of picnic shelters and playgrounds, trails, and a children's water-spray park.

GPS Trailhead Coordinates and Directions

N39° 03.121'   W84° 22.630'

Withrow Nature Preserve is on the east side of Cincinnati between the Ohio River and OH 125. From I-275, take the Five Mile Road exit and head south on Five Mile less than 1 mile to the park entrance on the left (south) side of the road. Follow the entrance road to the parking area.

CINCINNATI

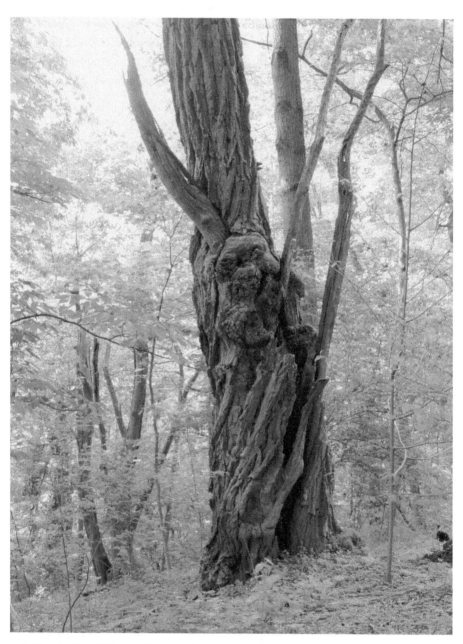

California Woods Nature Preserve (see page 162)

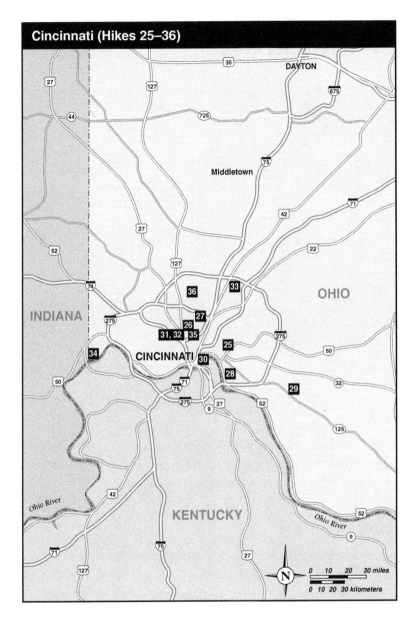

25 Ault Park

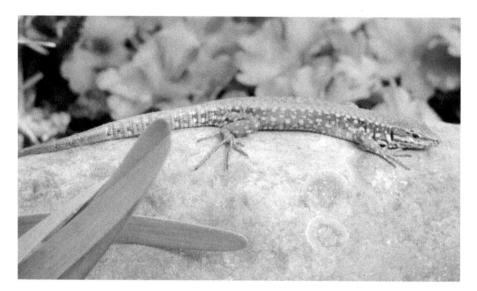

Exotic common wall lizards can be found in the garden areas at Ault Park. These lizards are known locally as Lazarus lizards.

In Brief

Located on Cincinnati's lower east side, Ault Park offers a variety of events and festivities throughout the year, including a Fourth of July celebration. Several hiking trails in this urban park make it easy to accidentally take a side trail.

Description

Ault Park, the fourth-largest park in Cincinnati, was named after Ida May and Levi Addison Ault, who were active in the development of Cincinnati Parks. In 1911 the Aults began giving land to Ault Park, donating a significant amount of the 224 acres that make up the park today.

Observatory Avenue ends at Ault Park. Follow Ault Park Drive around the observatory and park in the lot on the north side of the formal gardens and pavilion area.

Look to your left for a small picnic area. The entrance to the trail system is to the right of the picnic area. The series of trails covered in this hike will take you through a good portion of the park's 223 acres.

Once you enter the woods, the trail leads downhill. At 0.16 mile you'll descend a series of large, stone steps that take you farther into the valley of sugar maple, American beech, white oak, and Ohio buckeye trees.

LENGTH & CONFIGURATION 3.7-mile loops	**ACCESS** Daily, 6 a.m.–10 p.m.; free
DIFFICULTY Easy–moderate	**MAPS** USGS *Cincinnati East;* Ault Park map
SCENERY Woods and gardens	**WHEELCHAIR ACCESSIBLE** No
EXPOSURE Shaded	**FACILITIES** Picnic areas
TRAFFIC Moderate–heavy	**CONTACTS** Cincinnati Parks, 513-352-4080; **cincinnatiparks.com/index.php /ault-park**
TRAIL SURFACE Gravel and soil	
HIKING TIME 2.5–3 hours	**COMMENTS** Ault Park offers a variety of events throughout the year, including dances, wine and jazz festivals, and a Fourth of July celebration. Visit the website to see what might interest you.
DRIVING DISTANCE 20 minutes from downtown Cincinnati	
SEASON Year-round	

Within 0.2 mile, you'll encounter a series of spur trails and be able to see several footbridges over small, intermittent streams. Stay to your left and don't leave the trail that you're on.

The trail intersects with the T (Tree) Trail and a footbridge at 0.25 mile. Stay on the trail you're on and take the next series of stone steps down to a small bridge at 0.27 mile. Cross the bridge and turn to your right to follow the Valley Trail along the gravel path through this lower area. There's a small creek to your right. This portion of the trail is completely shaded by the dense canopy.

You'll come to a trail intersection at 0.56 mile (the footbridge on your right connects to the Tree Trail). Continue on the gravel and stone trail that you've been on and continue on the Forest Loop Trail.

At 0.69 mile, the trail joins with the Ridge Trail, which is marked with blue paint. Take the Ridge Trail by heading to your left and uphill before you get to the railroad overpass.

The narrow, single-person path leads uphill. As you walk up the ridge, be sure to look to your right. The view of this lush green valley and forest canopy warrants a few peaceful moments. Multiple trails intersect with the Ridge Trail, so be careful to stay on this main trail or you'll wind up getting turned around.

Ridge Trail intersects with Bur Oak (orange colored) Trail at 0.83 mile. Follow the Bur Oak Trail and avoid taking side trails. At 1.1 miles you'll encounter a tree that measures 17 feet in circumference. I won't spoil it for you by identifying it, but if you're unable to figure it out walk a little farther. A sign marker at 1.24 miles, in the open area near Observatory Avenue, will tell you.

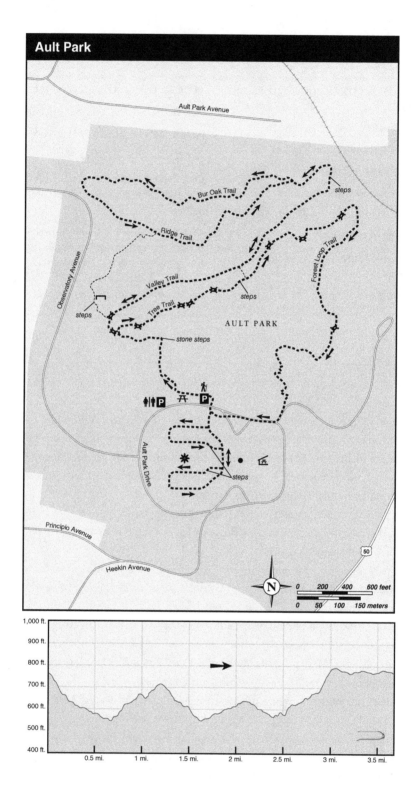

Ault Park

AULT PARK

Ault Park Avenue

Bur Oak Trail

steps

Ridge Trail

Forest Loop Trail

Observatory Avenue

Valley Trail

Tree Trail

steps

steps

stone steps

Ault Park Drive

Principio Avenue

Heekin Avenue

50

N

0   200   400   600 feet

0   50   100   150 meters

1,000 ft.
900 ft.
800 ft.
700 ft.
600 ft.
500 ft.
400 ft.

0.5 mi.   1 mi.   1.5 mi.   2 mi.   2.5 mi.   3 mi.   3.5 mi.

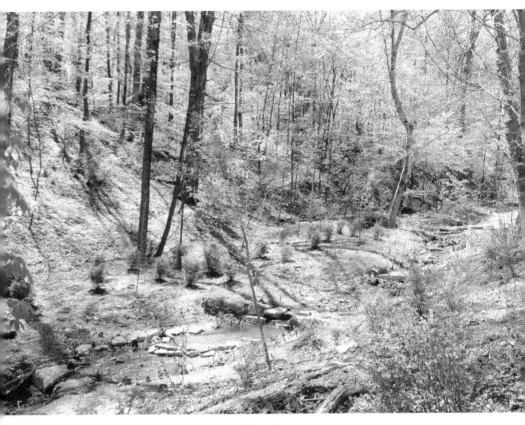

The creek area is a pleasant retreat at Ault Park.

Follow the trail around through the open area and look for the red post marking the Ridge Trail; reenter the woods by staying on Ridge Trail. At the intersection follow the Ridge Trail to the left and when it reconnects with the Valley Trail retrace your steps back along the Valley Trail to the intersection with the Tree Trail connector.

Follow the connector to your left to the Tree Trail, crossing the footbridge over the creek. Turn left onto the Tree Trail at 2.1 miles. This intersection is the same trail junction you passed earlier. You'll immediately cross another footbridge. The trail meanders through the woods and crosses several footbridges. As you walk along this lower portion of the trail in springtime, trilliums and spring beauties line the edges. You'll begin to head uphill and out of the valley at about 2.4 miles. At 2.5 miles the trail splits; stay on the trail you're on as it bends to the right and continues uphill.

You'll notice a lot of trail erosion, so watch your footing as you step over rocks and exposed roots.

Soon (at 2.8 miles), you'll come to a footbridge. Immediately after you cross you'll see an enormous red oak tree on the left side of the trail.

Continue uphill and the trail will exit the woods at about 3 miles. Take the road to your right and walk along the road (watch for traffic). When the pavilion area sidewalk starts, cross the road to your left, and follow the sidewalk to the garden on the left.

To your left is Ault Park Pavilion. This 1920s structure fell into disrepair with the passage of time, but in the 1980s the Ault Park Advisory Council and other civic groups carefully restored it to its previous grandeur. The Ohio Historical Society recognized the accomplishment in 1992.

At the apex of the formal garden you'll find a trellis area with benches. Here, you can rest and watch for the Cooper's hawks that use the open area of the formal garden for hunting small birds and mammals.

The formal garden area in front of the pavilion, maintained by the Adopt-A-Plot volunteer gardening program, includes roses, succulents, and a variety of flowers that attract butterflies and birds. When you're done enjoying the formal gardens, head north and follow the sidewalk to your vehicle.

Nearby Activities

Want to walk some more? You'll find several hikes nearby, including the hills of California Woods Nature Preserve and Eden Park (home to the Cincinnati Art Museum and nationally recognized Krohn Conservatory). Shopping opportunities abound in unique Hyde Park.

GPS Trailhead Coordinates and Directions

N39° 08.057'   W84° 24.713'

From I-71, near downtown Cincinnati, follow US 50 East for 4.6 miles. Turn left onto Delta Avenue and travel 1.5 miles, then turn right onto Observatory Avenue. Follow it 0.6 mile to Ault Park.

26 Buttercup Valley Preserve and Parkers Woods

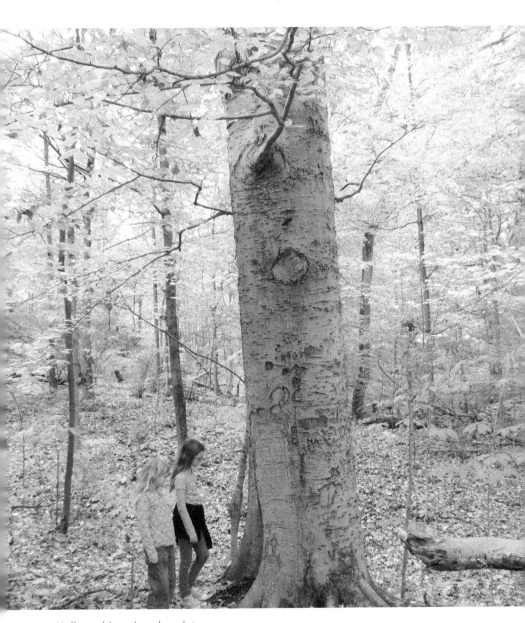

Hollowed American beech tree

LENGTH & CONFIGURATION 2-mile loop	**SEASON** Year-round
DIFFICULTY Easy–moderate	**ACCESS** Daily, sunrise–sunset; free
SCENERY Forest	**MAPS** USGS *Cincinnati West*; Buttercup Valley Preserve and Parkers Woods map
EXPOSURE Shade	**WHEELCHAIR ACCESSIBLE** No
TRAFFIC Moderate–heavy	**FACILITIES** None
TRAIL SURFACE Gravel, dirt, and sidewalk	**CONTACTS** Cincinnati Parks, 513-352-4080; **cincinnatiparks.com/index.php /buttercup-valley** or **cincinnatiparks.com /index.php/parker-woods**
HIKING TIME 1.5 hours	
DRIVING DISTANCE Less than 10 minutes from Cincinnati	**COMMENTS** Look for big tulip poplars, red and white oaks, and American beeches.

In Brief

Step out of the urban chaos and into a beautiful forest of mature tulip poplar, sugar maple, red and white oaks, and black cherry trees. This forest is unusual because, between earlier settlers and more recent development, it is amazing that any of the trees survived. The trail winds through the woods occasionally popping back out into civilization before ducking back into the forest.

Description

Set in the midst of the Cincinnati metro area is a small nature preserve that has managed to remain untouched since pioneer times. As you make your way deeper into the woods, you'll see evidence of this in the statuesque tulip poplars, red and white oaks, American beech, and sugar maples.

The land was acquired a parcel at a time beginning in 1973. The Buttercup Valley was a gift from the Greater Cincinnati Tree Council, with the help of conservationists and thousands of schoolchildren who aided in collecting funds to purchase the land. The total acreage was increased in 1974 by the Greater Cincinnati Tree Council and a Land and Water Conservation Fund grant from the Federal Bureau of Outdoor Recreation, bringing the acreage of Buttercup Valley Preserve and Parkers Woods to a little more than 25 acres. In 1979, the Buttercup Valley Trail was designated a National Recreation Trail by the U.S. Department of the Interior.

One set of trailheads is at the end of Stanford Drive. The parking at this location is along the curb. Once you have secured your vehicle, walk to the end of the street and to the large Buttercup Valley Preserve sign in the grassy opening.

Buttercup Valley Preserve and Parkers Woods

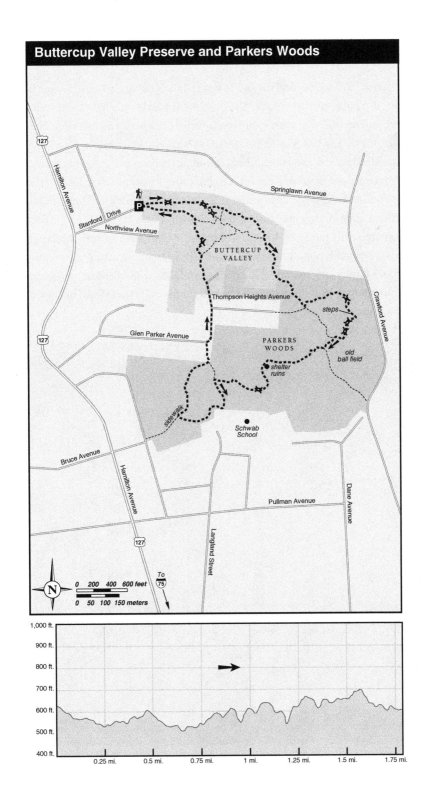

As soon as you step beyond the sign, two trailheads come into view. Follow the singletrack of Trail B into the woods. The trail begins a little roughly with silver maples, box elders, and redbuds but soon improves. Invasive bush honeysuckle is being eradicated from this area, which is great because bush honeysuckle can quickly take over a forest, crowding out common forest flora, including saplings and wildflowers.

Large tendrils of grapevine thread into the canopies of the trees. Look for wild ginger as you cross the footbridge under the canopy of shagbark hickories and box elders. Watch your footing over the exposed roots.

As the trail exits the bend, look for tulip poplar trees, also known as yellow poplar, tulip, canoewood, popple, and whitewood. Tulip trees are actually a member of the magnolia family and are one of the tallest, straightest, and lightest hardwoods found in North America. Pioneers used tulip trees for everything from lining wells to building homes.

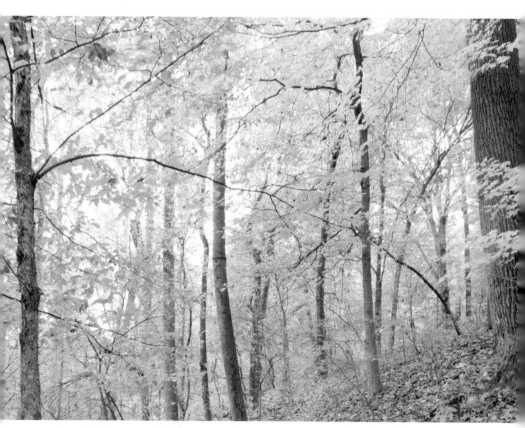

Woodlands at Buttercup Valley Preserve

When pioneers first arrived tulip trees were highly sought after and subject to widespread unregulated logging, which is one reason why it is unusual to find such fine specimens.

Cross the footbridge and stop at this point and enjoy the view of the valley. American beech trees are found throughout this woodland. There are many outstanding beech trees along this portion of the trail. To identify them look for very smooth, silver-colored bark and serrated-edge, glossy green leaves. If you are out in winter, beeches typically keep a few bright, golden-hued leaves throughout the season.

Take the Trail B Loop Trail to the left at the intersection 0.14 mile into the hike. The trail leads downhill through the spicebush, sugar maple, tulip, and sassafras. Stay on the main trail and don't accidentally veer off onto one of the many deer trails. Watch your footing on the heavily eroded trail.

At 0.23 mile, you'll encounter an area with lots of pawpaws and plenty of grapevine. Grapevine is a large rope-looking vine which is fun for the kids to play on as a swing. Be careful if you do this and make sure you don't accidentally pull a large limb out of a tree and onto your head.

This trail enters a lowland area adjacent to the edge of a creek. Watch your step over the plethora of walnuts on the ground. Don't cross the creek; the trail continues uphill to the right on an extremely narrow and steep footpath.

When you reach the trail junction at 0.35 mile, continue to the left and head toward the large trees. After the trail makes a sharp right, you'll see the marker for Trail B. At the intersection, follow Trail B left to Parkers Woods. Take your time and enjoy the serenity of the upland woods of 60- to 80-foot-tall sycamore, tulip, and sugar maple trees surrounded by wild ginger and the saplings of sugar maple and beech.

Follow the trail into a valley area. You'll need to work your way around fallen trees and down the hill. In the bottom of the valley, walk around the concrete drainage basin, and continue on the trail up the half-log steps.

At 0.4 mile into the hike the trail makes a hard left at the enormous hollowed beech tree. (This is an easy turn to miss.) You'll soon see locusts, black cherry, American elms, and sassafras trees. Continue on the Loop Trail to your left when you reach the intersection with Thompson Heights Trail.

When you reach the B and B Loop Trails intersection, follow the B Loop Trail to the left and downhill through an open forest of black cherry, hickory, and walnut saplings. The trail leads down log steps and in the valley area there are tulips, oaks, and basswood trees.

Over the next 300 feet, cross three small footbridges before continuing on the trail straight ahead through the trail intersection. At the Crawford Avenue and Trail B intersection, follow the Trail B to your right and pass several beech trees.

At 1.12 miles pass the remains of a shelter under the canopy of sugar maples and red oaks. Cross the bridge at 1.2 miles before ascending the steps. When you reach the next trail intersection follow the trail to your left and to the parking lot of Schwab School. Continue along the edge of the woods. You'll see a small sign for Parkers Woods and an old asphalt path. Follow it back into the forest.

You are greeted by forest of black and red oaks, sugar maples, black cherries, and hickory trees. In the valley area at 1.41 miles the trail passes by an extremely large sycamore tree. Sycamores have a distinct platy yellow, green, and gray bark that peels away and sloughs off the tree to expose a ghostly white bark.

At 1.5 miles into the hike you pop off the footpath and onto a sidewalk. Follow the sidewalk to your right and uphill under redbuds and sugar maples. Continue following the sidewalk to Glenn Parker Avenue. You'll exit the woods near the corner of Glenn Parker Avenue and Langland. Langland is to your right. This short street heads up a slight hill passing the Parkers Woods Preserve sign on the right.

At the next street corner, Langland and Thompson Heights Avenue, take a left and follow the narrow asphalt driveway. When you reach the end of the road, look to your left and you'll see the Buttercup Valley Preserve Trail A entrance.

Stay on Trail A and at 1.81 miles pass through the intersection with a trail that leads to Northview Avenue. When you reach the intersection with Stanford Drive and Trail A, follow the trail to your left. You'll exit the woods at the trailhead for A. Make your way across the grassy area and back to your vehicle.

Nearby Activities

More hiking trails are just a hop, a skip, and a jump away. Spring Grove Cemetery is literally right next door. Mount Airy Forest, LaBoiteaux Woods, and Winton Woods are a short drive away. Restaurants can be found further north on US 27. The closest outfitters are REI and Benchmark Outfitters.

GPS Trailhead Coordinates and Directions
N39° 10.470'   W84° 32.426'

From I-75 North take the Exit 6/Mitchell Avenue exit. Turn left onto West Mitchell and then turn left onto Spring Grove Avenue. Continue on Spring Grove and take slight right onto Blue Rock Street. Turn right onto Hamilton Avenue. Turn right onto Stanford Drive and park at the end of the street.

27 Caldwell Preserve

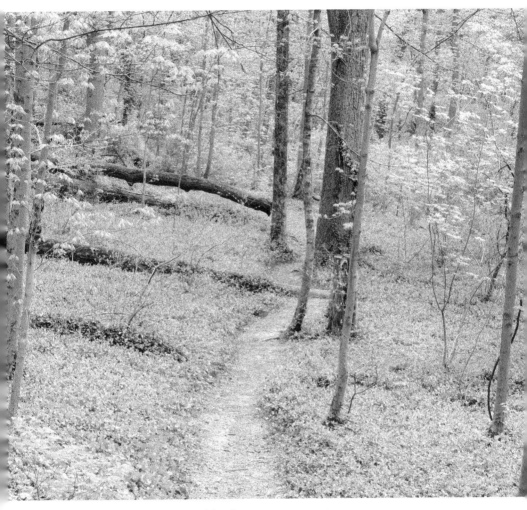

Spring beauty abounds at Caldwell Preserve.

In Brief

Caldwell Preserve is a great place to take your family hiking. Several beautiful valley overlooks are peppered throughout the preserve. The Ray Abercrombie and Ravine Creek Trails are very scenic, and the Paw Paw Ridge Trail provides some solitude. Be sure to venture behind the nature center on the paved trail to the platform overlooking the valley.

LENGTH & CONFIGURATION 2.78-mile series of loops	**ACCESS** Daily, 6 a.m.–10 p.m.; free
DIFFICULTY Moderate	**MAPS** USGS *Cincinnati East;* Caldwell Preserve map
SCENERY Woods, valleys, and streams	**WHEELCHAIR ACCESSIBLE** No
EXPOSURE Shaded	**FACILITIES** Nature center when open
TRAFFIC Moderate–heavy	**CONTACTS** Caldwell Preserve Nature Center, 513-761-4313; **cincinnatiparks .com/index.php/caldwell-preserve**
TRAIL SURFACE Soil	
HIKING TIME 1–1.5 hours	
DRIVING DISTANCE 20 minutes from downtown Cincinnati	**COMMENTS** You'll find beautiful views and well-kept trails at Caldwell Preserve. Although there is a fair amount of traffic, expect some solitude while you hike.
SEASON Year-round	

Description

Caldwell Preserve began in 1915, when J. Nelson Caldwell donated 89.3 acres to Cincinnati Parks as a memorial to his father, Major James Nelson Caldwell, who was one of this valley's early pioneers.

Caldwell's trail system is designated by the U.S. Department of the Interior as a National Recreation Trail. Hartwell Boy Scout Troop 14 constructed the earliest path, Ray Abercrombie Trail, in 1976.

After parking in the lot, look along the tree line to the left for the entrance to Ray Abercrombie Trail and step into the woods. You'll see strikingly white sycamore trees in the valley to the right.

The trail proceeds through a forest of black locusts, tulip poplars, and flowering dogwoods undergoing succession. This path sees heavy traffic, including dog walkers and people out for a day hike with their kids.

The older forest is composed of red oaks and sugar maples. Look to the right into the valley and waterway below. The water's ambient sounds do an excellent job of blocking most of the noise from the surrounding metro area.

A little more than 300 feet into the hike is an intersection. Follow the A/red/ Abercrombie Trail and head down a series of railroad-tie steps. The steps have fairly high rises, so be sure of your foot placement.

At 0.1 mile, the trail intersects with Meadow Trail, which leads back uphill and to the far side of the parking lot. Stay on the A/red/Abercrombie Trail and cross the footbridge.

Caldwell Preserve

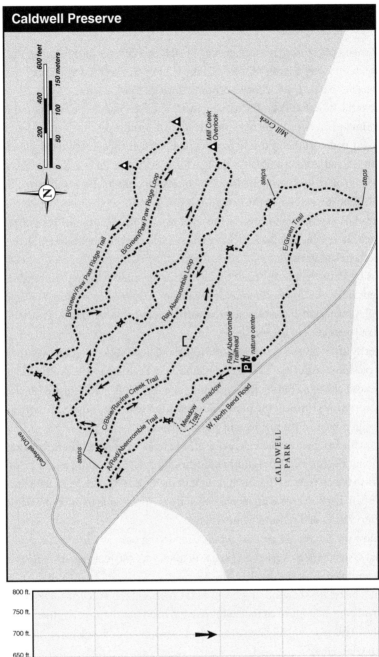

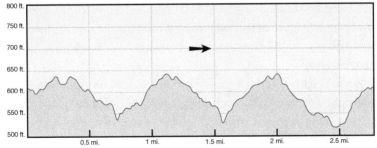

After you pass through a nice grove of black cherry trees near 0.3 mile, the trail leads downhill along a series of steps. To the left is a creek. If the trains are moving you'll be able to hear train whistles echoing through this low area.

Cross the bridge at 0.4 mile, passing by C/blue/Ravine Creek Trail to the right and continuing on A/red/Abercrombie Trail. In 0.1 mile take the A/red/Abercrombie Loop to the right. At the next trail intersection 260 feet ahead, take the trail to the left side of the A/red/Abercrombie Loop. The forest is American beech and red and white oak trees. If you're lucky, you might see woodpeckers, nuthatches, and tufted titmice.

Take four steps down to the bridge at 0.7 mile and four steps back up to continue on the trail. Pass a connector trail to the right at 0.8 mile. This is a fairly open woods with black cherry and shagbark hickory trees. Take a few moments to enjoy the view from the bench at 0.9 mile.

Pass by all the connector trails by staying on the main A/red/Abercrombie Loop, but do go check out the overlook. Pass the earlier A/red/Abercrombie Trail split and at 1.1 miles turn right at the intersection with the connector trail to B/green/Paw Paw Ridge Trail over the old access road.

Shortly after, cross a series of footbridges and head slightly uphill over the top of several erosion-control steps. The trail connects to the B/green/Paw Paw Ridge Trail, which leads back to an old service road and then downhill. The B/green/Paw Paw Ridge Loop winds through the park's oldest section of forest, a mix of American beech, tulip poplar, sugar maple, and pawpaw trees.

Cross the bridge over a creek ravine at 1.42 miles. The area suffers from a significant amount of erosion. Cross another footbridge at 1.48 miles and take a close look at the massive beech trees to the left and right of the trail. The path leads up a few steps into an open, flat-top area with lots of beech trees. The ravine to the right is filled with black cherry trees and red and white oaks.

Follow the B/green/Paw Paw Ridge Loop to the right at 1.6 miles through the white oaks, shagbark hickories, and sugar maples. Just 250 feet ahead are massive trees and a beautiful view of the creek ravine.

You'll be treated to another view of Mill Creek and the valley at 1.89 miles. After you've had your fill, return to the main trail and head uphill to yet another overlook at 1.96 miles. This overlook highlights a perfect example of drainage patterns in the southern Ohio area.

When you reach where the B/green/Paw Paw Ridge Loop split earlier, follow the trail to the right. Follow this trail back through the woods and downhill to the C/blue/Ravine Creek Trail you passed earlier. This is the intersection of the A/red/Abercrombie Trail and C/blue/Ravine Creek Trail near the bridge at 2.47 miles. Turn left on C/

blue/Ravine Creek Trail and follow the creek. Several blue clay deposits are visible along the creek.

Take a break on the benches at 2.65 miles. Pass the connector trails to your left by following the C/blue/Ravine Creek Trail to the right; it eventually leads to the nature center. Cross the bridge at 2.8 miles and head uphill.

The valley is significantly sheltered from urban noise and is very tranquil. A bridge crosses the ravine at 2.87 miles. At 3 miles, start heading uphill over a series of steps.

At the top of the hill at 3.1 miles, C/blue/Ravine Creek Trail connects to the figure eight–shaped E/lime-green Trail. Take the E/lime green Trail to the right. When this trail joins with itself, continue to the right passing the trail that connects to the amphitheater and then take the trail to the left, which leads to the back of the nature center. Walk around the nature center and return to your car in the parking lot.

Nearby Activities

The Cincinnati Museum Center and Cincinnati Zoo & Botanical Garden are located in downtown Cincinnati. My daughters' favorite is the Trading Post at the Cincinnati Museum of Natural History at the Cincinnati Museum Center. Bring in seashells, rocks, or fossils to trade for other specimens.

GPS Trailhead Coordinates and Directions

N39° 12.094'   W84° 29.543'

In Cincinnati, take I-75 North to Exit 9/Paddock Road/Seymour Avenue. Turn left on Paddock Road. Then turn left onto West North Bend Road. The entrance to the preserve is on the right.

28 California Woods Nature Preserve

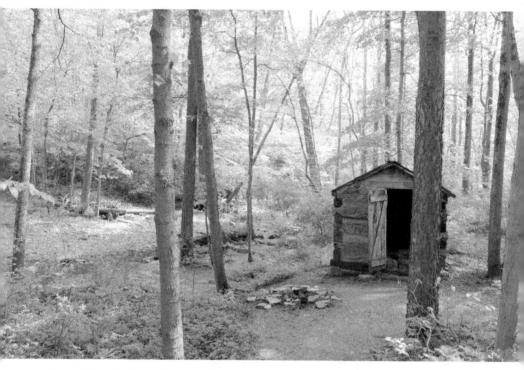

Log cabin at California Woods Nature Preserve

In Brief

Nestled into Cincinnati's lower east side, California Woods Nature Preserve offers a variety of trails, from easy to moderate, through valleys, hillsides, meadows, and forests. Your children will love exploring the hands-on displays at the nature center.

Description

The California Woods Nature Preserve, with 113 acres of forest and 1 acre of prairie, provides the perfect spot to quickly get away from it all. A variety of trails crisscross the property. The ones I have chosen for this hike will take you through a significant portion of the property, giving you a chance to see some of the delightful flora and fauna this preserve hides within its boundaries.

LENGTH & CONFIGURATION 3.7-mile series of loops	**ACCESS** Daily, 6 a.m.–10 p.m.; free
DIFFICULTY Easy–moderate	**MAPS** USGS *Newport;* California Woods Nature Preserve map
SCENERY Woods, ravines, and meadow	**WHEELCHAIR ACCESSIBLE** No
EXPOSURE Shade and sun	**FACILITIES** Restrooms and water when nature center is open
TRAFFIC Moderate–heavy	
TRAIL SURFACE Soil	**CONTACTS** Cincinnati Parks, 513-352-4080; **cincinnatiparks.com/index.php /california-woods**
HIKING TIME 3 hours	
DRIVING DISTANCE 20 minutes from downtown Cincinnati	
SEASON Year-round	**COMMENTS** This is a great place to take children for hiking and exploring nature.

When you turn into the nature preserve property, follow the road until you reach the nature center. Park in the open lot and secure your vehicle. This lot, with the open-grid paving stones, was once a pool. The nature center used to be the pool house, but over the years both its purpose and appearance have evolved.

In front of the California Woods Nature Center is a hummingbird–butterfly garden. Here you can get ideas for landscaping your own backyard. Near this area are rock garden plants, clearly identified, growing along the flat-stone borders.

The nature center's restroom, water, and facilities are available when it is open. Inside the nature center, you can comfortably let your kids explore the many artifacts on display, including antlers, turtle shells, fossils, and much more. This is one of my favorite nature centers because it is designed specifically for children and allows them to fully interact with the displays without fear of breaking something.

Exit the nature center and walk left to the stream with a low-flow dam and a bridge. Cross the bridge and follow the paved access road slightly uphill. On the left side of the trail at 0.1 mile is a small log cabin.

The trails are well maintained. This is a popular destination for hikers, bird-watchers, and wildflower enthusiasts, so odds are that you'll meet plenty of interesting people while you're out hiking.

After the log cabin, continue following the path uphill. Take the turnoff on the right at 0.18 mile. This area of the forest is dominated by sugar maples, but also has Ohio buckeye, black cherry, sycamore, and white oak trees as well as many spring wildflowers. The trail exits the road to the right and enters the forest and leads uphill over several railroad-tie steps, which gives you an excuse to slow down and enjoy the woods.

At another intersection at 0.34 mile, the trail forks. Stay to the right, on Ridge Loop Trail, which meanders through a forest with tulip trees. When you return to the

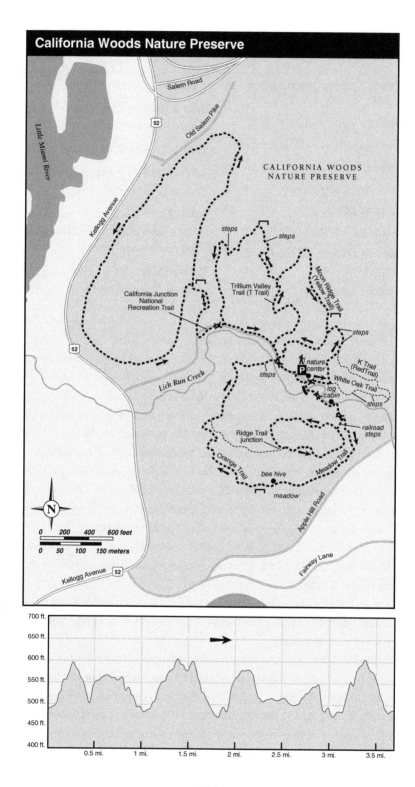

California Woods Nature Preserve

Salem Road

52

Old Salem Pike

Little Miami River

Kellogg Avenue

52

CALIFORNIA WOODS
NATURE PRESERVE

steps

steps

Moon Ridge Trail
(Yellow Trail)

California Junction
National
Recreation Trail

Trillium Valley
Trail (T Trail)

steps

nature
center

K Trail
(Red Trail)

Lick Run Creek

steps

White Oak Trail

log
cabin

steps

railroad
steps

Ridge Trail
junction

Orange Trail

bee hive

Meadow Trail

Apple Hill Road

meadow

N

0   200   400   600 feet

0   50   100   150 meters

Kellogg Avenue   52

Fairway Lane

700 ft.

650 ft.

600 ft.

550 ft.

500 ft.

450 ft.

400 ft.

0.5 mi.   1 mi.   1.5 mi.   2 mi.   2.5 mi.   3 mi.   3.5 mi.

intersection where you first turned off, retrace your steps to the asphalt road and then follow it to the right.

At 0.57 mile, you'll see the trailhead marker for Meadow Trail. The first part of this trail is sandy, allowing a perfect opportunity to look for animal tracks. As you continue, the trail will open into a meadow. A beehive is located at 0.76 mile, behind a hedge of brambles. In the middle of the meadow, 200 feet from the beehive, is a concrete bench beautifully decorated with tiled dragonflies. Here you can sit peacefully and watch hummingbirds and butterflies in the meadow.

Along the edge of the woods is the trail marker sign for the Orange Trail. Follow the one-person-wide footpath of the Orange Trail into the woods. Several trails crisscross in this area. If you find yourself going down a treacherously steep hill, turn around and retrace your steps. You likely took a wrong turn.

Stay on the Orange Trail and continue on it past the junction with the connector to the Ridge Trail. Stay on the Orange Trail to the left and follow it downhill.

At 0.96 mile, steps lead downhill and into an open field. A bridge crosses Lick Run Creek. When you reach the road, turn right and walk back to the nature center.

On the far side of the nature center building, nearest the waterway with the low-flow dam, look for the Twin Oaks/O/Brown Trailhead along the edge of the plantings. This trail meanders uphill and next to the creek. Stay on the O Trail, passing the junctions with the K/Red Trail at 1.1 and again at 1.2 miles.

Listen for downy and pileated woodpeckers. Brown creepers and nuthatches also work along the bark of the trees. Look for these small birds hunting along the crooks and crevices of the tree's bark.

At the trail junction of the Moon Ridge/M/Yellow and Twin Oaks/O/Brown Trails, remain on the M Trail to the right and pass by enormous red oak trees. (The M Trail to the left heads back to the nature center.) Cross several footbridges.

Stop and rest on the bench at 1.3 miles and look down the trail for the large sycamore tree. Most of this hike is serene, with only birds and a few butterflies for company. But this nature preserve is close to Lunken Airport, so you'll hear the occasional plane.

When you reach the junction of M Trail and Trillium Valley National Recreation/T/White Trails at 1.4 miles, continue on the T Trail to the right. (The T Trail straight ahead takes you back to the nature center.) In the springtime wildflowers, especially trilliums, Dutchman's-breeches, and spring beauties, are abundant throughout this area.

When the T Trail splits (you can go either way; the trail rejoins in a few feet), take the path to the right to see the large sycamore tree, which has similar characteristics to those of sign trees. Created by American Indians and seen mainly in the eastern forests of the United States, sign trees have a distinct "Z" or "4" shape and were formed by bending and tying down a pliable sapling. White oaks were frequently, but not always, used. Sign trees are also known as marker, trail, message, water, thong, or buffalo trees. The trees were used as trail markers or to point to a resource or territory boundary. To find out more or to report a possible sign tree go to **mountainstewards.org.**

Continue on the trail until it reconnects and follow it to the right.

A bench at 1.6 miles offers a pleasant view of the forest. A deer exclusion area is located on the left, 245 feet from the bench. This valley is used to measure the effects of deer damage on the nature preserve's vegetation. You can readily see the damage that deer have done to the wildflower population outside the exclusion area.

Cross the footbridge 210 feet from the exclusion area. The trail continues downhill and crosses a bridge. Take the trail to the road and turn right. The California Junction National Recreation Trail/J/Blue Trailhead sign is on the right side of the road 230 feet away.

Follow this trail up a fairly steep hillside. At the top of the hill, enjoy a peaceful moment on the bench at 1.9 miles. The J Trail is a loop; follow it to the right and continue hiking through the open wooded area.

At 2.2 miles, both sides of this trail are lined with wild ginger. Here, Kellogg Avenue becomes visible. Continue on this trail until you reach the bench again.

Retrace your steps downhill to the road. Follow the road to the left. Pass the first entrance to the T Trail on the left, and at 3.1 miles turn left at the second entrance to the T Trail. Follow the trail up the steps. This trail is thick with spring wildflowers.

When you reach the T and M Trails intersection at 3.3 miles, follow the M Trail to the right (partly retracing some of your earlier steps). At the M and O Trail junction, follow the M Trail downhill to the right. Continue on the trail around the building, down the stone steps, and to the road. Turn left to return to your vehicle.

Nearby Activities

Find more trails at Great Parks of Hamilton County's Woodland Mound and Withrow Nature Preserve, as well as Cincinnati Parks' Ault Park. The Eastgate Mall area has a little bit of everything, including Jungle Jim's (an eclectic grocery store)—bring your appetite and your wallet. Roads Rivers and Trails in Milford is the closest outfitter.

GPS Trailhead Coordinates and Directions

N39° 04.595'   W84° 24.935'

From Cincinnati, take I-471 South and merge onto I-275 East. Travel 1.9 miles and take Exit 72/Kellogg Avenue/OH 52 West. Turn west onto Kellogg Avenue and travel 1.3 miles to the entrance of California Woods Nature Preserve on the right side of the road.

29 Cincinnati Nature Center's Rowe Woods

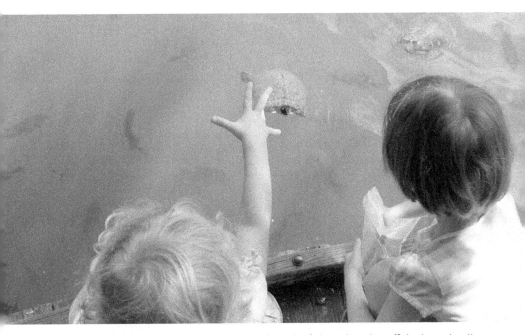

Purchase fish food at the nature center to feed the fish and turtles off the boardwalk. Maybe you'll get lucky and see the snapping turtles.

In Brief

Cincinnati Nature Center is a gem. Plenty of trails, ranging from wheelchair-accessible to difficult, take hikers through different habitats. In addition to the coffee shop, library, gift shop, and bird-viewing area, the nature center has friendly naturalists and hands-on interactive activities.

Description

In spring, Rowe Woods is filled with the dainty blooms of thousands of daffodils, which possibly descend from the thousands of bulbs Mary and Carl Krippendorf and family planted on their property in the early 1900s. Mary and Carl enjoyed sharing their love of nature with friends and family.

They lived in the building that is now the Krippendorf Lodge for 64 years until they died within one month of each other in 1965. After their deaths, friends and family

LENGTH & CONFIGURATION 8.9-mile loop

DIFFICULTY Difficult

SCENERY Forest, ponds, prairie, restored stream, and creeks

EXPOSURE Shade and full sun

TRAFFIC Moderate–heavy

TRAIL SURFACE Soil, mowed, gravel, and mulch

HIKING TIME 7 hours

DRIVING DISTANCE 30 minutes from Cincinnati

SEASON Year-round

ACCESS November–January: Daily, 8 a.m.–5 p.m.; February: Daily, 8 a.m.–6 p.m.; March and September: Daily, 8 a.m.–7:30 p.m.; April: Daily, 8 a.m.–8 p.m.; May and August: Daily, 8 a.m.–8:30 p.m.; June and July: Daily, 8 a.m.–9 p.m.; October: Daily, 8 a.m.–6:30 p.m. Adults and children age 13 and older, $8; children ages 4–12, $3; active military and seniors age 65 and older, $6; children age 3 and younger and members, free

MAPS USGS *Batavia, Madeira, Withamsville,* and *Goshen*; Cincinnati Nature Center map

WHEELCHAIR ACCESSIBLE Stanley M. Rowe All-Persons' Trail

FACILITIES Restrooms and drinking water at Cincinnati Nature Center

CONTACTS Cincinnati Nature Center, 513-831-1711; **cincynature.org**

COMMENTS Bring a bag and a couple of quarters for turtle food.

rallied to protect the land from development. Karl Maslowski, Stanley Rowe Sr., Rosan Krippendorf Adams, and Kay Nyce signed the articles of incorporation for the Cincinnati Nature Center (CNC) Association. Today CNC's 1,657 acres of natural and agricultural land is composed of two sites: Rowe Woods and Long Branch Farm and Trails.

CNC is one of the top 10 nature centers in the country, and it continually succeeds in fulfilling its mission statement ("to enrich lives by inspiring passion for nature through experience, education, and stewardship") via excellent staff, displays, trails, the *Newsleaf* newsletter, and ongoing educational programming and events.

Park your vehicle in the gravel lot and walk to the nature center at the bottom of the slight hill. Be sure to plan time to explore the center. If you have small children, they'll enjoy the hollowed-out log and playhouse. Adults will enjoy the small café and wonderful reading room and library. The enormous bird-viewing area is a great place to sit and sketch the birds at the feeders.

Outside the door to the right of the bird-viewing area is a turtle food dispenser. Buy a handful and stash it in your bag before returning inside the Cincinnati Nature Center and leaving through the doors near the front desk and to the left (if you are facing the front doors). On the deck to the right is an outdoor nature center, complete with skulls, fossils, rocks, paper wasps' nests, and much more.

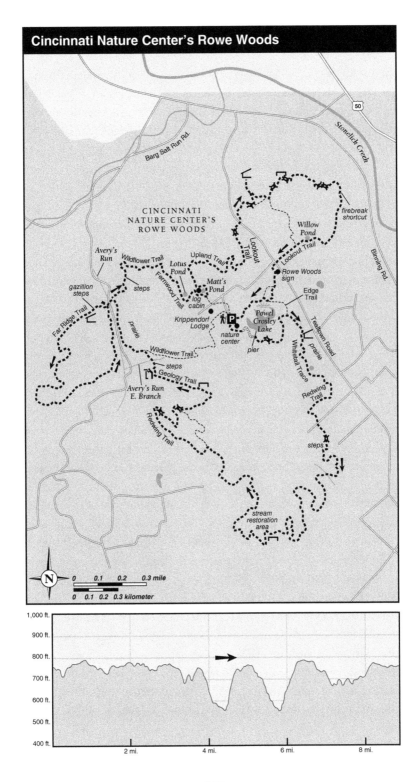

Continue forward to the mulched path and turn left. At the split in the trail, follow Edge Trail to the left and around the back of the nature center. When it joins with a wooden boardwalk, turn right and follow Edge Trail along the boardwalk down to the edge of Powel Crosley Lake. The boardwalk skirts the edge of the lake over the water. This is where the turtle food comes in handy. Just don't get your hands too close to the water, as at least two enormous snapping turtles are regulars.

The boardwalk ends; at the trail intersection, turn left. In about 150 feet, take the side trail to the left that leads to a small pier. Return to Edge Trail and head downhill. Pass Geology Trail and cross the bridge. The forest includes chinquapin, red, and white oaks; honey locusts; and sugar maples.

Pass by the first trailhead for Whitetail Trace, a bench, and the shelter house. At 0.5 mile, turn right onto the second trailhead for Whitetail Trace and into a forest dominated by sugar maples. At 0.69 mile, the trail takes a hard right at the edge of a prairie. At the junction, in 200 feet, follow Whitetail Trace to the left and into the woods. Watch for waterfowl, dragonflies, and songbirds on the small pond to your left.

Sassafras and redbuds line the edges of the trail before it joins with Redwing Trail at 1.1 miles. Turn left onto Redwing Trail, which follows the ridges of several beautiful hillsides of shagbark hickories, red oaks, and sugar maples. Cross a footbridge at 1.28 miles. This area is well insulated from urban noise.

Cross on the flat rocks over a small stream at 1.51 miles, then walk through an area dense with pawpaw and honeysuckle. At 2.66 miles, cross the stream and enter a stream restoration area. The kiosk explains the partnership, scope, and results of the project.

Continue on Redwing Trail uphill as it passes along the edge of an open field and a forest of sugar maples, hackberry, and sassafras. Pass the shortcut at 3.26 miles. Sugar maples dominate the forest, which also includes a few black cherry and hackberry trees. The understory is virtually nonexistent as the trail weaves up and down hills through the serene, picturesque woods.

You'll reach a junction at 3.82 miles with the other end of the shortcut. Follow Redwing Trail to the left and over a bridge. Turn left onto Geology Trail at 4.02 miles and follow the ridge 0.25 mile to the small gazebo-style overlook. Take the boardwalk trail around the hillside and check out the rocky outcropping at the observation deck below. Return to the main trail, follow the steps downhill, and cross Avery's Run East Branch.

At 4.32 miles, Geology Trail intersects with Wildflower Trail. Keep left to stay on Wildflower Trail. The open prairie is to the right, and the wood line and stream to the left.

At the junction, turn left onto Far Ridge Trail at 4.49 miles. When the trail splits, take the right side and walk up more than a gazillion steps. (OK, I may have rounded

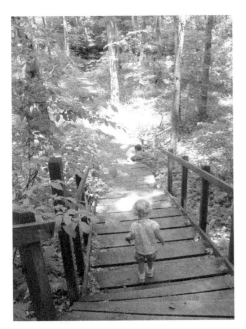
Steps along Geology Trail lead to the creek.

up . . . a little.) Halfway up the hill is a small flat area where a shelter house used to be. This is a good place to catch your breath and take in the view of the upland woods and valley.

At the top of the hill, the trail flattens out a bit and passes through an incredible white oak, ash, and sugar maple forest. The loop trail passes over a swath of flat stones before crossing the creek again and rejoining Wildflower Trail.

Turn left and follow Wildflower Trail over several steps and through a predominately sugar maple forest, which is stunning in the fall. At 6 miles, turn right at the intersection with Fernwood Trail, which leads to Upland Trail.

Pass by Lotus Pond and turn left at the end of the pond onto the Discovery Trail. Enjoy the view of the pond from the boardwalk and turn left onto the recycled lumber boardwalk. Look for the "Sun=Free Energy" education station. The trail soon transitions to gravel; follow it to the Abner Hollow Cabin and Matt's Pond.

From here you can see portions of the PlayScape nature playground off to the right. It is one of the first nature-based playgrounds in the United States. This is a great place to spend a day.

Follow the trail down the short hill to the right of the log cabin and take the raised boardwalks to crisscross over Matt's Pond. Return to the gravel Discovery Trail (the cabin will be to your left), turn left, and cross the footbridge, and after the kiosk for "Who Goes There," turn right and follow the connector trail through the prairie. At the next intersection, turn right onto the Upland Trail. Cross the gravel road.

Stay on the Upland Trail. Pass the shortcut and stay on the main trail through an incredibly beautiful upland woods with several large sycamore trees. At 6.76 miles, turn left onto Lookout Trail and follow it north across Tealtown Road.

At the trail split near the bridge, turn left and head to the shelter house to enjoy a rest. Return to the main trail and turn left. The trail passes over a shortcut and several footbridges as it weaves through the forest and eventually through prairie before crossing back over Tealtown Road at 8.4 miles.

Immediately behind the Rowe Woods entrance sign, the trail continues back into the woods, eventually intersecting with Edge Trail at 8.6 miles. Turn left and follow the trail to the boardwalk overlooking the Marsh Pond. This is a great place to see bullfrogs and enormous dragonflies.

Follow the boardwalk through, and at the end turn left and retrace your steps on the Edge Trail. Pass the intersection with the Lookout Trail and cross a footbridge before stopping at the bird blind. Walk around the back of the nature center and continue on the trail to your vehicle.

Nearby Activities

East Fork State Park, California Woods Nature Preserve, and Withrow Nature Preserve offer additional trails. Milford's downtown shops have plenty of dining and shopping opportunities, including Roads Rivers and Trails outfitters.

GPS Trailhead Coordinates and Directions

N39° 02.735'   W84° 13.679'

On the east side of Cincinnati, follow I-275 to OH 32 East. Travel east 1.4 miles on OH 32 and turn north onto Glen Este–Withamsville Road (Meijer is on the corner). At the T-intersection, turn right onto Old OH 74/Batavia Pike. At the next traffic light, turn left onto Tealtown Road. Follow the road 2.9 miles and turn left into Cincinnati Nature Center's Rowe Woods.

30 Eden Park

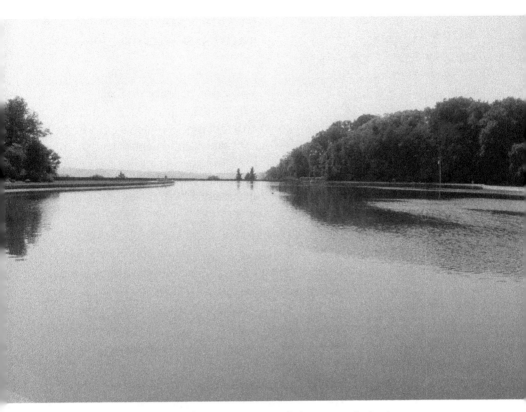

At the right angle, Mirror Lake appears to go all the way to the horizon.

In Brief

Eden Park offers an array of activities, including a playhouse, amphitheater, conservatory, art museum, outdoor sculptures, and gardens. Plan to spend a few hours or an entire day enjoying this wonderful park.

Description

Eden Park's creation began in 1859. The park encompasses 186 acres near downtown Cincinnati. The Cincinnati Art Museum, Cincinnati Art Academy, Playhouse in the Park, Murray Seasongood Pavilion, and Irwin M. Krohn Conservatory are all located on the property.

LENGTH & CONFIGURATION 3.1-mile loop	**ACCESS** Daily, 6 a.m.–10 p.m.; free
	MAPS USGS *Newport*; Eden Park map
DIFFICULTY Easy	**WHEELCHAIR ACCESSIBLE** Paved portions
SCENERY Woods, art, water features, and conservatory	
	FACILITIES Restrooms and drinking water at the art museum and conservatory
EXPOSURE Sun and shade	
TRAFFIC Heavy	
TRAIL SURFACE Paved, soil, and gravel	**CONTACTS** Cincinnati Parks, 513-352-4080; **cincinnatiparks.com/index.php/eden-park**
HIKING TIME 1.5–2 hours	
DRIVING DISTANCE 10 minutes from downtown Cincinnati	**COMMENTS** Break free of the hustle and bustle and enjoy a nice, leisurely hike around Mirror Lake and through the Krohn Conservatory.
SEASON Year-round	

Begin this hike at the Cincinnati Art Museum's parking area. Head south of the building, following the sidewalk downhill to the street crossing. Eden Park is peppered with sculptures, artwork, and specialty gardens.

Cross the street at the bottom of the hill and walk along the paved path to the left, which leads to the large sycamore trees in front of the Seasongood Pavilion. The pavilion was built in 1959 to commemorate former mayor Murray Seasongood.

Walk to the right of the pavilion and pass under the conical bald cypresses with feathery-looking leaves. The path leads to the entrance to Mirror Lake at 0.42 mile, on the left. Mirror Lake is a raised body of water surrounded by a concrete edge. The lake's decorative fountain is peaceful and beautiful.

Follow the concrete pathway around the lake and back to the entrance. Turn left and follow the concrete path downhill and past the service entrance, to the corner of Park Side Place and Martin Drive at 0.9 mile. On the adjacent corner is the Cincinnati Art Club and Gallery.

Take the trail to the left and continue uphill. The enormous wall resembling a fort is a remnant of the old reservoir wall. At the entrance to the walkway along the top of the wall, take a moment and walk down to the end and enjoy the view. The touches of elegant stone and ironwork are a wonderful and surprising treat.

Return to the trail and continue following it to the left. At 1.3 miles, the trail passes the restful Hinkle Magnolia Garden, which includes a fountain and small gazebo.

Return to the trail and follow it uphill to the intersection of Eden Park Drive and Martin Drive. Take the trail to the right and continue to the Krohn Conservatory. (This is where you're going to need to budget some extra time.)

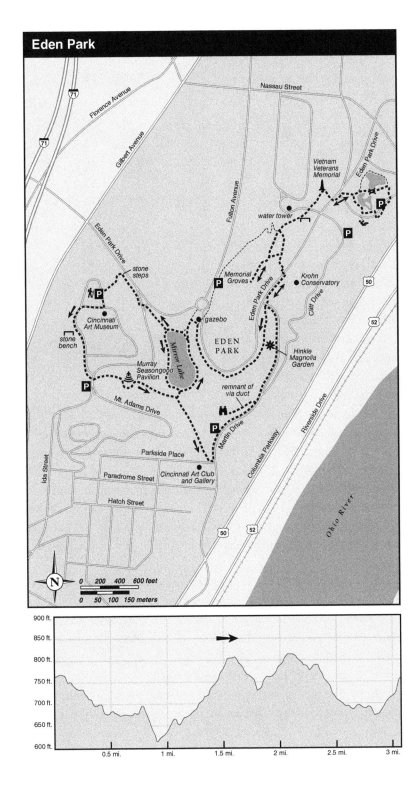

Built in 1933, the Krohn Conservatory is nationally recognized as a showcase for more than 3,500 plant species from around the world. In addition to the gardens, the conservatory hosts many programs throughout the year, including a butterfly show, holiday display, and bonsai gardening.

The hike continues directly across from the front of the Krohn Conservatory. Look across the road to the stone path that leads uphill and into the area with memorial plantings of trees, commemorative stones, and plenty of benches to take in the fabulous scenery. The Presidential Grove began in 1882 and is the largest of the memorials.

Also in this area, at 1.6 miles, is the 172-foot-tall water tower. Built in 1894,

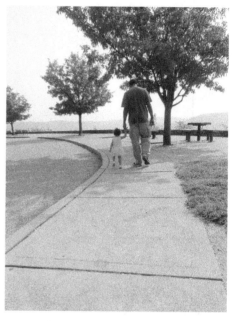

Enjoy the paths around Twin Lakes, or find a bench for great views of the Ohio River.

the tower is currently used by the City of Cincinnati as a communications facility. Look for the gargoyles on the top of the tower. Continue on the footpath down to the Vietnam Veterans Memorial at 1.7 miles.

Cross the street to the Twin Lakes area. Continue on the concrete path and stay to the right. Follow the path by the concession stand. The trail leads to an overlook area and views of the Ohio River and the northern Kentucky hillside. The sycamore tree leaning over the pond, bronze statues, stone bridge, and waterfalls make this area delightful.

Continue walking around the Twin Lakes to the stone bridge. Cross the stone bridge and follow the path to the trail that leads along the edge of Eden Park Drive. Look down Eden Park Drive toward Krohn Conservatory and to the Melan Arch Bridge, built with concrete in 1894. This bridge was an engineering accomplishment that garnered worldwide attention. The stone eagles that guard the bridge are from the Chamber of Commerce building that was destroyed by a fire in 1911.

Cross the road and return to the path that leads uphill to the water tower. At the tower, continue on the trail to the left and retrace your steps to the Hinkle Magnolia Garden. When you reach the garden's gazebo at 2.5 miles, continue on the trail to the right, which parallels Eden Park Drive.

Follow this trail uphill to Spring House Gazebo, at 2.8 miles. This gazebo replaced a straw-shack springhouse built in 1904. The spring was thought to have medicinal qualities, and people carted away 100 barrels of water daily. Unfortunately, contamination shut down the spring in 1912.

From Spring House Gazebo walk to the edge of Mirror Lake parallel to Eden Park Drive. Cross the lawn to the steps and take the steps to the road. Follow the trail across the road as it borders Eden Park Drive. The trail turns left away from the road and climbs a series of large, cut-stone steps.

Once you reach the top, you'll be back in the Cincinnati Art Museum parking area. This is a good time to take a few minutes and enjoy the variety of artwork at Cincinnati Art Museum, including the 1851 painting *Blue Hole* by Robert S. Duncanson. This oil on canvas depicts a portion of the Little Miami River in Clifton Gorge. The Clifton Gorge State Nature Preserve hike is included in this book.

Nearby Activities

You must try Graeter's Ice Cream. Hungry for lunch? Dine under the canopy at Mecklenburg Garden or enjoy lunch at the Cincinnati Art Museum's restaurant. The Cincinnati Zoo & Botanical Garden is also close by just in case you want to feed a giraffe.

GPS Trailhead Coordinates and Directions

N39° 06.901'   W84° 29.823'

From I-71 North take Exit 2 (to the left) for Eden Park Drive. Stay on Eden Park Drive to Eden Park. In Eden Park follow the signs to Cincinnati Art Museum.

31 Mount Airy Forest:
Furnas, Twin Bridge, Beechwood, Red Oak, and Ponderosa

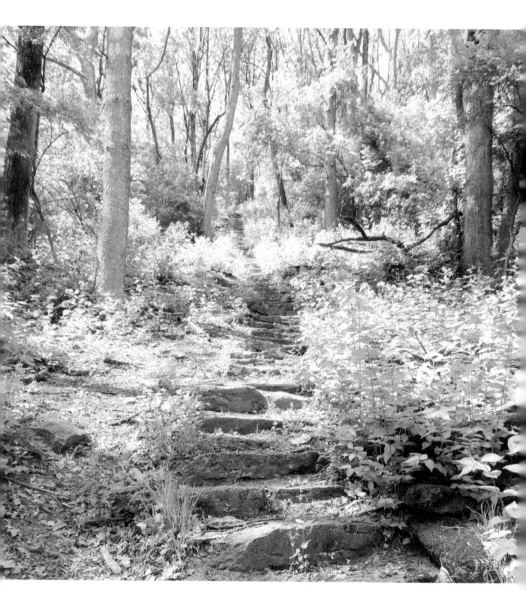

The Stone Steps at Mount Airy Forest will stretch your legs.

LENGTH & CONFIGURATION 4.6-mile loop	**MAPS** USGS *Cincinnati West;* Mount Airy Forest map
DIFFICULTY Moderate–difficult	**WHEELCHAIR ACCESSIBLE** The trail to the tree house is accessible and follows universal design principles.
SCENERY Woods, ravines, tree house, and lots of stone steps	
EXPOSURE Shaded	**FACILITIES** Restrooms and water located throughout park
TRAFFIC Moderate–heavy	**CONTACTS** Cincinnati Parks, 513-352-4080; **cincinnatiparks.com/mt-airy-forest**
TRAIL SURFACE Soil with exposed rocks and roots	
HIKING TIME 4 hours	**COMMENTS** Mount Airy Forest is in an urban setting. Make sure you complete this hike before daylight ends; it's not a good idea to hang out in this neighborhood after dark. Portions of Mount Airy Forest are closed during deer archery season; check the website for up-to-date information.
DRIVING DISTANCE 10 minutes west of downtown Cincinnati	
SEASON Year-round	
ACCESS Daily, 6 a.m.–10 p.m.; free	

In Brief

Mount Airy Forest is a park bustling with activity. The trails pass through beautiful valleys that offer serenity in the midst of urban chaos. The Stone Steps challenge your calf muscles, but you can let your mind wander and just relax and enjoy the hike.

Description

This beautiful, 1,469-acre wooded park just minutes from downtown Cincinnati is designated by the U.S. Department of the Interior as a National Recreation Trail. For more information about the park's history, please refer to the next profile, Mount Airy Forest: West Fork Road, Diehl Ridge, and Elm Ravine.

Plan to spend a few hours or an entire day at this beautiful park and arboretum. The park has multiple picnic shelters, lodges, trails, and playgrounds, as well as the arboretum to explore. But don't expect the trails to be quiet, as Mount Airy Forest is under a portion of the flight path for Cincinnati/Northern Kentucky International Airport.

Enter the park from US 27 and follow Trail Ridge Road to parking/picnic location 20. All park locations are numerically labeled, and the trails are color-coded. The trails at Mount Airy Forest are very popular and receive a significant amount of foot traffic each year. Some portions of the trail are eroded and have exposed rocks and roots, or are so compacted that in wet weather they're very slippery and difficult to navigate.

Mount Airy Forest: Furnas, Twin Bridge, Beechwood, Red Oak, and Ponderosa

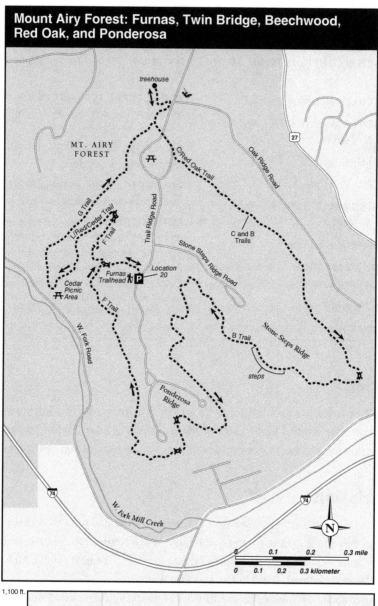

treehouse

MT. AIRY FOREST

Oak Ridge Road

27

C/Red Oak Trail

G Trail

L/Red/Cedar Trail

F Trail

Trail Ridge Road

C and B Trails

Stone Steps Ridge Road

Location 20

Furnas Trailhead

P

Cedar Picnic Area

W. Fork Road

F Trail

B Trail

Stone Steps Ridge

steps

Ponderosa Ridge

74

W. Fork Mill Creek

74

N

| 0 | 0.1 | 0.2 | 0.3 mile |
| 0 | 0.1 | 0.2 | 0.3 kilometer |

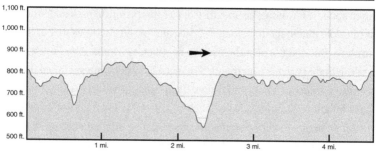

Park in location 20. Near the 20 post is the lime-green-topped trail marker for Furnas Trail, labeled F. Walk past the trail post and into an American beech, sugar maple, Ohio buckeye, and red oak forest. Watch your step over the exposed roots in the well-worn path. Ground cover is virtually nonexistent, meaning that this area is under pressure from the deer population. Throughout the hike, you may need to cross over the trunks of several large downed trees.

Cross a bridge at 0.1 mile. In 130 feet is the intersection of Furnas Trail with the White Square and Diamond trail. Take Furnas/F Trail to the right and then cross another bridge.

Pass through a valley area at 0.2 mile. The valley opens to the left and the structure of the woods begins to change to shagbark hickory, sugar maple, white oak, and American beech trees.

Cross over a bridge at 0.33 mile. The trail passes through a valley area near a trail intersection. Take the trail to the left and cross another bridge within 25 feet. The canopy is mostly sugar maples. The limestone rocks on the other side of the bridge are chock-full of Ordovician fossils typical of the Cincinnati Arch area. Just look at the fossils because collecting is prohibited.

Try to make as little noise as possible while you hike, and watch for movement ahead of you on the edges of the trail. Odds are good that you will see a white-tailed deer at some point on this path. Do not try to feed or pet wild animals—they didn't get the memo about not biting the hand that feeds them.

At 0.41 mile, the trail heads uphill through walnut, sugar maple, and Ohio Buckeye trees. Furnas Trail intersects with Cedar/Red/L Trail and White Square and Diamond Trail. Follow Red/L Trail to the left. Look for the large sinkhole to the right.

The trail exits near Cedar Picnic Area and sign for the Cedar/Red/L Trail at 0.63 mile. Continue on the trail near the large sycamore tree. Hang a hard right and walk up the hill away from the bridge. Pass by the red and white oak trees. The tree in the middle of the path is a shagbark hickory.

The trail weaves back uphill through the woods. The road on the left is West Fork Road. At 0.77 mile, you'll come upon an open area at the top of a hill. The surrounding woods include red oak, locust, and sugar maple trees. Cedar/Red/L and Twin Bridges/Purple/G Trails meet at 0.88 mile. Follow the Purple/G Trail straight ahead. At 0.9 mile, pass the trail to the left, which is the Yellow/H Trail to the tree house. Continue straight ahead on the G Trail. This portion of the trail appears to be an old road.

The forest understory becomes dense with sugar maple saplings and a few oaks at 0.97 mile. The trail exits at 1.14 miles near a tower and the Pine Ridge Picnic Area. Walk to the traffic circle, which is Trail Ridge Road. Turn left and follow Trail Ridge Road to the tree house.

At 1.3 miles is the entrance to the tree house. The path and the tree house itself follow universal design principles, allowing full access for everyone. Return to the traffic circle and playground area and walk to the left side to the entrance to the C/ Red Oak Trail at 1.5 miles. Descend the stone steps embedded with fossils.

Park managers are eradicating invasive bush honeysuckle from Mount Airy Forest. Along this portion of the trail you'll see the results of their efforts. This is important work, because nonnative bush honeysuckle crowds out native species. It damages the forest structure by preventing the growth of native bush and tree saplings as well as wildflowers.

At 1.8 miles, the B/Ponderosa and C/Red Oak Trails intersect. Follow the C to the left through several intersections with the B Trail and through the beautiful ravine area with lots of redbuds at 1.9 miles.

Cross the footbridge over the creek at 2.3 miles. Follow the trail next to the sign post, into the woods, and uphill via the irregular stone steps to the Stone Steps Ridge. (The steps begin at 2.4 miles and end 0.3 mile later.)

At the trail intersection at 2.5 miles, follow the B/Ponderosa Trail to the left and pass the ash, sugar maple, and chinquapin oak trees, leading to the Ponderosa Shelter. The forest transitions at 2.8 miles to one dominated by sugar maple and red oak trees, with the occasional white pine. The trail is marked with white blazes on the trees. Be wary of taking spur trails.

At the trail intersection at 3 miles, take the trail straight ahead, passing a few sink-holes, to the Ponderosa Ridge Area. Stay on the main trail and don't follow any side trails. The trail passes through a ravine with plenty of stinging nettles. Cross the series of footbridges near 3.1 miles.

The forest is dominated by sugar maples. At the trail intersection, take the trail to the left to the Ponderosa Shelter. Cross over the large, flat stones embedded with fossils at 3.4 miles.

The trail opens in the Ponderosa Shelter area. Pass the shelter, cross the grassy area, and walk to the water pump along the edge of the woods with locust and redbud trees. Look to the right along the wood line for the F/Furnas Trail colored lime green and the D/Quarry Trail colored blue. The trailhead for these two trails is 3.5 miles into the hike.

Cross a small footbridge at 3.6 miles. At the trail intersection at 3.7 miles, follow the trail straight ahead and through a wonderful valley. Cross another footbridge at 3.8 miles—you are walking along the edge of a ravine.

Follow the white blazes on the trees. At the trail intersection to the left of location 22, take the trail to the left and cross over the bridge. At 4.2 miles, continue straight ahead at the trail junction. Cross over several more footbridges. At the trail

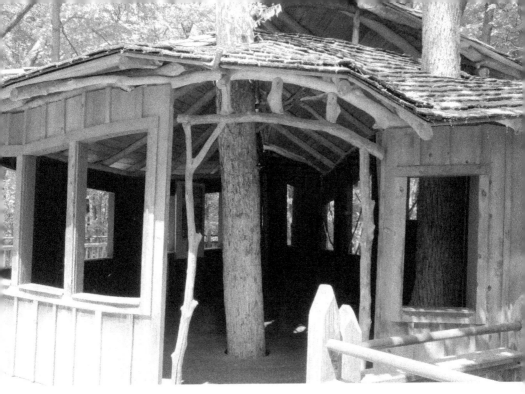

This tree house was specifically designed to be accessible to all.

intersection at 4.4 miles, continue following F/Furnas Trail straight ahead. Cross a footbridge and pass under the canopies of locust, elm, and hackberry trees. Cross the bridge and head up the stone steps. When you see the small trail to your right follow it to retrace your earlier steps back to your vehicle.

Nearby Activities

Mount Airy Forest has an excellent arboretum. Additional hiking trails can be found on the property, as well as at Caldwell Preserve, Spring Grove Cemetery, and Winton Woods. The Cincinnati Museum Center and the Cincinnati Zoo & Botanical Garden offer plenty of fun family activities.

GPS Trailhead Coordinates and Directions

N39° 10.112'   W84° 34.154'

From Cincinnati, take I-75 North to I-74 West and exit onto US 27 North. Follow US 27 North for 2.3 miles. Turn west (left) onto Trail Ridge Road and follow it less than a mile to location 20 on the right.

32 Mount Airy Forest:
West Fork Road, Diehl Ridge, and Elm Ravine

In Brief

Mount Airy Forest, near downtown Cincinnati, has several amenities and is designated by the U.S. Department of the Interior as a National Recreation Trail.

Description

Mount Airy Forest began in 1911 when the Cincinnati Park Board purchased 168 acres of land near Colerain Hill. This was the beginning of the first municipal reforestation project in the United States.

The property that was originally forested had been cleared for agricultural use. But years of poor grazing and agricultural practices resulted in the land succumbing to severe erosion and poor soil composition.

After the 1911 purchase, rehabilitation of the farmland began immediately. More than 1,000 acres were acquired over the next 10 years, and over time more acreage has been added. Today, Mount Airy Forest encompasses more than 1,469 acres. The once-barren land now includes 700 acres of reforested hardwoods, 200 acres of forested evergreens, 269 acres of wetlands, 170 acres of meadows, and a 120-acre arboretum.

Mount Airy Forest is Cincinnati's largest park, boasting a multitude of picnic areas, playgrounds, pavilions, and bridle trails. The arboretum displays more than 5,000 plants. The park's lush wooded ridges and valleys make it hard to believe that downtown Cincinnati is only 10 minutes away.

Mount Airy Forest's trails are designated as a National Recreation Trail by the U.S. Department of the Interior and are also a nationally designated trail by the Boy Scouts of America.

After parking in the small lot and securing your vehicle, walk along the edge of the woods nearest the road and toward the bridge. The architecture of the area's bridges is quite beautiful, though some have been defaced by graffiti.

Although the beginning of this trail earns a solid 10 in the ugly-duckling category of trails, the rest of the trail earns a solid 10 in beauty and tranquility.

Look for the post labeled E for the trailhead, which is on the edge of the forest near the bridge. This narrow path heads uphill and into the forest. While this area did

LENGTH & CONFIGURATION 1.9-mile loop	**ACCESS** Daily, 6 a.m.–10 p.m.; free
DIFFICULTY Moderate	**MAPS** USGS *Cincinnati West;* Mount Airy Forest map
SCENERY Woods and streams	**WHEELCHAIR ACCESSIBLE** No
EXPOSURE Shaded	**FACILITIES** No
TRAFFIC Light	**CONTACTS** Cincinnati Parks, 513-352-4080; **cincinnatiparks.com/mt-airy-forest**
TRAIL SURFACE Soil, exposed rocks, and roots	**COMMENTS** This is just one of many trails at Mount Airy Forest, which also includes an exceptional arboretum. Mount Airy Forest is in an urban setting. Make sure you complete this hike before daylight ends; it's not a good idea to hang out in this neighborhood after dark.
HIKING TIME 45 minutes–1 hour	
DRIVING DISTANCE 10 minutes from downtown Cincinnati	
SEASON Year-round	

have a tremendous amount of bush honeysuckle crowding the trail and the native plants, you can see where efforts have been made to eliminate this obnoxious plant. Bush honeysuckle invasions will grow so dense that the forest floor is not visible. This causes wildflowers and native trees species to die out, which in turn reduces the habitat that the songbirds and other wildlife need to survive. Watch your step over several large rocks as the trail leads uphill before flattening out.

At 0.2 mile, you'll climb several steps, and within 0.1 mile the honeysuckle's density lessens and the roadway is visible to the right. Within a few hundred feet the honeysuckle transitions to an understory of aromatic spicebush and pawpaw trees along the hillside. (Spicebush leaves smell like lemon furniture polish, while pawpaw leaves smell like lemon-scented diesel fuel.)

At 0.36 mile, the sloping hillside, narrow trail, ghostly white sycamores, aromatic spicebush, and insulation from the roadway noise begin to show a glimpse of the swan that the ugly-duckling trail blossoms into.

Use the flat stones to cross the ravine at 0.4 mile. In springtime, or when there has been abundant rain, this trail will most likely be muddy, and some portions of it might not be passable due to moving water.

The roadway and waterway are visible in the ravine below the trail at 0.55 mile. Another invasive plant, garlic mustard, grows along the edges.

At 0.6 mile, a waterfall flows over what appears to be an old dam down in the ravine where West Fork Mill Creek flows. The white noise from this waterfall helps to cancel out the urban noise.

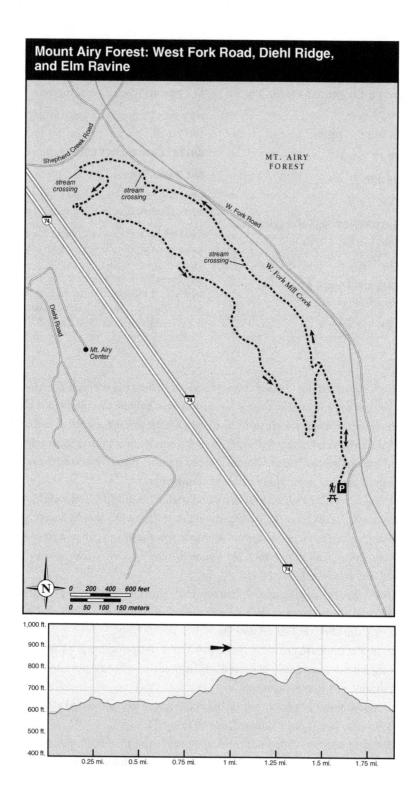

Mount Airy Forest: West Fork Road, Diehl Ridge, and Elm Ravine

Shepherd Creek Road

stream crossing

stream crossing

MT. AIRY FOREST

74

W. Fork Road

stream crossing

W. Fork Mill Creek

Diehl Road

● Mt. Airy Center

74

74

N

| 0 | 200 | 400 | 600 feet |

| 0 | 50 | 100 | 150 meters |

1,000 ft.
900 ft.
800 ft.
700 ft.
600 ft.
500 ft.
400 ft.

0.25 mi.   0.5 mi.   0.75 mi.   1 mi.   1.25 mi.   1.5 mi.   1.75 mi.

At 0.7 mile, the trail leads down a steep, rocky hill. Cross the creek bed using the limestone rocks. If you are grace-challenged, use a long stick as a cane to balance while crossing the stream. The trail leads up the hill straight ahead.

The trail makes a sharp U-turn and heads uphill at 0.8 mile. At 0.87 mile, you'll encounter a series of steps meant to decrease erosion along the steep portion of the trail. Cross the stream at 0.9 mile. Take a right and travel up the streambed for 10–15 feet. The trail continues on the other side of the streambed, where it turns left and proceeds uphill.

White blazes 10 feet up on the tree trunks mark the trail. At 1.1 miles, the trail is mostly flat. Continue following the path marked by the white blazes.

Along the hillside near 1.2 miles are red and white oaks, a nice spot to stop and enjoy the beauty of the woods and the serenity of the trail and ravine.

After a large hill at 1.4 miles, the trail flattens into open woods with red oak, sugar maple, and hackberry trees. Continue following the trail until it reconnects. Turn right and retrace your earlier steps to exit the trail.

Nearby Activities

Downtown Cincinnati, Cincinnati Museum Center, Cincinnati Zoo & Botanical Garden, and Newport Aquarium are just minutes away from this enormous park. Additional hiking opportunities include Mount Airy Forest: Furnas, Twin Bridge, Beechwood, Red Oak, and Ponderosa; Buttercup Valley Preserve & Parkers Woods; Spring Grove Cemetery; Caldwell Preserve; and Winton Woods.

GPS Trailhead Coordinates and Directions

N39° 09.775'   W84° 34.372'

From Cincinnati, take I-74 West to the West Fork Road exit. Off the ramp, take a right onto Montana Avenue. Then take an immediate left onto West Fork Road. Follow West Fork Road less than 0.5 mile. The parking area for this hike is on the left side of the road.

33 Sharon Woods

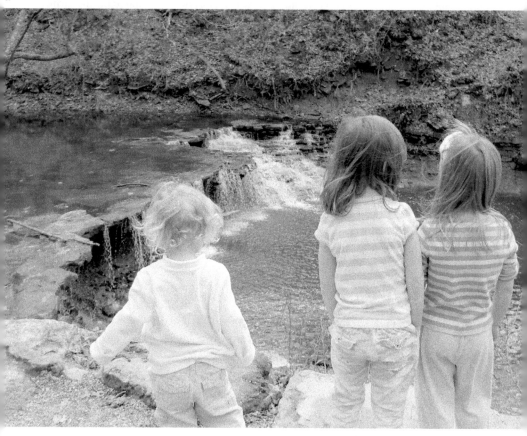

Friends taking in the view of one of Sharon Woods' many waterfalls

In Brief

Sharon Woods offers a variety of activities, including playgrounds, a harbor, and a marina that rents a variety of boats. The trail system is well maintained and has a fair amount of traffic. This park is also well known for an incredible holiday light show.

Description

Sharon Centre's interactive nature displays, indoor playground, and Nature Niche Store offer plenty of places to explore. From the parking area, walk north to the paved trail behind Sharon Centre's outdoor playground and Pavilion Grove.

LENGTH & CONFIGURATION 5.3-mile series of loops	**MAPS** USGS *Glendale;* Sharon Woods park map
DIFFICULTY Moderate	**WHEELCHAIR ACCESSIBLE** Paved portions and around lake
SCENERY Woods and lake	
EXPOSURE Shaded and sun	**FACILITIES** Water and restrooms at harbor and Sharon Centre
TRAFFIC Heavy	
TRAIL SURFACE Paved	**CONTACTS** Great Parks of Hamilton County, 513-521-7275; **greatparks.org /parks/sharon-woods**
HIKING TIME 2.5–3 hours	
DRIVING DISTANCE 20 minutes from downtown Cincinnati	**COMMENTS** The gorge area is beautiful. There are plenty of activities at Sharon Woods to keep kids entertained for hours.
SEASON Year-round	
ACCESS Daily, sunrise–sunset; annual vehicle permit, $10; daily vehicle permit, $3	

Before crossing a bridge 200 feet into the hike, explore the Heritage Village Museum area to the right. Cross the stone-arch bridge and stop for a few minutes to enjoy the view of the waterfall before continuing on the paved trail.

The trail crosses a road at 0.2 mile and heads uphill, where red oak and sugar maple trees border the path. At 0.49 mile you'll see several white pines on the left side of the trail; at 0.55 mile you'll pass a historic cemetery. Follow the trail to the right downhill at 0.57 mile (immediately after the cemetery).

If you're with your kids, they'll be happy to see a playground area to the right at 0.63 mile. Cross the road at 0.67 mile and walk to the entrance for Richard H. Durrell Gorge Trail in a small vehicle pull-off area. The Gorge Trail is well known for its abundance of Ordovician fossils. Collecting fossils and going off-trail are prohibited.

Overhead on the Gorge Trail is a tall canopy of black cherry, hackberry, and white oak trees. The shade provided by the trees, in addition to the low-lying gorge, makes this trail a pleasant retreat in summer. Benches and an overlook area await at 0.82 mile. Cross the bridge at 1.07 miles.

The overlook at 1.19 miles provides a scenic view of Sharon Creek. The waterfall cascades into a deep basin at 1.34 miles. This area suffered a substantial landside in 1996 due to the saturated clay and the shell limestone bedrock giving way.

The trail climbs uphill over several steps before reaching the road. Cross the road and continue on the trail to the left that is the closest to the lake. Walk on the boardwalk extending along the edge of the lake. The boardwalk transitions to a paved trail near the harbor. On the parking area side of the harbor is a universal playground which includes basic spray features. During warmer weather the harbor rents paddleboats,

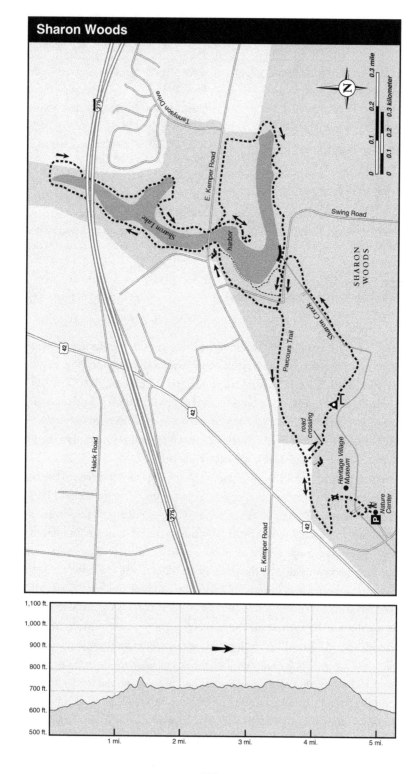

kayaks, rowboats, and bicycles. Pass the harbor and continue on the trail, taking it through the stone-arch tunnel under the Kemper Road bridge. After the tunnel, watch the lake for waterfowl. This portion of the hike is shaded by sugar maples and red and chinquapin oak trees. At 1.7 miles, sit on the bench and enjoy the tranquility of the bridge and lake.

Sycamores border the lake, stretching their ghostly white gnarled limbs over the water to provide a cool spot for fish. Another bench at 1.9 miles lends a portal view of the lake through the branches of birch and sugar maple trees.

Before the trail passes under I-275, you will pass a footbridge that connects to the trail on the opposite side of the lake. Staying on the paved trail, go under I-275 at 2.2 miles. This is a unique auditory experience, with the ghostly drone of the cars passing overhead and echoing through the passageway. Immediately after the overpass is another bench in an open area.

The trail passes over a small bridge at 2.2 miles where Sharon Creek enters the park. The trail continues into an area with sycamores. Sycamores are easily identified by the tan, green, and gray platy bark that peels away from the tree, exposing the white bark. Sycamore trees are found in areas with wet soils.

The trail passes back under I-275 at 2.4 miles. Numerous benches along the side of the lake offer panoramic views of the lake.

The trail passes back through the tunnel under Kemper Road. When the trail splits 3 miles into the hike, continue on the trail to the right and follow it to the Harbor Overlook area. Harbor Overlook is a shaded retreat where you can sit and enjoy the peaceful view of the lake.

Return to the main trail and continue on it to the right, which passes through a parking area at 3.4 miles before reentering the beech and red and chinquapin oak forest. Follow this trail as it meanders through the shady woods bordering the lake on the right. Several benches are scattered through this wooded area. Continue following this trail as it passes over the dam at 4.2 miles.

When the trail splits on the other side of the dam, take the trail to the left that parallels Swing Road. This trail leads uphill, crosses the entrance road, and reenters the forest at 4.4 miles. At the T-intersection, follow the Parcours Trail to the left, continuing uphill and into the forest. Try out the fitness moves on the parkour equipment by following the directions on the signs. The Parcours Trail ends at the trail intersection 4.8 miles into the hike. Continue on the paved trail straight ahead. Do not turn on the trail to the left, which leads to the playground you passed earlier and the Gorge Trail.

The trail splits again at 5 miles. Take the trail to your left and retrace your earlier steps back to the Sharon Centre and your vehicle.

Nearby Activities

Additional hikes include Caesar Creek State Park, Fort Ancient State Memorial, Winton Woods, and Caldwell Preserve. Kings Island and The Beach are within 20 minutes of this hike. You'll find ample shopping at the Tri-County Mall and in the Kings Mill area.

GPS Trailhead Coordinates and Directions

N39° 16.725'   W84° 24.171'

From the north side of Cincinnati, on I-275, take Exit 46/US 42 South. Drive 0.8 mile to the entrance to Sharon Woods on the east (left) side of the road.

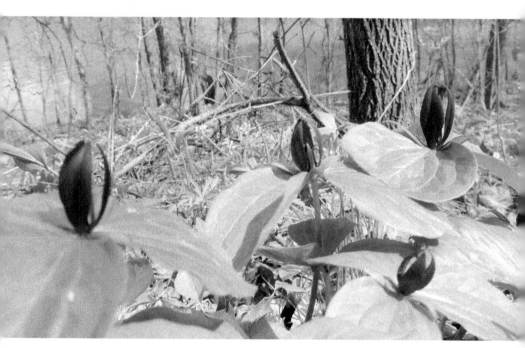

Trillium sessile, *or toadshade, abounds along the trail around Sharon Lake.*

34 Shawnee Lookout

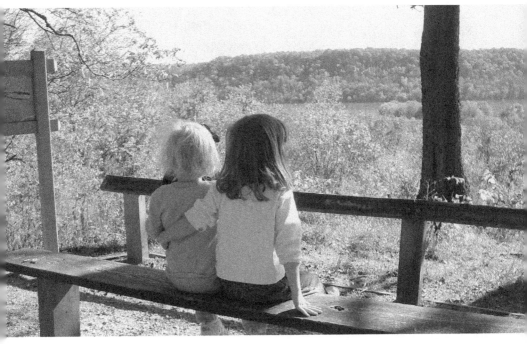

The overlook at Shawnee has impressive views of the confluence of the Ohio and Great Miami Rivers.

In Brief

Shawnee Lookout is another gem of the Great Parks of Hamilton County. Covering 1,515 acres and more than 14,000 years of American Indian history, this park offers incredible overlooks of the Ohio and Great Miami Rivers and the confluence as well as the oxbow of the Great Miami River.

Description

On the far west side of Cincinnati and inside the I-275 loop, Shawnee Lookout is an excursion into thousands of years of American Indian history, plus the overlooks provide incredible panoramic views of the Great Miami and Ohio Rivers and Valleys. This park is also bordered by the 263-acre Uhlmansiek Wildlife Sanctuary and the Oxbow Wetlands. In fact, 914 acres of adjacent wetlands are protected through conservation easements. This is an important resting area for migrating waterfowl.

LENGTH & CONFIGURATION Miami Fort: 1.4-mile balloon; Little Turtle: 2.0-mile balloon; Blue Jacket: 1.25-mile balloon

DIFFICULTY Moderate

SCENERY Ohio River overlooks and historic American Indian earthworks

EXPOSURE Mostly shaded

TRAFFIC Moderate

TRAIL SURFACE Gravel, bare ground, and wooden steps

HIKING TIME 1–1.5 hours each

DRIVING DISTANCE Less than 15 minutes from I-275 and OH 50 interchange

SEASON Year-round

ACCESS Daily, sunrise–sunset; annual vehicle permit, $10; daily vehicle permit, $3

MAPS USGS *Hooven;* at **greatparks.org** or on-site at the museum

WHEELCHAIR ACCESSIBLE No

FACILITIES Restrooms and water at ranger station, visitor center, and near the Blue Jacket Trailhead

CONTACTS Great Parks of Hamilton County, 513-521-7275; **greatparks.org /parks/shawnee-lookout**

COMMENTS The museum details the unique history of the American Indian tribes who lived in the area. Steep Miami Fort Trail has a multitude of steps and fantastic vistas. Meandering Little Turtle Trail offers several places to rest and enjoy the view of the Ohio River.

The journey begins at the Shawnee Lookout visitor center, where interpretive signs, maps, and archaeological exhibits highlight the history of the American Indian tribes that once lived in this area.

Continue on the entrance road, passing Little Turtle (2 miles long) and Blue Jacket (1.25 miles long) Trails, as well as the historic Springhouse School and Log Cabin. You'll find ample picnic and playground areas throughout the park. Continue on the entrance road to the turnaround and parking area for the Miami Fort Trailhead. The hike begins with Miami Fort Trail and will include Little Turtle Trail. If you want additional mileage, add Blue Jacket Trail (directly across the road from Little Turtle).

A large information sign and bench clearly mark the Miami Fort Trailhead. Walk up the steep, gravel-covered trail with steps for erosion control. The climb ends with a delightful seating area and view of the Great Miami River far below—a prime spot to catch your breath after the 0.2-mile climb.

Small camps and habitation sites have been discovered within the fort's walls, but historians theorize that the original builders of the fort probably lived in the valleys below. The valley overlook takes in views of the Great Miami River basin framed by a patchwork of green and gold farm fields. Follow the trail to the left and enter the pleasant open area shaded by ash and walnut trees.

Continue up a small hill that leads to an overlook with millstone benches, which sit next to the Daniel Carter Beard memorial commemorated on a large boulder. From this vantage point it is very easy to see the power plant stacks as well as hear heavy

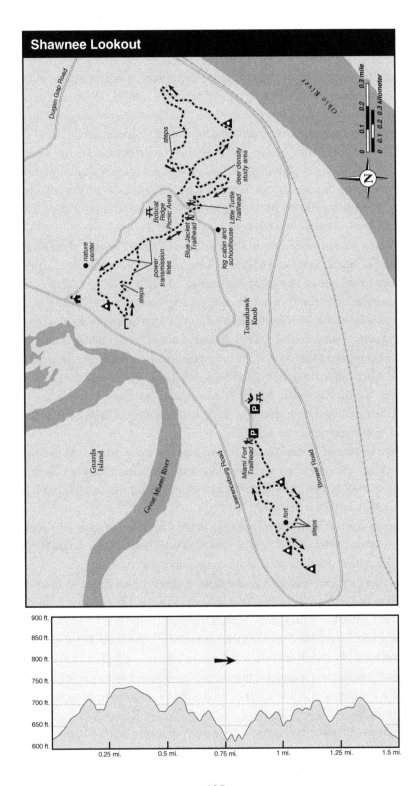

equipment from far below. Despite the modern-day sounds and structures, the view from the stone benches shows the grace and beauty of the Ohio River as it curves and eventually is joined by the Great Miami River. This area was once home to the Hopewell American Indians, who typically lived in family groups.

At the end of a handful of steps, the trail winds to the right and enters a lovely upland forest with plenty of shagbark hickory trees. Ignore the multiple spur trails as the trail meanders by several large white oaks. It then descends into the valley by way of about 50 steep steps down. At the small footbridge there is only one thing left to do—climb nearly 50 steps to ascend out of the beautiful valley.

When the trail reconnects to itself, go left for 0.2 mile. This part of the hike is slightly uphill. Black cherry and hackberry trees compete along the edges of the trail, which then opens into an impressive overlook.

During the 1700s, the Shawnee, Wyandot, Mingo, and Miami tribes, as well as others, populated the area. The benches at the end of the overlook allow you to enjoy the views and ponder what the river valley and confluence of the Great Miami and Ohio Rivers far below might have looked like before the area was seen by European settlers.

The American Indian tribes of this area used the ridge as a strategic position during battles, and they hunted in the area. Burial mounds and earthworks from a variety of area tribes are found throughout this park. In fact, historical finds date the use of this area by humans as early as AD 270.

Retrace your earlier steps along the trail, pass the trail junction, and continue straight ahead. The trail edges along the ridge lined with elm, hackberry, black cherry, and red oak trees. It then leads downhill and into a younger wooded area, with plenty of walnut trees, so watch your step.

Throughout this hike, several openings in the tree canopies allow for a peek at the valleys and farm fields below. The trail joins back together, and you should keep going straight, then head down the steep slope to the parking area.

Take the entrance road back to the parking area for Blue Jacket and Little Turtle Trails. Park and walk to the edge of the playground area. The entrance to Little Turtle Trail is marked with a large interpretive sign.

The 2-mile-long Little Turtle Trail is named after Chief Little Turtle of the Miami tribe, known to have spent some time in the area 200 years ago. The gravel-and-dirt trail is wide enough for two people to walk side by side for most of the hike. The hike will take 1.5–2 hours, depending on how much time you spend enjoying the Ohio River overlooks.

Brambles of blackberries and multiflora rose border the trail for 0.3 mile before the trail opens into a meadow. In the forest, the fenced-off area is a study plot for measuring deer density. Expect to see and hear a variety of birds, including chickadees, nuthatches, cardinals, and woodpeckers. Trees include box elder, ash, black cherry, and black locust.

A junction appears at approximately 0.5 mile. The trail to the left leads out of the forest and to the Water Hole Meadow and Shelter. Continue on Little Turtle Trail to the right. The habitat changes to a forest with black cherry and hackberry trees and a prairie area. At 0.8 mile, the Ohio River is visible from the ridge. Plan to spend a few minutes at the scenic overlook and bench 70 yards farther along the trail. Watching the river and the occasional barge traffic flowing past is an oddly serene and enjoyable experience.

Red oaks, sugar maples, and sycamores provide ample shade as the trail meanders down- and uphill to the next scenic overlook a little more than 100 yards away from the last. A good breeze flowing in off the Ohio River keeps you cool, especially as you climb the series of steps leading uphill.

The trail eventually flattens out and leads up to yet another overlook at 1.2 miles. This overlook is very open and free of trees due to the natural widening of the Ohio River. Throughout Shawnee Lookout are numerous burial mounds, such as Site 39 at 1.3 miles. Please respect these sacred burial mounds by viewing them from the trail only.

The trail begins a steep descent and after 45 yards flattens into a valley area where it meanders along a creek bed with moss-covered rocks and fallen trees. Of course those who travel down must travel back up. Climb up the steps until you reach the four-way junction you crossed at the beginning of the hike.

Retrace your steps from here back to your vehicle. If you would like to do an additional hike, try the Blue Jacket Trail, which is named after Chief Blue Jacket of the Shawnee tribe. This 1.25-mile loop trail meanders up- and downhill and offers several places to rest and enjoy the woodland views.

Nearby Attractions

Great Parks of Hamilton County's Miami Whitewater and Mitchell Memorial Forests are within a few miles of Shawnee Lookout. For even more hiking options, try Cincinnati Park Board's Mount Airy Forest, Buttercup Valley Preserve & Parkers Woods, and Spring Grove Cemetery.

GPS Trailhead Coordinates and Directions

N39° 07.242'   W84° 48.504'

Shawnee Lookout is located along the southwest side of Cincinnati near the Ohio River and the Indiana state line. From I-275 on the far west side of Cincinnati, take Exit 16/US 50 (Ohio Scenic Byway) East. Follow US 50 East for 3.4 miles and turn right to head south on Lawrenceburg Road. Follow Lawrenceburg Road 2.25 miles to the park entrance. Follow the entrance road past the museum, golf course, log cabin, and playground areas to the turnaround and parking area at the Miami Fort Trailhead.

35 Spring Grove Cemetery

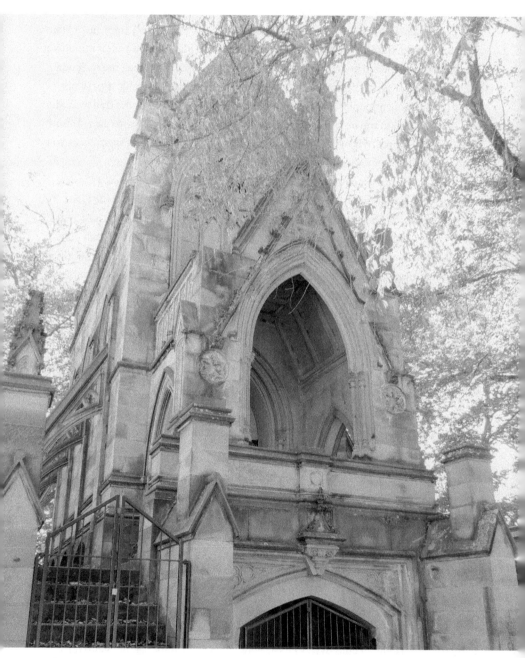

The Gothic Revival–style Dexter Mausoleum and Chapel was constructed circa 1866.

LENGTH & CONFIGURATION 4.2-mile figure eight	8 a.m.–8 p.m.; Tuesday–Wednesday and Friday–Sunday, 8 a.m.–6 p.m. Closed January 1, July 4, Thanksgiving, and December 25; free
DIFFICULTY Easy–moderate	
SCENERY Woods, lakes, and gardens	**MAPS** USGS *Cincinnati West;* Spring Grove Cemetery map
EXPOSURE Mostly full sun	
TRAFFIC Moderate	**WHEELCHAIR ACCESSIBLE** Yes
TRAIL SURFACE Paved	**FACILITIES** Restrooms and water at visitor center
HIKING TIME 2 hours	
DRIVING DISTANCE 15 minutes from downtown Cincinnati	**CONTACTS** Spring Grove Cemetery, 513-681-PLAN (7526); **springgrove.org**
SEASON Year-round	**COMMENTS** Landscape designers from around the globe have studied the beautiful, well-planned landscape of Spring Grove Cemetery.
ACCESS September–April: Daily, 8 a.m.– 6 p.m. May–August Monday and Thursday,	

In Brief

Spring Grove Cemetery's grounds are impeccable. The arboretum has a wide collection of native and exotic plants. Several State and National Champion Trees are located on the property as well.

Description

The Cemetery of Spring Grove began with the dedication of its original 220 acres in 1845. The name was officially changed in 1987 to the Spring Grove Cemetery and Arboretum. The cemetery continues to serve Cincinnati as a beautiful final resting place for loved ones.

The grounds contain an enormous collection of native and exotic plants. Trees ranking as State and National Champions, as well as the Centenarian Collection (100-plus-year-old trees), are also found throughout the property. Today, the cemetery covers 733 acres, of which 400 are landscaped and maintained. It is the second-largest cemetery in the United States.

Spring Grove Cemetery began with a recurrence of a cholera epidemic and concerns over proper internment facilities. Members of the Cincinnati Horticultural Society created a cemetery association with the goal of finding a suitable location to create a parklike setting to bury the dead. The planners researched and visited renowned cemeteries throughout the United States and Europe. Spring Grove Cemetery's

Spring Grove Cemetery

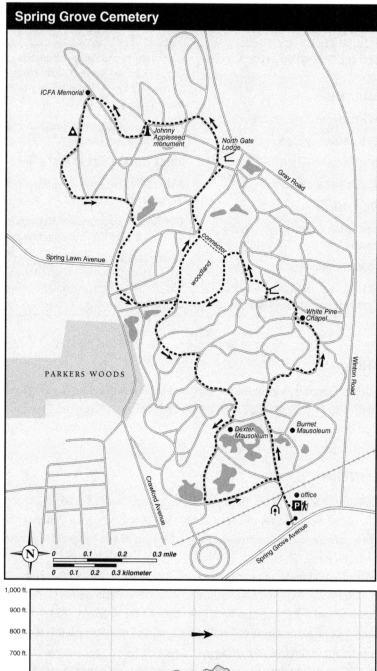

ICFA Memorial

Johnny Appleseed monument

North Gate Lodge

Gray Road

Spring Lawn Avenue

connector

woodland

White Pine Chapel

Winton Road

PARKERS WOODS

Dexter Mausoleum

Burnet Mausoleum

office

Crawford Avenue

Spring Grove Avenue

N

| 0 | 0.1 | 0.2 | 0.3 mile |
| 0 | 0.1 | 0.2 | 0.3 kilometer |

1,000 ft.
900 ft.
800 ft.
700 ft.
600 ft.
500 ft.
400 ft.

1 mi.   2 mi.   3 mi.   4 mi.

exquisite landscape speaks to the amount of thoughtful consideration that went into designing the grounds. It was designated as a National Historic Landmark in 2007, joining four other cemeteries that hold this distinction. (These landmarks are designated by the U.S. Secretary of the Interior and meet the criteria of having exceptional value or quality in illustrating or interpreting the heritage of the United States.)

Enter through the main entrance from Spring Grove Avenue, take the first right, and park in the customer parking lot adjacent to the Historic Office. This office was built in 1863 by James Keys Wilson. India Boyer, one of America's first female architects, created the east addition, which was completed in 1955. Take time to admire the intricate details of the stonework, especially near the roof.

Before you start down the road to the bridge overpass, stop in the customer service center to the right and peruse the brochures covering the history, wildlife, and plant species found here. If you're a history buff, be sure to pick up a copy of "Spring Grove Cemetery: Self-Guided History, Art and Architecture Walking Tour," by Blanche Linden-Ward.

Walk a few hundred feet down the main road to reach the tunnel under the bridge. This is the Cincinnati–Hamilton–Dayton Railroad Bridge. The train once caused numerous delays in funeral processions and taxed the patience of visitors. Even though the tracks were laid in 1850, the bridge was not constructed until 33 years later.

Pass under the bridge and go straight. On the right side of this road is the Civil War Section, where more than 1,000 soldiers are laid to rest. This area also has State Champion Trees, the Veteran Section, and Cedar Lake, which is edged with bald cypress trees.

It's easy to see why this cemetery was the place to go on the weekends in the 1800s. The ornate statues, exquisite landscaping, and picturesque lakes and ponds provide a tranquil respite.

At 0.37 mile you can see the Burnet mausoleum, where Judge Jacob Burnet, US senator and author of Ohio's first constitution, rests. The mausoleum is set into the hillside and has a façade and doors of white marble. Continue following the roadway to the right. Turn to the left at 0.66 mile and pass under a large sycamore.

Take two immediate rights and then follow the bend in the road to the left. At 0.69 mile, the trail passes in front of the White Pine Chapel, built in 1859.

Turn right at 0.71 mile. From this vantage point, you can see over the treetops and view the Cincinnati skyline. An old shelter house is at 0.89 mile.

At 1.06 miles, follow the road to the left and into the shaded Woodland Area. Take the road downhill under the canopy of sugar maple, sycamore, and Ohio buckeye trees. The edges of this path are covered in wild ginger and ferns.

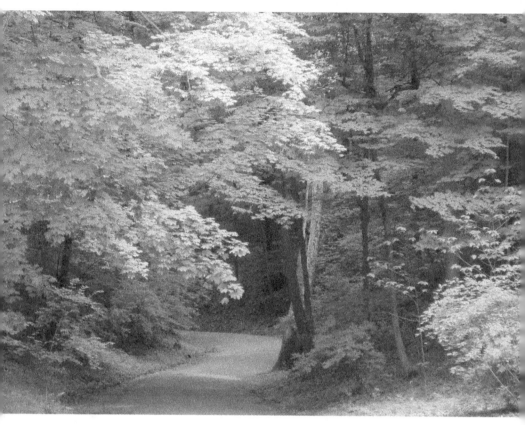

A tranquil path through a woodland area

Exit the woods at 1.3 miles, turn right at Section 118, and follow the woods around. When you reach the corner with the ponds adjacent to you, turn left at the corner of Sections 115 and 114.

At the next intersection at 1.36 miles (Sections 115, 122, 124, and 114) turn right. When the road comes to a T-intersection at 1.47 miles turn left (Sections 114, 125, and 140) and then take an immediate right (Sections 125 and 140). Continue following this road as it curves around. When it intersects with four roads, take the road that is relatively straight ahead and passes between Sections 135 and 141.

The Johnny Appleseed statue at 1.62 miles honors John Chapman's missionary work in this area. Chapman didn't absentmindedly drop apple seeds. He collected seeds from cider mills, grew the seeds into saplings, transplanted the saplings into nurseries, and maintained the nurseries. Over his lifetime he distributed apple seeds and trees throughout much of Ohio, Indiana, Pennsylvania, Illinois, and Kentucky.

Follow the road and take a right at the Cremation Garden. Follow this route by staying to the right at the intersections. The International Cemetery and Funeral Association Memorial is 2 miles into the hike. As you walk along the roadway, be sure to look up and enjoy panoramic views of the Cincinnati skyline.

The road comes to at T at 2.4 miles, near another pond (Sections 126 and 123). Take the road to the right, and at the next T take the road to the right again (Sections 68, 122, and 121). Follow this road to a four-way intersection at 2.68 miles, adjacent to two ponds. Turn left at this intersection and pass the large, pink-granite Taft tombstone.

When you reach the intersection with the Woodland Area, turn right. You'll find ornately carved tombstones throughout this area. Continue on this road to the next intersection at 2.91 miles, then turn right (Sections 48, 75, and 49).

The trail you are on joins with a portion of Spring Grove Cemetery's self-guiding walking tour. Go straight through the intersection at 3.09 miles. At the edge of Geyser Lake is the Dexter mausoleum, which is a private family Gothic Revival mausoleum and chapel constructed around 1866. At the intersection at 3.22 miles, turn right and 200 feet ahead is a convoluted intersection. Remain on the road that is straight ahead.

Ornate statues, monuments, mausoleums, sarcophagi, lakes, and immaculately maintained landscaping make this area very beautiful and serene. Continue on this road to the T-intersection and take a left. This road takes you back to the main road. At that intersection, take a right, pass underneath the bridge, and retrace your steps to your vehicle.

Nearby Activities

Discover more hiking trails at Buttercup Valley Preserve & Parkers Woods, LaBoiteaux Woods, and Mount Airy Forest. The Cincinnati Museum Center, Cincinnati Zoo & Botanical Garden, and Newport Aquarium are just minutes away. Plenty of fine-dining opportunities await your taste buds in the downtown Cincinnati area, as well as along the Ohio River in Newport.

GPS Trailhead Coordinates and Directions

N39° 09.899' W84° 31.375'

From downtown Cincinnati, take I-75 North to Exit 6/Mitchell Avenue. Turn left and follow Mitchell Avenue northwest 0.3 mile. Turn left on Spring Grove Avenue and travel south 0.6 mile. Turn right into the main entrance.

36 Winton Woods

In Brief

Winton Woods offers hiking trails, boat rentals, Parky's Farm, golfing, disc golf, and picnic areas. Check out the event schedule for the park, as the Great Parks of Hamilton County's naturalists provide excellent programs.

Description

Winton Woods was initially known as West Fork Lake. The lake was created in accordance with the Flood Control Act of 1946 and is managed by the Louisville District of the U.S. Army Corps of Engineers with the primary goal of reducing flood damage downstream from the dam.

The park began with 905 acres that were leased from the federal government. In 1939, Hamilton County Park District changed the name from West Fork Lake to Winton Woods. Winton is a historical reference to Winton Road, which was constructed in 1798 as part of a military road; prior to that it was used as a pathway by American Indians.

Today the heavily used urban park encompasses 2,555 acres, including two state-dedicated natural areas: Spring Beauty Dell and the Greenbelt Area.

Winton Woods has a disc golf course, fitness trail, campsites, picnic areas and shelters, golf courses, and—the favorite with kids of any age—Parky's Farm, which is an educational farm and play area.

From Winton Road, turn right into the park. Park admission is available via a daily or annual pass. The very affordable annual pass allows access to any of the Great Parks of Hamilton County.

After the gatehouse, take the first left. The building for the Winton Woods office and ranger station is to the right. Straight ahead and to the left is a large parking area. Secure your vehicle and walk toward the Winton Woods office.

Inside the Winton Woods office are several living displays to help people understand the native wildlife found in Winton Woods and around the Cincinnati area. Throughout the year, talented naturalists on staff host excellent nature programs.

To the left of the office are several playground swings. The paved trail is between the swings and the office building. You won't find an official trailhead sign at this point—just a sign and bag dispenser reminding you to clean up after Fido, but you'll know you're on the right path because this trail is paved and wide enough for a vehicle. Walk up the hill toward the building and away from Winton Road.

LENGTH & CONFIGURATION 3.03-mile balloon	**MAPS** USGS *Green Hills;* Winton Woods park map
DIFFICULTY Easy	**WHEELCHAIR ACCESSIBLE** Yes, paved portion
SCENERY Winton Lake, wetland, and woods	**FACILITIES** Restrooms, nature center, boat rentals, disc golf, and educational farm
EXPOSURE Full sun, shaded	
TRAFFIC Moderate–heavy	**CONTACTS** Great Parks of Hamilton County, 513-521-7275; **greatparks.org /parks/winton-woods**
TRAIL SURFACE Paved, soil	
HIKING TIME 1.5 hours	**COMMENTS** Great Parks of Hamilton County's inexpensive annual pass is a must-have. Take the kids to Parky's Farm to play and pet farm animals. Winton Woods also has boat rentals, camp-grounds, an equestrian riding center, and two golf course facilities.
DRIVING DISTANCE 20 minutes from downtown Cincinnati	
SEASON Year-round	
ACCESS Daily, sunrise–sunset; annual vehicle permit, $10; daily vehicle permit, $3	

The paved trail passes a small pond. At 0.1 mile a bench overlooks the pond area. The trail is bordered by a prairie, and in the summertime a multitude of butterflies, skippers, and songbirds utilizes the prairie's resources.

Use the picnic shelter at 0.4 mile to sit in the shade and enjoy the scenery. As you continue, you'll find another picnic area at 0.55 mile.

The trail crosses a parking area at 0.72 mile. Pick up the trail on the other side. Note that this portion of the trail is not paved and therefore is not fully accessible.

This trail leads down to a wetland restoration area. If it has been raining, the trail's lower portion will most likely be underwater. When you reach the fork in the trail, take it. To the right, that is.

Expect to hear the staccato of woodpeckers as well as the chatter of many song-birds and insects. For a more prolonged concert, take a seat on the bench at 0.92 mile and listen to the sounds of the wetland area.

Immediately after the bench, the trail rejoins itself. Follow the portion that leads to the right and back up to the parking area. Cross the road at 1.03 miles. The King-fisher Trail trailhead sign is to the left of the playground equipment.

The 1-mile-long Kingfisher Trail, a single-person-wide gravel path that leads through wetlands and forest, is the most popular hike at Winton Woods.

When the trail splits at 1.1 miles, take the trail to the left. This trail leads to the Kingfisher wetland, which is fed by the West Fork of Mill Creek.

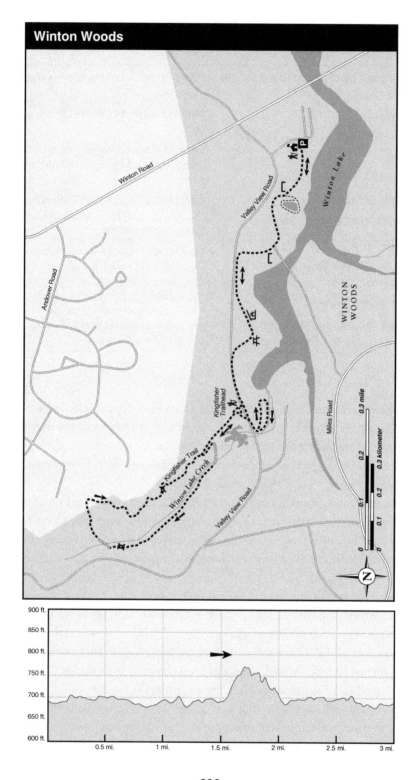

Winton Woods

Winton Road

Andover Road

Winton Road

Valley View Road

Winton Lake

WINTON WOODS

Miles Road

Kingfisher Trailhead

Kingfisher Trail

Winton Lake Creek

Valley View Road

0.3 mile
0.2
0.1
0
0.3 kilometer
0.2
0.1
0

900 ft.
850 ft.
800 ft.
750 ft.
700 ft.
650 ft.
600 ft.

0.5 mi.   1 mi.   1.5 mi.   2 mi.   2.5 mi.   3 mi.

The boardwalk at 1.23 miles helps to keep hikers' feet dry as they enjoy the song-birds in the wet woods. Look for the tracks of raccoons, white-tailed deer, and wild turkeys in the muck.

Take the stairs at 1.51 miles, and in 260 feet cross the bridge. At 1.9 miles you'll see a sinkhole created when the limestone rock under the surface was dissolved by acidic water, resulting in a cave-in.

The bridge at 1.96 miles overlooks a small valley area. Railroad-tie steps at 2.1 miles lead downhill and into an open field area. This area is actively managed to keep it as a field. Bluebirds, song sparrows, and other birds use this area as nesting and feed-ing grounds. The trail rejoins itself at this point as well. Take the portion of Kingfisher Trail that leads to the left and exit Kingfisher Trail.

Cross the road, take a left onto the paved trail, and retrace your steps to the pond at 2.83 miles. Turn to the right and take the trail down to the man-made pond. At the edge of the pond, watch for frogs leaping to the safety of the water.

Return to the trail and turn right to retrace your steps back to your vehicle.

Nearby Activities

Get a better view of the lake by renting a canoe or kayak at Winton Woods Lake. Out-door gear wonderland, also known as Bass Pro Shops, is located at the Cincinnati Mall. The enormous grocery/specialty store Jungle Jim's is off OH 4—be sure to bring your appetite and your wallet. For more hiking opportunities, try Caldwell Preserve, Sharon Woods, Gilmore MetroPark, or Spring Grove Cemetery.

GPS Trailhead Coordinates and Directions

N39° 15.381'   W84° 31.185'

From I-275 and I-75 on Cincinnati's north side, take I-275 West 4.8 miles. Exit at Exit 39/Winton Road and turn south onto Winton Road. Travel 3.6 miles and turn into the park entrance to the west.

INDIANA

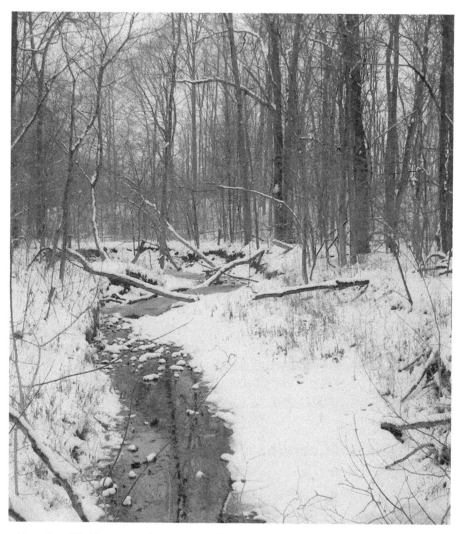

Mary Gray Bird Sanctuary (see page 225)

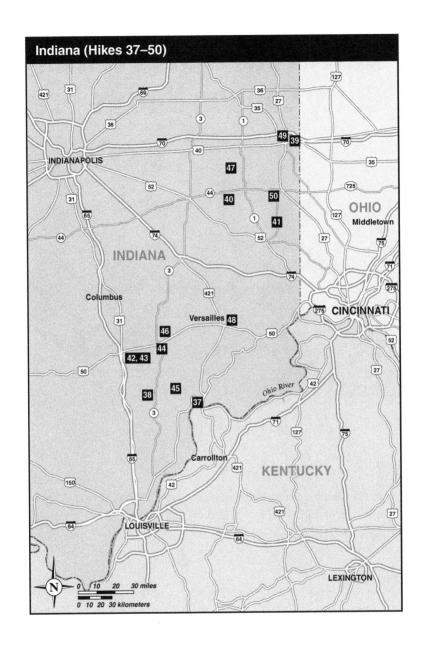

37 Clifty Falls State Park and Clifty Canyon Nature Preserve

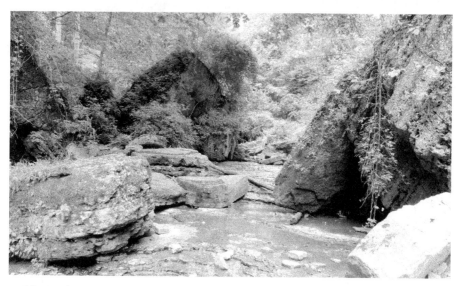

Clifty Creek

In Brief

By far one of the most beautiful hiking locations in the Tri-State area is Clifty Falls State Park and Clifty Canyon Nature Preserve. It just also happens to be one of the most difficult and rewarding.

Description

Clifty Falls State Park and Clifty Canyon Nature Preserve offer incredible hiking trails, exquisite views, and interesting places to explore. At Clifty Inn, you'll find plenty of relaxing spots to sit and watch the river roll by as you grab a bite to eat in the restaurant.

Park in the nature center's parking area. Inside the center are multiple displays about the history, flora and fauna, and geology of this beautiful park. Naturalists are available to answer questions and can provide you with up-to-date trail information.

Before you hike this trail, make sure you have plenty of water, snacks, a map, a small flashlight, this book, and your cell phone.

Please seek a naturalist's advice on the current condition of the trails before heading out; Trail 2 may be flooded or a landslide might have wiped out a portion of a trail.

210

LENGTH & CONFIGURATION 6.1-mile balloon

DIFFICULTY Difficult

SCENERY Creek bed, cliffs, forest, observation tower, tunnel, and falls

EXPOSURE Shaded

TRAFFIC Moderate–heavy

TRAIL SURFACE Exposed bedrock, loose river stones, soil, boardwalk, and gravel

HIKING TIME At least 6 hours

DRIVING DISTANCE 1.5 hours southwest of Cincinnati

SEASON Year-round, but Trail 2 may flood in spring and might be hazardous during the icy winter months.

ACCESS Daily, sunrise–sunset; Indiana residents, $5 daily vehicle permit; out-of-state residents, $7 daily vehicle permit

MAPS USGS *Clifty Falls* and *Madison West;* Clifty Falls State Park map

WHEELCHAIR ACCESSIBLE No

FACILITIES Restrooms and drinking water at Clifty Inn, nature center, and most shelters.

CONTACTS Clifty Falls State Park, 812-273-8885; **in.gov/dnr/parklake/2985.htm**

COMMENTS Do not go in closed-off areas such as near Big Clifty Falls or the Tunnel.

A landslide destroyed a portion of Trail 1 in 2008, and the trail was closed while it was being repaired.

The best times to view the waterfalls are from December to June. Clifty Inn typically offers winter packages and is a great place to stay during any season.

If you're hiking during the warmer months, bring along sandals and a small towel. At several spots on Trail 2 it is easier to walk through the water than around it. But be wary of the depth because there are several deep pools.

From the nature center, walk south along the boardwalk to Trail 1. Then follow Trail 1 downhill over the exposed bedrock to the observation tower. Take the two flights of stairs up to the top of the tower and enjoy the view of the Ohio River and Clifty Falls State Park.

Return to the base of the observation tower and follow the trail downhill. The hillside is stabilized with a retaining wall. Sugar maples and red oaks dominate the canopy, and you can see fossils in the rocks beneath your feet.

The boardwalks at 0.55 mile help prevent further damage to the soil structure. The trail passes through an area filled with wild ginger and spicebush. At the multiple trail intersection at 0.76 mile, follow Trail 2 and the connector trail to Trail 8 to the left.

Follow Trail 2 as it continues up Clifty Creek. There are no markings for this trail—it simply follows Clifty Creek north to Clifty Falls.

Trail 2 is a challenging trail—a lot more difficult than it appears on paper—that might be flowing, dry, flooded, or have intermittent pools depending on the time of year. Multiple-sized stones are strewn about Big Clifty Creek, and making your way

Clifty Falls State Park and Clifty Canyon Nature Preserve

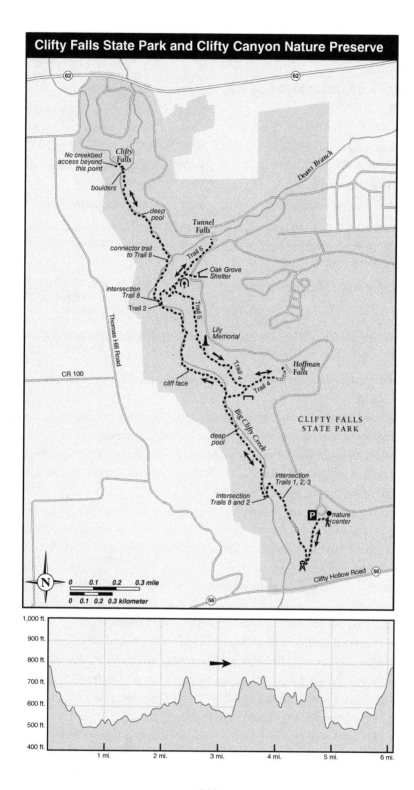

No creekbed access beyond this point

Clifty Falls

boulders

deep pool

Tunnel Falls

Deans Branch

connector trail to Trail 8

Trail 5

Oak Grove Shelter

intersection Trail 8

Trail 2

Trail 5

Lily Memorial

Hoffman Falls

Trail 4

Trail 4

cliff face

Thomas Hill Road

CR 100

Big Clifty Creek

deep pool

CLIFTY FALLS STATE PARK

intersection Trails 1, 2, 3

intersection Trails 8 and 2

P

nature center

Clifty Hollow Road

N

0   0.1   0.2   0.3 mile

0   0.1   0.2   0.3 kilometer

1,000 ft.
900 ft.
800 ft.
700 ft.
600 ft.
500 ft.
400 ft.

1 mi.   2 mi.   3 mi.   4 mi.   5 mi.   6 mi.

212

along the creek bed will test your patience, balance, agility, and stamina. Even experienced hikers should budget about an hour per mile, including extra time to backtrack and try different routes around large rocks, islands, and deep pools.

The shale and limestone in Clifty Falls contain marine fossils some 425 million years old. The stones beneath your feet are fossilized corals from the sea that once covered the Greater Cincinnati area. Several of the corals are larger than a basketball, and the honeycomb structures are readily visible.

At 1.12 miles, a deep pool of water allows you to rest and enjoy the view while cooling off. The stones along the creek begin to get larger as you get closer to Clifty Falls. In fact, at 1.71 miles large chunks of dolomite are scattered along Clifty Creek. Continue on Trail 2 and be sure to look at the moss- and fern-covered boulders near 2.4 miles.

Trail 2 terminates before you reach Clifty Falls. Please, for your safety, do not go farther back along the streambed. Clifty Falls is 60 feet tall, and the rock ledge is not stable. Large chunks of rock break off and crash to the bottom.

Besides the human company, you won't be alone on this hike, as you may startle a white-tailed deer or wild turkey. Listen closely to the calls of a multitude of songbirds and insects.

The old stair structure that used to connect Trails 2 and 7 still partially stands, but it has been decommissioned due to the structural problems of tacking a staircase to the side of an unstable cliff (it tends to fall down). *Do not* attempt to get from Trail 2 to Trail 7 using the skeletal remains of the structure. Attempting it is foolhardy and may cost you your life.

Take a break on one of the many large chunks of dolomite and enjoy the peace and quiet of the end of Trail 2. Return down Trail 2 by following the creek bed back to the intersection with Trail 5 at 3.2 miles. Trail 5 is to your left. This narrow path weaves uphill through the woods. Be careful not to accidentally follow one of the multiple user-made spur trails that radiate from the main trail.

At 3.4 miles is a trail junction where Trail 5 comes to a T. Turn left, staying on Trail 5 to follow it to Tunnel Falls. At 3.5 miles, look for the tunnel opening that passes all the way through the hillside. Known as John Brough's Folly, it was meant to eventually become a railroad tunnel passageway, eliminating the problem of the drastic elevation change and allowing the railroad to pass through Clifty Canyon. However, economic troubles caused construction to stop.

The 600-foot tunnel is closed to help prevent the spread of white-nose syndrome, a disease devastating bat populations. Bats are integral to our food supplies, and this emergent disease is spreading fast through bat populations in eastern North America.

White-nose syndrome is a fungal disease that has killed more than 5.7 million bats and is spreading. Do your part to protect bats by staying out of caves and hibernacula and, if you must go in, follow decontamination procedures.

Continue following Trail 5 as it skirts the edge of a steep hillside. At the northern end of Trail 5 at 3.6 miles, you'll reach a great place to view the 83-foot-tall Tunnel Falls, the tallest at Clifty. Retrace your steps and pass straight through the intersection with the trail that leads to Oak Grove Shelter unless you need to take a restroom break or refill your water bottle. (Drinking water is available seasonally.) Continue south on Trail 5, heading toward the Lily Memorial area and Trail 4.

At 3.9 miles you'll reach the other opening to the tunnel. During the summertime, stand at the opening and enjoy the cooler breeze from the tunnel. At 4 miles pass the stairs that lead to the Lily Memorial and continue on Trail 4.

Make your way along the hillside through the woods dominated by shagbark hickory, red oak, and sugar maple trees. Continue on Trail 4 to Hoffman Falls. The stone path is replaced by a boardwalk at 4.7 miles. Here you can view the 78-foot-tall Hoffman Falls.

Retrace your steps until you reach the intersection at 4.9 miles. Continue on Trail 4 as it leads down to Trail 2 (the creek). Follow it until you reach Trail 2. Turn left and retrace your steps along Trail 2 to Trail 1. Take Trail 1 to the observation tower and then to the nature center parking area and your vehicle.

Nearby Activities

Pennywort Cliffs Preserve and Hardy Lake in Indiana and General Butler State Resort Park in Kentucky offer great hiking trails. Historic Madison, Indiana, offers shopping, wine tasting, and incredible dining.

GPS Trailhead Coordinates and Directions

N38° 44.676'   W85° 25.162'

From Cincinnati, take I-71 South and take Exit 44/Carrollton/Worthville. Turn right onto KY 227, travel 3.3 miles and turn left onto US 42. Travel 2.7 miles and bear right onto KY 36. Travel 10 miles and turn right onto US 421 and take the bridge over the Ohio River. Turn left onto IN 56. Travel 2.5 miles and turn right into the park.

38 Hardy Lake State Recreation Area

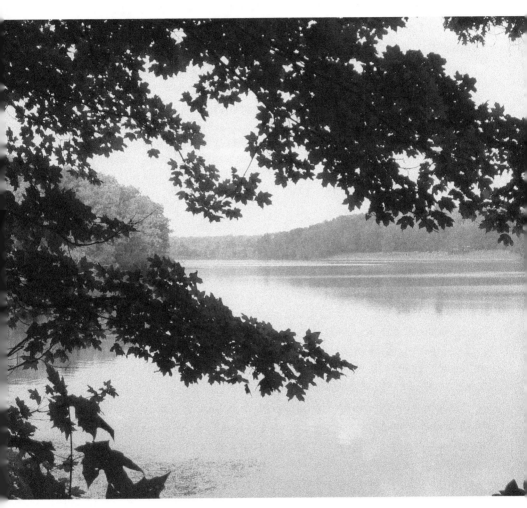

Calm morning along Hardy Lake's Island Trail

In Brief

The trails at Hardy Lake take you through a forest of sugar maple, beech, and oak trees as well as pine stands. The trails skirt the edges of the lake, providing multiple wildlife-viewing opportunities.

215

LENGTH & CONFIGURATION 3.1-mile loop	out-of-state residents, $7 daily vehicle permit
DIFFICULTY Easy	**MAPS** USGS *Deputy;* Hardy Lake map
SCENERY Woods, fields, and lake	**WHEELCHAIR ACCESSIBLE** No
EXPOSURE Shaded and full sun	**FACILITIES** Restrooms and water at picnic area
TRAFFIC Moderate	
TRAIL SURFACE Soil and mowed paths	**CONTACTS** Hardy Lake, 812-794-3800; **in.gov/dnr/parklake/2958.htm**
HIKING TIME 1.5–2 hours	
DRIVING DISTANCE 2 hours west from Cincinnati	**COMMENTS** During the summer, look for juicy black raspberries along the edges of the trails and pack industrial-strength insect repellent to slow down the deer-flies. The hike is a pleasant escape with wonderful views of the lake.
SEASON Year-round	
ACCESS Daily, sunrise–sunset; Indiana residents, $5 daily vehicle permit;	

Description

Hardy Lake was created in 1970 when Quick Creek was dammed for water supply and recreation. At 2,449 acres (which include the 741-acre lake), it is Indiana's smallest state-operated reservoir. This area has much to offer visitors, including trails, archery practice trails, a beach, boat ramps, and electric and primitive campgrounds, as well as fishing, hunting, and picnicking areas.

After passing through the main gate, follow Hardy Lake Road to the trailhead parking lot, which is the first parking area to the left. The trailhead for Cemetery and Island Trails is on the west side of the parking lot.

Trails pass through a state recreation area's wildlife unit and are open for hunting. Be aware of hunting seasons and show courtesy to others. To be safe, wear a blaze-orange jacket and cap, stay on the trail, and never imitate the sound of a wild animal such as the grunt of a deer or the gobble of a turkey.

Cemetery Trail enters the woods near the sign for the Whitsitt Wildlife Unit. Be sure to watch for activity in the nesting box on the back of the sign. The narrow soil path weaves under the canopy of sugar maples, red oaks, and a few white oaks, as well as near spicebush and mayapple.

Pass through an open area and then over a footbridge at 0.17 mile. Continue on the main trail and at 0.22 mile pass by McClain Cemetery, which dates back to the 1700s. The narrow exposed soil path leads downhill through an area of American beech, oak, and shagbark hickory trees. This is a classic example of an oak–hickory climax forest structure.

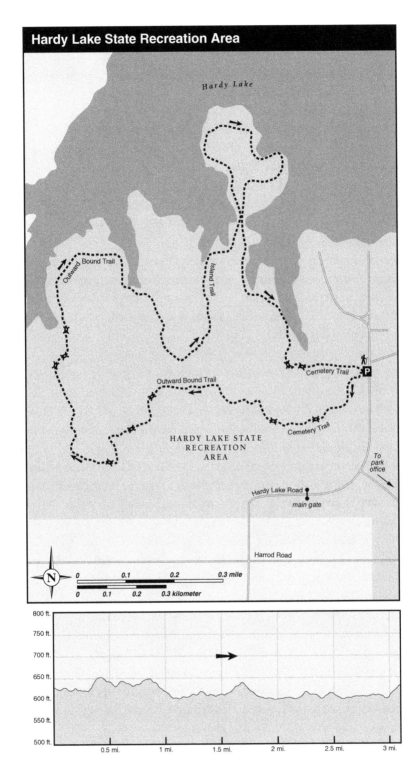

Hardy Lake State Recreation Area

Hardy Lake

Outward Bound Trail

Island Trail

Outward Bound Trail

Cemetery Trail

Cemetery Trail

HARDY LAKE STATE
RECREATION
AREA

P

To
park
office

Hardy Lake Road
main gate

Harrod Road

N

| 0 | 0.1 | 0.2 | 0.3 mile |

| 0 | 0.1 | 0.2 | 0.3 kilometer |

800 ft.
750 ft.
700 ft.
650 ft.
600 ft.
550 ft.
500 ft.

0.5 mi.   1 mi.   1.5 mi.   2 mi.   2.5 mi.   3 mi.

Cross footbridges at 0.27 and 0.31 mile. There is relatively little ground cover under the high canopy of the sugar maples. Be careful not to take a spur trail near 0.42 mile. Stay on the main trail to the left, which is marked with hiker icons. This trail passes by some beautiful large red oak trees. Cross straight ahead over the access road at 0.47 mile and follow the marked trail for Outward Bound Trail, which skirts the edge of the lake and coves where wildlife-viewing opportunities abound.

The trail reaches an open area at 0.48 mile. Watch out for the abundant poison ivy. Jerusalem artichoke is easily identified by its miniature sunflower-like blooms. There are also plenty of deerflies during the warmer months. The trail's edges are dense with greenbrier and small sassafras trees.

Cross yet another footbridge at 0.59 mile, and in 0.1 mile, cross an access road. The trail continues across the road. Follow the markers for the hiking trail and pass between the sentinel shagbark hickory trees. Cross another footbridge at 0.68 mile over a stream. This area is dominated by shagbark hickory trees, which are easy to identify by their peeling gray bark.

Listen and watch for a variety of songbirds, such as chickadees, nuthatches, and towhees, flitting through the canopies of the white oak and beech trees. In the early morning this is a birder's nirvana. Cross the large bridge over the top of the creek at 0.79 mile. The white oaks with woodpecker holes in them are good places to look for smaller birds that are using the cavities for nests. You may also see numerous deer throughout this area. The trail is marked with white blazes.

The trail enters into a serene open valley at 1 mile. At the access road crossing, at the fork in the trail, take the trail to the right labeled with the hiker medallion and look for small white blazes. Basswood, sugar maple, oak, and shagbark hickory trees provide ample shade. Within 0.1 mile, cross a long footbridge through the wet area. At the end of the bridge is a trail junction. Follow the trail to the left.

Cross another footbridge at 1.15 miles. The cove to the left is filled with lotus and water lilies. Here, stop and listen to the frog calls and watch dragonflies skim the water's surface.

At 1.4 miles, shagbark hickory and sugar maple trees dominate the woods. In spring, look for mayapples in this area. The trail crosses over a few more footbridges before intersecting with another access road at 1.56 and 1.72 miles.

At the trail junction at 1.74 miles, turn left to follow Island Trail through a stand of red cedars. (Look for the green markers.) At 1.8 miles, pass through the open grassy area. Cross over an access lane and continue straight across to the sign for the Island Trail. Look for wild turkey dusting spots along the trail.

In summer the open meadow area is complete with wildflowers, such as yarrow and goldenrod, and plenty of juicy blackberries. Be careful when you pick the berries—the plants have thorns, and blackberries and poison ivy typically grow near each other, so watch your step.

At 1.96 miles, pass over the firebreak and remain on the trail straight ahead. Pass the fork at 2.03 miles and continue following the green markers. This area is dominated by sweet gum trees. At 2.05 miles follow the trail to the left. This portion of Island Trail loops up into the peninsula. Follow along the edge of the lake and into the woods of red cedar trees. This portion of the hike is eerily serene, with the sounds of the lake, woods, and birds drowning out the noise of everyday life.

To fully appreciate the wetland area at 2.13 miles, time your hike to arrive here early in the morning. That's the best time to watch the wildlife. Bring a field cushion to sit on, find a comfortable tree, sit at the base of it, and try not to move. The tree will help to conceal you, and if you sit still you'll be able to see a variety of waterfowl, songbirds, Neotropical migrants, wild turkeys, and deer going about their day.

Pass by the large beech at 2.25 miles. Continue uphill and into a younger forest. In the open area, at 2.4 miles, the lake is visible to the left through the red pine and red cedar stand. At the end of the loop in the Island Trail at 2.46 miles, follow the split to the left through shagbark hickory, white oak, and sugar maple trees.

At 2.87 miles the trail borders the cove and enters into a forest of shagbark hickory, white oak, and red cedar trees. Cross the footbridge at 2.96 miles. At the trail junction at 2.98 miles, follow Cemetery Trail to the left. At 3.04 miles cross a footbridge before entering into an open area bordered to the right with dogwoods and poison ivy.

Continue on Cemetery Trail to the main trailhead, the parking area, and your vehicle.

Nearby Activities

Muscatatuck National Wildlife Refuge, Clifty Falls State Park, and Pennywort Cliffs Preserve offer more hiking and wildlife-viewing opportunities. Madison, Indiana, has plenty of specialty shops, restaurants, gourmet coffee and candy stores, and wineries to keep you occupied.

GPS Trailhead Coordinates and Directions

N38° 46.802'   W85° 42.167'

From I-275 on the west side of Cincinnati, take US 50 West 47 miles. Turn south (left) onto IN 3 and travel slightly less than 20 miles. Turn right onto IN 256 and travel 3 miles. Turn right onto North Hardy Lake Road and follow it 2.7 miles to the main entrance.

39 Hayes Arboretum

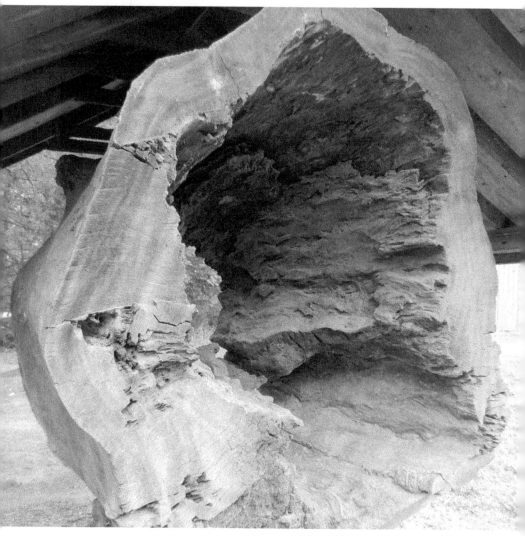

One of the many educational exhibits at Hayes Arboretum

In Brief

Hayes Arboretum is a wonderful escape from urban existence, even though a mall and a retail row are just a few hundred feet away. The arboretum has several nice hikes as well as a driving tour of the property. Events are offered throughout the year. Check the website for more information.

LENGTH & CONFIGURATION 3-mile series of loops	**ACCESS** March–October: Tuesday–Saturday, 9 a.m.–5 p.m.; November–February: Open only for scheduled events; free
DIFFICULTY Easy–moderate	
SCENERY Woods, streams, springhouse, and pond	**MAPS** USGS *New Paris;* Hayes Arboretum map
EXPOSURE Mostly shaded except for a portion of the red trail	**WHEELCHAIR ACCESSIBLE** No, but there is an auto tour
TRAFFIC Moderate	**FACILITIES** Restrooms and drinking water in the nature center
TRAIL SURFACE Soil	**CONTACTS** Hayes Arboretum, 765-962-3745; **hayesarboretum.org**
HIKING TIME 1.5–2 hours	
DRIVING DISTANCE 1 hour northwest of Cincinnati	**COMMENTS** The auto tour trails are also open to foot traffic. Hayes Arboretum is a great place to explore nature.
SEASON Year-round	

Description

Hayes Arboretum is a 466-acre natural area that actively involves people in nature. With multiple educational opportunities, including a nature center housed in a barn, experiencing and learning about nature is a breeze. Living classrooms include an oak–tulip tree experiment in hardwood reforestation, a pond in succession, and a natural springhouse. The trees for the oak–tulip experiment were planted in 1922 and 1923.

Follow the main entrance road to the nature center parking area. The nature center lends rustic appeal and provides plenty of space to explore the multiple exhibits and the bird-viewing area.

Hayes Arboretum's auto tour allows you to share the beauty and grace of this wonderful natural area with someone who is not able to hike. Access tokens can be purchased in the nature center.

Once you've finished exploring the nature center, head outside. Walk around to the south of the building toward the stone garden, which is made up of several large boulders. This is an interesting spot for the weekend geologist to explore.

Continue on around behind the nature center. To the left is a large archway entrance to the three color-coded trails. Take the blue and yellow trail to start.

Cross the gravel road. This trail climbs uphill as it enters into a beautiful sugar maple and red and white oak forest. At 0.25 mile, you'll find a bench at the top of the hill before the trail descends again. Along this portion of the hike, look for wild turkeys—especially in spring.

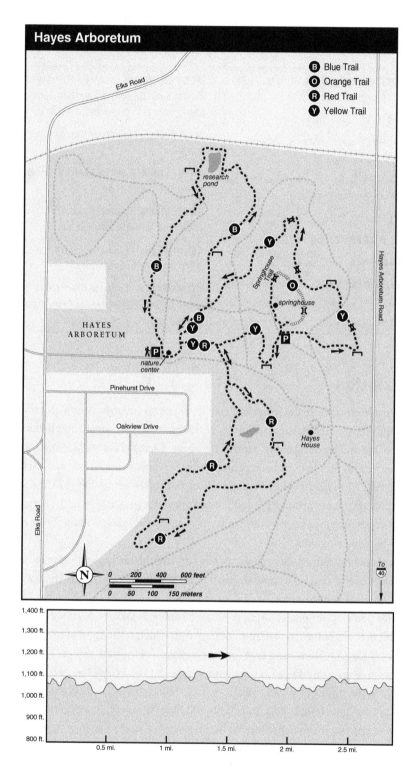

Hayes Arboretum

B Blue Trail
O Orange Trail
R Red Trail
Y Yellow Trail

Elks Road

research pond

Springhouse Trail

springhouse

HAYES ARBORETUM

nature center

Pinehurst Drive

Oakview Drive

Hayes House

Elks Road

Hayes Arboretum Road

To 40

N

0   200   400   600 feet
0   50   100   150 meters

1,400 ft.
1,300 ft.
1,200 ft.
1,100 ft.
1,000 ft.
900 ft.
800 ft.

0.5 mi.   1 mi.   1.5 mi.   2 mi.   2.5 mi.

At 0.37 mile, cross the old road, and when the trail splits, follow the blue trail to the left. After 0.1 mile from the intersection, the trail heads downhill to another trail intersection near the Research Pond. Continue on the blue trail around the Research Pond. This pond is going through succession and over time will eventually fill in.

At 0.57 mile, a bench awaits near a nice spot to watch the activity on the pond. Take a few moments to closely examine the pond via the boardwalk before continuing on the blue trail.

Follow the blue trail across the road. At this point, the trail is a one-person-wide footpath through the woods. At 0.66 mile, a bevy of spring wildflowers edges the trail. Keep an eye out for slow-moving rocks (also known as box turtles) in spring.

At 0.87 mile, the trail returns to the nature center area. Take time to check out the large section of a tree trunk under the shelter. Walk behind the nature center and reenter the trail area.

This time, continue on the red trail to your right. One mile into the hike, the red trail crosses an old road. Continue on the red trail as it enters an upland woods composed of white oaks and sugar maples. In 160 feet, the trail crosses a gravel road. Follow the red arrows, and at 1.14 miles, the trail enters an open area.

Follow the path uphill to a bench underneath a sugar maple tree. Directly behind the tree is a sundial that was custom-made in France for this latitude. Walk toward the sundial, climb the stone steps, and continue on the red trail at 1.22 miles. Don't follow the sidewalk; look for the trail marker along the wood line. Follow the red arrows to stay on the trail.

Watch out for the multiple spur trails along this section of the hike. Stay to the right to remain on the red trail, which enters an open, grassy meadow at 1.4 miles. This area has little shade. A bench at 1.6 miles sits adjacent to a classification notice of Forest Stewardship by the Indiana Department of Natural Resources Division of Forestry.

The trail intersects with yet another trail at 1.72 miles. The trail is easy to stay on, just keep following the red trail markers. When the red trail loops back to its beginning, continue on this trail back to the junction with the yellow trail at 1.9 miles.

At the trail intersection, take a sharp right to follow the yellow trail. The relatively flat trail winds through the woods and crosses a gravel road before reaching another gravel road with a parking lot at 2 miles. Enter the parking lot and walk to your left to follow the Springhouse Trail. Take the Springhouse Trail to the springhouse, complete with flowing water. Continue on the Springhouse Trail and cross the footbridge at 2.23 miles and take the steps uphill. Wild ginger borders both sides of the trail along this area.

Springhouse Trail is wonderfully quiet and serene. In spring the forest is blanketed by an enormous variety of wildflowers. The narrow trail is reminiscent of walking through a maze or labyrinth and gives you time to enjoy the scenery and reflect.

The narrow path winds uphill through a variety of spring wildflowers shaded by white pine trees. Cross another footbridge at 2.3 miles and look for animal tracks in the muddy area surrounding the small waterway.

The boardwalk returns you to the graveled parking area. In the parking area, turn left and look for the entrance to the yellow trail. It's about 50 feet ahead, near the end of the parking area.

Enjoy some more peace and quiet at 2.47 miles by sitting on the bench while an array of songbirds flits around in the canopies of the white oak, tulip poplar, and sugar maple trees. The trail crosses a gravel road at 2.49 miles. After crossing the road, yet another opportunity to relax and enjoy the sights and sounds of the woods awaits. This area has minimal urban noise even though it is close to a major roadway and a shopping area.

Continue on the yellow trail to the right until you reach the large footbridge over a dry creek bed at 2.57 miles. Here, the forest transitions to one dominated by American beech trees.

In spring in this beautiful forest, look for wildflowers such as trilliums and spring beauties. The bridge crosses the creek at 2.76 miles. Cross the old roadway and continue uphill on the yellow trail.

The yellow trail crosses another road at 2.89 miles and enters the oak–tulip experiment area. Tulip poplar trees have a tight bark with gray and yellow tones. Here, the yellow trail merges with the blue trail. Follow the yellow and blue trail back to the nature center and return to your vehicle.

Nearby Activities

The usual medium-size-city restaurants and retail stores line US 40. Additional hiking opportunities in the area that are featured in this book are Mary Gray Bird Sanctuary, Shrader–Weaver Nature Preserve, Whitewater Memorial State Park, and Mounds State Recreation Area.

GPS Trailhead Coordinates and Directions

N39° 50.325'   W84° 50.893'

From Cincinnati's west side at the intersection of I-275 and US 27, follow US 27 North 48 miles to Richmond, Indiana. Turn right onto US 40, travel east 2 miles, and turn left onto Elks Country Club Road. After 0.1 mile, turn right into Hayes Arboretum.

40 Mary Gray Bird Sanctuary

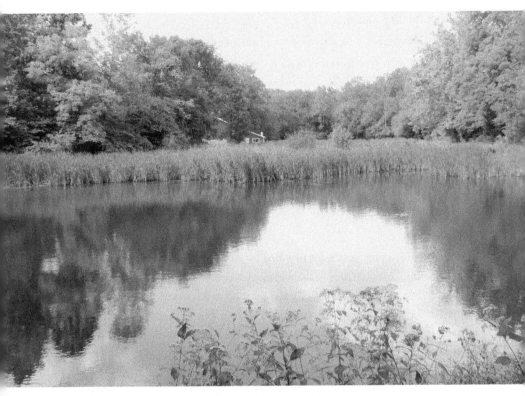

Goldfinches flit around the ponds at Mary Gray Bird Sanctuary.

In Brief

Nestled in the scenic rural landscape is the Mary Gray Bird Sanctuary, which offers more than 700 acres of forest, meadow, prairie, and pond habitats to explore, plus a spectacular variety of songbirds, birds of prey, and waterfowl to spy upon.

Description

In memory of their daughter, Mary, Alice Greene Gray and Congressman Finley H. Gray donated 600 acres of land to establish the Mary Gray Bird Sanctuary. Since the initial series of donations in the 1940s, the sanctuary has grown to more than 700 acres of rolling forests, as well as spacious meadows and prairies. In addition to the multitude of small wooded streams, several ponds dot the landscape.

LENGTH & CONFIGURATION 3.6-mile loop	**ACCESS** Daily, sunrise–sunset; free
DIFFICULTY Easy–moderate	**MAPS** USGS *Alpine;* property maps available at kiosk on site
SCENERY Prairie, forest, and ponds	**WHEELCHAIR ACCESSIBLE** No
EXPOSURE Open in prairie areas and shaded in woods	**FACILITIES** Latrine, water, and picnic shelters
TRAFFIC Light–moderate	**CONTACTS** Mary Gray Bird Sanctuary, 765-827-5109; **indianaaudubon.org /marygraybirdsanctuary**
TRAIL SURFACE Soil	
HIKING TIME 2–3 hours	
DRIVING DISTANCE 15 minutes south of Connersville, Indiana	**COMMENTS** Great destination for birding enthusiasts, plus the public is welcome to attend several of the nature programs offered throughout the year.
SEASON Year-round	

The diversity of habitats leads to a long list of wildlife living in the Mary Gray Bird Sanctuary. When I visited during the winter, I interrupted a pair of coyotes hunting in the open prairie, startled several deer, and listened to the sounds of nuthatches, brown creepers, and many different woodpeckers. The sanctuary is even livelier in spring and summer, when nesting songbirds return to the area. Visitors can regularly spot pileated woodpeckers, dark-eyed juncos, and white-eyed vireos, as well as cerulean and prairie warblers, orchard orioles, and summer tanagers.

Park in the lot near the kiosk at the end of the entrance road. The kiosk has property maps, Indiana Audubon Society information, and checklists for birds and mammals.

Walk around the kiosk to the entrance road and turn to the southwest (so that your back is to the buildings). The entrance becomes a limited-access service road. Stay on the service road until you reach the open prairie right behind the small stand of trees. In summer, the prairie is painted a crisp yellow with thousands of goldenrods.

Take the Prairie Trail (7) to the right and head along the edge of the prairie and the woods. Several bluebird nesting boxes line the edge of the trail to the right. Approximately 0.1 mile into the hike, the Prairie and Beech Trails (Trails 7 and 2, respectively) connect. Take the Beech Trail (2) into the woods and over a small footbridge.

At the next trail junction, remain on the Beech Trail (2), which heads left and downhill. This area is full of black cherry, ash, sugar maple, beech, American hornbeam, and hackberry trees. The trail leads back uphill and reaches a junction with the Cornus Trail (8E). Remain on the Beech Trail (2).

The creek winds through the forest valley. Pass the bridge to Woods Loop Trail (9) and remain on the Beech Trail (2). The low-lying areas are filled with wide, tall

Mary Gray Bird Sanctuary

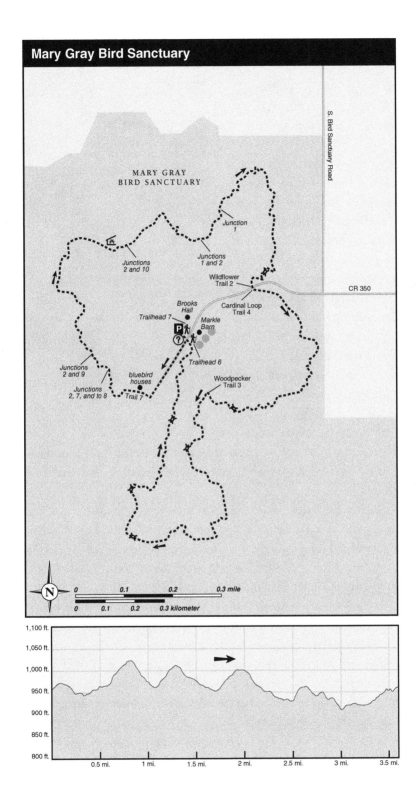

American beech trees, cottonwoods, and sugar maples. Along the left side of the trail at 0.5 mile is a hollowed-out beech.

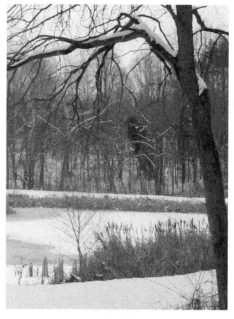

Forty yards beyond this is a fallen beech tree that has been cut to allow access along the path—count the number of growth rings to determine the tree's age. Along this stretch of the trail is a massive American beech tree.

Cross the metal footbridge at 0.6 mile. The trail climbs steadily uphill for 0.25 mile. During this section, red and white oak, beech, sugar maple, and tulip trees, plus a good variety of saplings and understory plants, combine to create a textbook example of a secondary forest.

Winter hikes at Mary Gray are peaceful.

After 0.7 mile, the woods open into a meadow dotted with a few large trees. Remain on the Beech Trail (2) through the open meadow area. Purple ironweed, goldenrod, thistles, and grasses attract butterflies and birds.

At 0.8 mile, a small pavilion sits atop one of the high points of the hike. Walk through the pavilion and straight ahead to continue on the trail. At the pavilion, you can take a break and enjoy the view. The junction of the Beech Trail (2) and Malus Trail (8A) is located at the pavilion. Remain on the Beech Trail (2) as it heads back downhill and past the junction of the Locust Trail (10).

As you continue on the Beech Trail (2), the trail leads to the bottom of the hill and back into the woods. Red and white oak, beech, sugar maple, and tulip trees line the edges of the trail through this secondary growth forest.

The trail narrows to the size of a deer path as it meanders back and forth until it reaches a steep path to a footbridge at 1 mile. Be careful of your step, especially if you're hiking in wet weather or during the fall season, when leaves can make footbridges and steep slopes treacherous.

When the Beech Trail (2) and Wildflower Trail (1) intersect 80 yards ahead, take the Wildflower Trail (1) to the left and cross the bridge over the creek. In 0.1 mile, the Wildflower Trail (1) will split with a trail labeled C G for Campground; stay on the Wildflower Trail (1). At the next trail intersection, follow the Wildflower Trail (1) to the left and slightly uphill.

Over the next 0.5 mile, the trail crisscrosses creeks and wooded hillsides lined with black cherry, white and red oak, shagbark hickory, tulip, and beech trees. Remain on the Wildflower Trail (1) to the entrance road.

Look 20 feet across the road and follow the signs for the Cardinal Trail (4), and at the Cardinal Trail (4) split, stay on the left, heading uphill. In 0.25 mile is the junction of the Cardinal Trail (4) and the Woodpecker Trail (5). Follow the Woodpecker Trail (5) to your left. You'll pass through an area with several downed trees.

One-half mile into the Woodpecker Trail (5) is a steep hill to a footbridge. When the trail joins the Tulip Poplar Trail (3), follow the Tulip Poplar Trail (3) to the left along the edge of the creek.

The trail leads up and down hills into an open forest and over several footbridges crisscrossing the creek. Tulip Poplar Trail (3) runs along the ridgelines, lending excellent views of the surrounding ravines. Eventually it heads back downhill and to a bridge, where it connects with the Wetland Trail (6) and Prairie Trail (7). At the opening take Wetland Trail (6) to the right, cross the bridge, and continue on the trail heading back toward the creek and into the woods.

Follow the trail to the left. Three-tenths of a mile after entering the woods again, the trail leads to an open area near the ponds. Take some time exploring the area around the ponds before heading northwest to the grassy field with picnic areas and to your vehicle.

Nearby Activities

While you are in the area, make time to hike the Shrader–Weaver Nature Preserve 7 miles northwest of Connersville. In Connersville, you can find restaurants, grocery stores, and gas stations. The Whitewater Valley Railroad hosts several themed events throughout the year.

GPS Trailhead Coordinates and Directions

N39° 35.381'   W85° 13.533'

From Connersville, Indiana, take IN 121 South and turn right on West County Road 350 South. Continue straight for 3 miles until the road ends at the entrance of Mary Gray Bird Sanctuary. Enter the sanctuary and drive past Brooks Hall and the Markle Barn. The parking area is to your right near the kiosk and latrine.

41 Mounds State Recreation Area

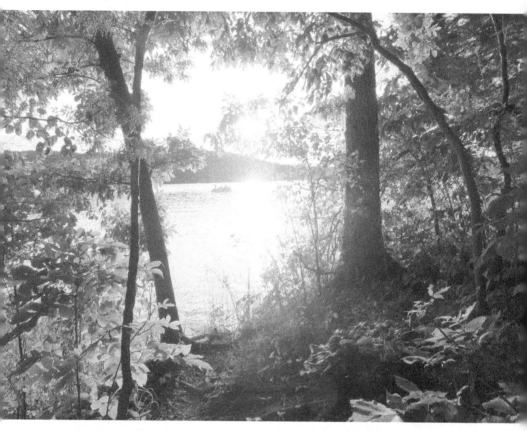

Serenity along Glidewell Trail

In Brief

Mounds State Recreation Area features the Glidewell Mound located off Trail 2. You'll definitely stretch your legs on the Glidewell long loop. This hike covers a portion of the 25-mile-long Adena Trace Loop.

Description

Indiana Department of Natural Resources properties charge a small admission fee, or you can purchase an annual pass, which is well worth the money.

LENGTH & CONFIGURATION 8.1-mile balloon

DIFFICULTY Difficult

SCENERY Woods, lake and backwaters, and Glidewell Mound

EXPOSURE Mostly shaded

TRAFFIC Light

TRAIL SURFACE Soil

HIKING TIME 6 hours

DRIVING DISTANCE 1.5 hours northwest of Cincinnati

SEASON Year-round

ACCESS Daily, sunrise–sunset; Indiana residents, $5 daily vehicle permit; out-of-state residents, $7 daily vehicle permit

MAPS USGS *Whitcomb;* Brookville Lake map

WHEELCHAIR ACCESSIBLE No

FACILITIES Drinking water and restrooms at main office, campground, and camp store; outhouse facility at pavilion near trailhead

CONTACTS Brookville Lake, 765-647-2657; **in.gov/dnr/parklake/2961.htm**

COMMENTS Plenty of nature-based activities are available in the Brookville Lake area, which includes Whitewater Memorial State Park and Quakertown and Mounds State Recreation Areas. The cut-through along US 27 about 1 mile south of Richmond is a well-known Ordovician fossil-hunting site.

Mounds State Recreation Area is on the southeast side of Brookville Lake, in the Whitewater River Valley. The lake's primary purpose is flood control, but it and the surrounding area were developed to offer recreational opportunities.

Brookville Lake's 12,000 acres include boat ramps, a beach, campgrounds, marinas, picnic areas, and fishing and hiking opportunities. The area is rich in prehistoric American Indian mounds. The Miami and Delaware tribes once lived along the Whitewater River.

Follow the entrance road and take the first left turn. This road leads past a service building. Turn left into the parking area near the shelter house. Across the road from the shelter house is the entrance to Trail 4. Cross the bridge over the ditch area and enter the Wildlife Wander Trail.

This hike is a wonderful escape from urbanization, cell phones, and to-do lists. Near the trailhead you'll find a kiosk with trail tips, such as bringing along plenty of water, basic safety rules, and how much time to plan for hiking various trails.

Immediately upon entering the forest you'll see a trail intersection; take the trail straight ahead. The gravel-covered path lies under the high canopy of the sugar maple–dominated forest. Identification stations are located throughout the woods. Station 4 is a red oak, and at station 5, 0.15 mile into the hike, are three shagbark hickory trees.

At the intersection of Wildlife Wander and Templeton Creek Trails at 0.25 mile, follow Templeton Creek Trail to the left. This wide soil path leads through a forest of shagbark hickory, red oak, and sugar maple trees.

Mounds State Recreation Area

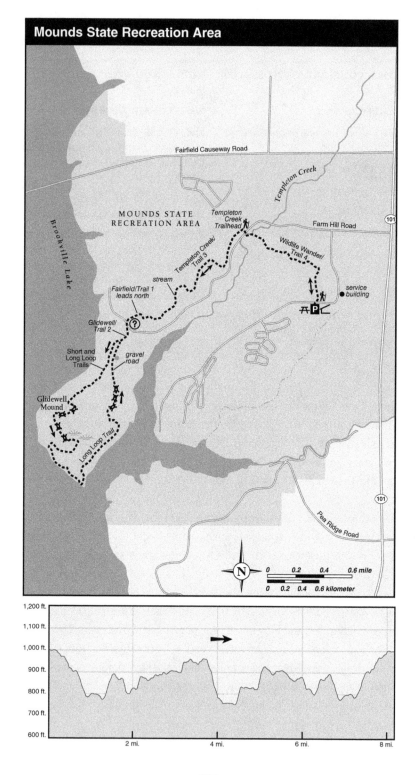

At 0.48 mile, use the flat stones to cross the creek. The forest transitions to one dominated by sugar maples, with a few elm trees. Begin a series of streambed crossings at 0.5 mile. Head downhill, and at 0.7 mile, enter an area with redbuds, dogwoods, and red cedars.

Pass through a stand of red cedars with reindeer fern ground cover at 0.77 mile. Reindeer fern is a small, delicate fern with a branching structure resembling a reindeer's antlers, and it is commonly associated with red cedars. At 0.83 mile the trail enters an upland woods dominated by sugar maples, with relatively no understory.

Use the concrete posts to cross the stream at 0.94 mile. Walk past the trailhead sign for Templeton Creek Trail (Trail 3) at 0.96 mile before walking around the riprap, crossing the road, and continuing on Templeton Creek Trail at 0.99 mile.

At 1.3 miles, the trail enters an open grassy area. In the summer this area might be overgrown and difficult to pass through without scraping your legs against the weeds. The trail ducks back into the forest at 1.33 miles, shaded by plenty of dogwoods.

At the trail intersection at 1.5 miles, follow the trail to the left with the orange blaze tape on the trees. This trail passes through an area with several hackberries and leads downhill.

The trail might be a little difficult to find at 1.7 miles, but follow the orange blaze marks on the trees as the trail takes a hard left. At 1.73 miles the trail takes another hard left and leads downhill. At 1.75 miles the trail is very eroded.

Cross the stream at 1.8 miles and enter a maple forest with elm and hackberry trees. The trail enters an open area at 1.86 miles, which wild turkeys frequent as a location to dust in. The dusting helps remove parasites.

Cross under the power lines at 2.2 miles. Follow the power lines uphill and pass Fairfield Trail (Trail 1), which leads to the right, and follow Glidewell Trail to the left. This is a gravel access road that leads down to a paved road. Cross the asphalt road at 2.4 miles, and look to the left for the Glidewell Trailhead (Trail 2) and kiosk.

This is part of the Adena Trace Loop. The Adena Trace is named after the American Indians who once inhabited the Whitewater River Valley. (A trace is a commonly used pathway.) You'll soon pass by an American Indian mound dating back 2,000 years.

Follow the gravel path behind the kiosk sign back into the woods. Be prepared to cross downed trees throughout this portion of the hike. At 2.5 miles is the entrance to Glidewell Trail. At the trail junction between the Short and Long Loops, follow the trail to the right, Long Loop Trail, off the gravel trail and weave through the woods of sugar maple, ash, and elm trees. At 2.6 miles, the trail takes a hard right and heads downhill. Follow the signs for the Short and Long Loops and cross over a few drainage areas.

At 2.91 and 2.97 miles, cross the footbridges in the shagbark hickory, sugar maple, and ash forest with a high canopy. The trail is very shaded and serene except for the occasional sounds from a lake. Cross another footbridge.

The Glidewell American Indian mound at 3.4 miles dates to 10 B C. Be respectful of the mound and do not disturb it or walk over the top of it. Cross over the footbridge at 3.5 miles. The trail is a single-person-wide footpath through the sugar maple–dominated forest. At the next trail intersection, turn right to stay on the Long Loop Trail.

The trail edges along the shoreline near 4.1 miles. You'll reach a grove of spiderwort and ginger near 4.3 miles. The trail leads up a steep hill and into a forest with a denser understory beneath a canopy of sugar maple, red oak, and ash trees at 4.72 miles. (At least what is left of the ash trees, thanks to the invasive emerald ash borer.) Cross the footbridges over the next 0.2 mile. Turn right when the trail intersects with a gravel road at 4.96 miles. Pass by a small pond at 5.12 miles and continue on the trail to the kiosk.

Retrace your steps to the overhead power lines and then along Templeton Creek Trail. Follow Templeton Creek Trail to Wildlife Wander Trail. Retrace your steps along Wildlife Wander Trail to your vehicle.

Nearby Activities

The Brookville Lake area includes Quakertown State Recreation Area and Whitewater Memorial State Park, both of which offer additional hiking and wildlife-watching opportunities. Mary Gray Bird Sanctuary and Shrader–Weaver State Nature Preserve are also nearby and offer serene hiking trails. If you are hungry, Brookville, Indiana, has plenty of nice restaurants.

GPS Trailhead Coordinates and Directions

N39° 29.722'   W84° 57.449'

From Cincinnati, follow I-74 West. Take Exit 169/Brookville/West Harrison, head west on US 52 (which merges with IN 1), and travel north 14.6 miles. Stay on IN 1 through Brookville, then turn right and follow IN 101 North 7 miles and turn left into Mounds State Recreation Area.

42 Muscatatuck National Wildlife Refuge: Chestnut Ridge Trail

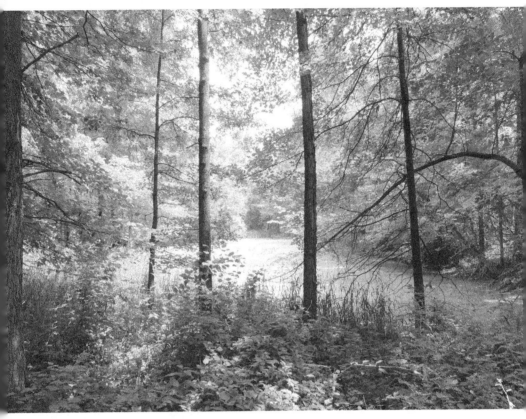

Quietly approach the pond along Chestnut Trail and you may see turtles and snakes.

In Brief

Muscatatuck National Wildlife Refuge offers adventures for everyone, including five hiking trails. Bring your camera and bird identification guides, as more than 280 species of birds have been identified on the refuge.

Description

Muscatatuck National Wildlife Refuge was established as Indiana's first National Wildlife Refuge in 1966 to provide resting and feeding areas for waterfowl during their

LENGTH & CONFIGURATION 0.5-mile loop	**SEASON** Year-round
DIFFICULTY Easy	**ACCESS** Daily, sunrise–sunset; free
	MAPS Chestnut Ridge map
SCENERY Woods, wetland, wet woods, and ponds	**WHEELCHAIR ACCESSIBLE** Yes
EXPOSURE Shaded	**FACILITIES** Nature center and shop, restrooms, and drinking water
TRAFFIC Moderate	**CONTACTS** Muscatatuck National Wild-life Refuge, 812-522-4352; **fws.gov/refuge /muscatatuck**
TRAIL SURFACE Paved, recycled plastic boardwalk, and gravel	
HIKING TIME 30–45 minutes	**COMMENTS** Plan to spend a weekend exploring the Muscatatuck National Wildlife Refuge. Five hiking trails and one driving trail provide many ways to view wildlife.
DRIVING DISTANCE 2 hours west of Cincinnati	

annual migrations. *Muscatatuck* is an American Indian word meaning "land of winding waters," and as one of more than 545 refuges of the National Wildlife Refuge system, its mission is to restore and preserve a mix of forest, wetland, and grassland habitat for fish, wildlife, and people.

This is a wonderful place to introduce children to hiking. Muscatatuck has a lot to see—if you slow down and take a close look. Be wary of the trail borders, as an ample supply of poison ivy dominates the edges. If you come in contact with poison ivy, use *cold* water and soap to wash it off immediately. If that isn't available, look for jewelweed (it looks like gangly impatiens), crush the stem, and rub the plant on the affected area. The plant's juices help to remove the oils from your skin. If you don't recognize jewelweed, don't guess! Find a place to wash the oils from the poison ivy off of your skin.

After entering the refuge, pass through a gate and take the first turn to the right to the Conservation and Nature Center. Follow the road back to the center and park in either lot.

Take some time to explore the nature center's kid-friendly exhibits, as well as the bird-viewing room. For the shopper in you, the well-stocked nature store in the Visitor Center is delightful. Immediately outside the nature store, you'll find maps at a self-serve kiosk on the wall to the right. Grab a copy of the Muscatatuck National Wildlife Refuge Chestnut Ridge Trail interpretive guide.

When you exit the front of the nature center, walk to the parking lot and look to your left. You will see the sign for the entrance to the Chestnut Ridge Trail. Immediately to the right of the sign is the trailhead.

Muscatatuck National Wildlife Refuge: Chestnut Ridge Trail

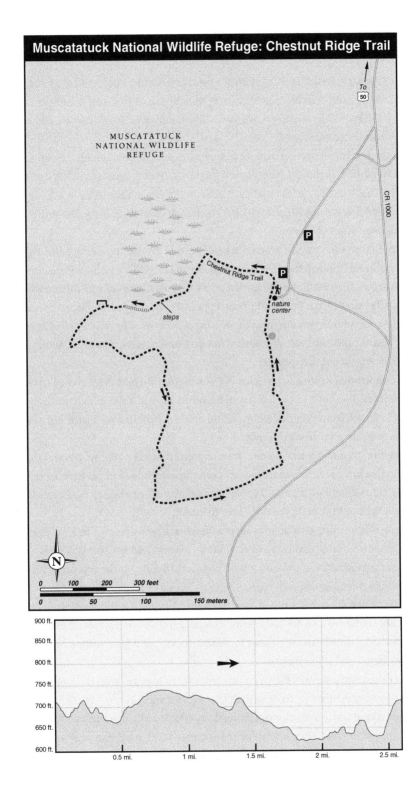

The Chestnut Ridge Trail is relatively short at 0.5 mile, but it covers a broad time frame of history and contains a great variety of habitats, as well as the animals that live in these habitats. While we hiked, we saw white-tailed deer, frogs, turtles, and a very unconcerned water snake.

This trail is excellent year-round. In spring, expect to be serenaded by an assortment of songbirds, including Neotropical migrants. In fact, Muscatatuck is a well-known birding location, celebrated each year on the second Saturday in May at the Wings Over Muscatatuck Migratory Bird Festival. Muscatatuck is recognized as a continentally important bird area.

Throughout the year, Muscatatuck hosts several events, including butterfly counts, National Public Lands Day Cleanup, National Wildlife Refuge Week, and the Log Cabin Day Festival. For more information, visit **fws.gov/refuge/muscatatuck**.

The Chestnut Ridge Trail's interpretive points cover the area's history as well as the plants and animals you are most likely to see and hear. The first 400 feet of the hike pass through a tulip- and oak-dominated forest. Chestnuts used to grow in this area, but a blight wiped out the species.

The enormous white oak tree that is 484 feet into the hike is estimated to be more than 100 years old. At this point, the trail becomes a boardwalk, which was built using "lumber" created from recycled plastics, and heads downhill over a series of steps. (The paved route goes along the ridge.)

Take the steps down into an old creek channel that keeps the woods wet during spring. In this low area, chestnut oak, hickory, musclewood, and pawpaw trees shade the multitude of wetland plants. The elevated boardwalk provides a bird's-eye view of the area without the fear of sinking into the mud.

Along this bottom-area boardwalk is a bench at a little over 0.1 mile, the perfect spot to get comfortable and listen to the chorus of frogs and songbirds. The boardwalk ends, and the trail leads uphill on a gravel path at 0.15 mile. At the top of the hill, the trail becomes paved again.

At the trail split at 0.17 mile, stay to the right. As you pass the man-made ponds throughout this area, look for waterfowl, herons, egrets, turtles, snakes, and songbirds. The pond at 0.2 mile is a nesting spot for wood ducks and is surrounded by chestnut oaks, pawpaws, and sugar maples.

Over the years, the area has been through many changes, with the landscape evolving from chestnut woods to farm fields to forest succession. At 0.34 mile, you'll see a spot where the forest joins open meadow, creating an edge habitat. Whenever one habitat borders another, a vital habitat is created. Edge habitats are excellent areas to look for various wildlife species, including songbirds.

Another good spot where two habitats meet is at 0.39 mile. This simple pond with the surrounding woods has many surprises—if you sit and wait. In fact, there is a handy bench to facilitate this process. (This is where we saw the water snake plus five turtles that were more interested in sunning than evading us.)

When the trail exits the woods take a few moments to watch for butterflies and birds utilizing the butterfly garden behind the split rail fence. Look for great spangled fritillaries as well as glimmering goldfinches.

The hike terminates at the nature center. More hiking adventures await, such as the Turkey, Bird, Wood Duck, and Hunt–Richart Lake Trails. The Hunt–Richart Lake Trail is profiled beginning on the next page.

When your feet are too tired to hike, you can choose an auto tour trail that leads past several of the controlled water structures. Expect to see egrets, cedar waxwings, great blue herons, and hundreds of ducks and geese. (Your vehicle makes a great blind for taking photos. Just be sure to turn off the engine, so your photos aren't blurry.)

Nearby Activities

Other hiking opportunities in this area include Versailles and Clifty Falls State Parks, Hardy Lake State Recreation Area, Selmier State Forest, and Pennywort Cliffs Preserve. Seymour, Indiana, is less than 5 miles away from Muscatatuck and offers the standard medium-size-city amenities.

GPS Trailhead Coordinates and Directions

N38° 57.579'   W85° 47.918'

This is by far one of the easiest locations to find. Take US 50 West out of Cincinnati and drive for about an hour and a half. The entrance to Muscatatuck is on the south (left) side of the road about 10 miles west of North Vernon.

43 Muscatatuck National Wildlife Refuge: Hunt–Richart Lake Trail

In Brief

The Hunt–Richart Lake Trail is an easy hike for families to enjoy as it weaves through open meadows and woods and along the shoreline. The observation blind provides plenty of wildlife-viewing opportunities.

Description

One of the most highly recommended hikes at Muscatatuck National Wildlife Refuge is the Hunt–Richart Lake Trail. It might have this distinction because of the excellent wildlife-viewing opportunities or the incredible scent of the flowering trees in spring, but either way, Hunt–Richart Lake Trail provides something for everyone.

For this hike, definitely bring along a camera, binoculars, bird-identification book, sunscreen, and insect repellent. Although the Hunt–Richart Lake Trail is short, it passes through several different habitats and has a fantastic bird blind that allows you to stop and watch wildlife.

As you drive to this trail, enjoy the view of Richart Lake from the dam. A 4-mile auto tour passes by beautiful wetlands with waterfowl, herons, egrets, and songbirds.

From the Hunt–Richart Lake Trailhead parking area, head to the right of the trailhead marker kiosk in the semi-open prairie area thicket. The trail is a mowed path. Standing water fills multiple low spots, which provide excellent amphibian breeding grounds in spring. Look closely for tadpoles in these small pools.

Continue on the trail as it heads uphill into a wooded area at 0.2 mile. The forest is a nice, cool break from the open field. The canopy of the woods is quite high, creating a cathedral feeling. Take a moment in the forest to stand perfectly still and listen to the sounds of the songbirds.

The upland woods of high-canopy sugar maples and oaks slowly begins to transition to a large, thick stand of sweet gum saplings to the left before entering into another prairie area at 0.3 mile. The deep roots of prairie plants allow them to survive harsh conditions.

The prairie is bordered by a fence to the left. Along the edges, expect to see roosting red-tailed hawks, and, in the open area, perhaps turkey vultures riding the thermal

LENGTH & CONFIGURATION 0.9-mile loop

DIFFICULTY Easy

SCENERY Woods, meadow, and lake

EXPOSURE Shaded and full sun

TRAFFIC Moderate

TRAIL SURFACE Gravel and grass

HIKING TIME 1 hour

DRIVING DISTANCE 1.5 hours west of Cincinnati

SEASON Year-round

ACCESS Daily, sunrise–sunset; free

MAPS USGS *Chestnut Ridge;* Muscatatuck National Wildlife Refuge Hiking Trails

WHEELCHAIR ACCESSIBLE No

FACILITIES Restrooms and water at nature center

CONTACTS Muscatatuck National Wildlife Refuge, 812-522-4352; **fws.gov/refuge /muscatatuck**

COMMENTS Plan to spend a weekend exploring the Muscatatuck National Wildlife Refuge. Five hiking trails and one driving trail lend plenty of access and opportunities to view wildlife.

currents of air. This is a favorite spot for bird-watchers and photographers because of the diversity of birds using the edge habitat.

In spring watch for brightly colored Neotropical migrants, including many warblers, flycatchers, tanagers, orioles, and vireos. The bird list for Muscatatuck National Wildlife Refuge is available at the nature center office, and each year Muscatatuck National Wildlife Refuge hosts a birding festival in early May.

In summer the prairie is active with butterflies, moths, and skippers. Along the edge of the prairie you may hear great blue herons squawking overhead on the busy flight path from one body of water to the next.

The trail leads down along the edge of the lake and to an overlook. Richart Lake was created in 1979 by impounding a small stream. The 90-acre lake provides habitat and is the source of water for the moist-soil units—the systematically flooded wetlands.

You'll find the Hackman Overlook by following the path along a short boardwalk. This overlook is a gazebo-style blind with plenty of benches and windows to secretly view the activity on the lake. Find a comfortable spot and spend as much time as you wish watching the birds on the lake. A good place to look for activity is along the edges, where herons and egrets are busy hunting. This is a good point to complete a tick check, especially after hiking through grassy areas.

Ospreys hunt this body of water. Ospreys were once decimated by the effects of a pesticide called DDT but have made a comeback with the help of several

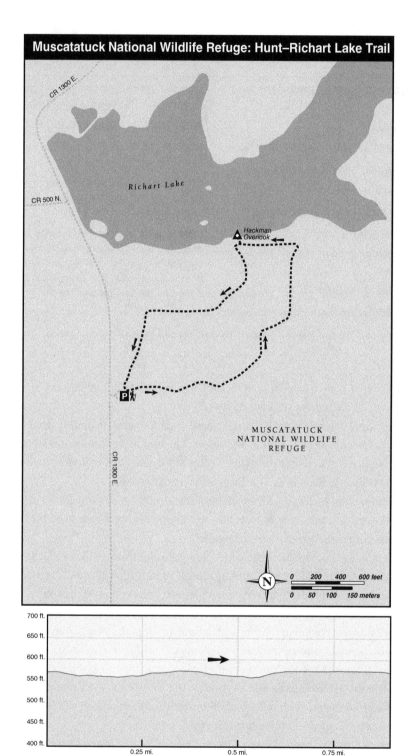

Muscatatuck National Wildlife Refuge: Hunt–Richart Lake Trail

CR 1300 E.

CR 500 N.

Richart Lake

Hackman
Overlook

P

MUSCATATUCK
NATIONAL WILDLIFE
REFUGE

CR 1300 E.

N

| 0 | 200 | 400 | 600 feet |

| 0 | 50 | 100 | 150 meters |

700 ft.
650 ft.
600 ft.
550 ft.
500 ft.
450 ft.
400 ft.

0.25 mi.   0.5 mi.   0.75 mi.

reintroduction projects throughout the Midwest, including the Indiana Department of Natural Resources' three-year reintroduction project.

Ospreys are a unique raptor, with wingspans that reach up to five feet across and a toe on each foot that can be positioned forward or in reverse. If you get the opportunity to see an osprey take a fish, the bird will often go under water and come back out shaking off the water much like a dog does. Once back in the air, ospreys carefully manipulate the fish to point headfirst to improve aerodynamics. Ospreys build their nests on old snags using a collection of branches, cattail fluff, and cornstalks.

Spring and fall migrations bring the greatest variety of waterfowl to the lake, including several threatened and endangered species. Spring (mid- to late March) and fall (late November) bring the greatest concentration of birds to the lake.

The Muscatatuck National Wildlife Refuge seasonally manages several moist-soil units, which means a multitude of wetlands are in this area. Wetlands are one of the most diverse habitats, and the ones at Muscatatuck are great examples. The best times to see the most wildlife are in the early-morning and late-evening hours.

After leaving the blind, return to the trail and continue to the right into the prairie. Look for butterflies and skippers flitting through this area. The field area is undergoing succession, pioneered by red cedar. Continue along the path to return to your vehicle.

Nearby Activities

Seymour, Indiana, is less than 5 miles from Muscatatuck and offers amenities common to most medium-size cities in the Midwest. If you are looking for more hiking trails, Big Oaks National Wildlife Refuge and Clifty Falls and Versailles State Parks are less than 90 minutes away.

GPS Trailhead Coordinates and Directions

N38° 57.054'   W85° 47.803'

This is by far one of the easiest locations to find. Take US 50 West out of Cincinnati and drive for about an hour and a half. The entrance to Muscatatuck National Wildlife Refuge is on the south side of the road about 10 miles west of North Vernon.

44 Muscatatuck Park

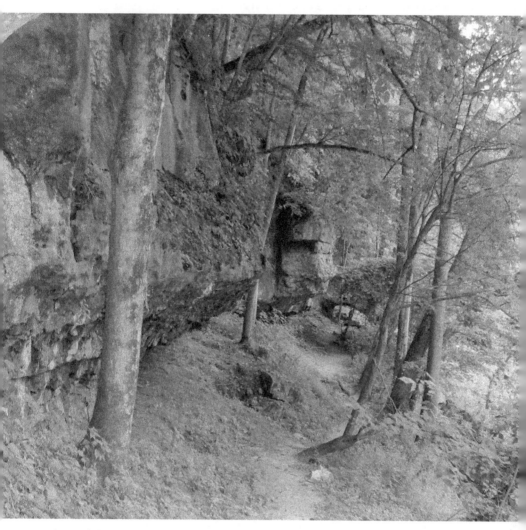

The trail skirts the edge of the Muscatatuck River.

In Brief

Muscatatuck Park includes the historic William Read home, Walnut Grove One-Room School, and Vinegar Mill. Trails crisscross the park, and the one that follows the river corridor provides a rugged journey. History buffs, nature lovers, and people who like to scamper over boulders will enjoy the many venues of this park.

244

LENGTH & CONFIGURATION 2.8-mile loop	**SEASON** Year-round
DIFFICULTY Moderate–difficult because of the portion of trail along the edge of the river	**ACCESS** Daily, sunrise–sunset; free
	MAPS USGS *Vernon;* Muscatatuck Park Trails Map
SCENERY Woods, wetlands, river, cliff outcrops, and boulders	**WHEELCHAIR ACCESSIBLE** No
EXPOSURE Mostly shade; some full sun	**FACILITIES** Water and restrooms in the pavilion area and at the Visitor Center Monday–Friday, 9 a.m.–4 p.m.
TRAFFIC Moderate	
TRAIL SURFACE Soil and exposed rocks and roots	**CONTACTS** Muscatatuck Park, 812-346-2953; **muscatatuckpark.com**
HIKING TIME 2.5–3 hours	**COMMENTS** Good boots, strong ankles, and a sense of humor are required for the latter portion of this trail.
DRIVING DISTANCE 1.5 hours west of Cincinnati	

Description

Muscatatuck Park began as Indiana's fourth state park in 1921—Vinegar Mills State Park. A year later the park was renamed Muscatatuck State Park. As with many state parks of this era, the Civilian Conservation Corps (CCC) and the Works Progress Administration (WPA) built park structures, roads, bridges, fire towers, and stone structures.

The park went through many transitions, including becoming a quail and pheasant farm that raised birds to reintroduce the species to Indiana. Other states also tried this method of releasing pen-raised birds into the wild, only to discover the hard way that the birds lacked survival skills and soon perished from exposure, predation, or disease. Muscatatuck Park dropped the project after six years.

The Jennings County Park Board was created in 1967 to manage the park in advance of the governor signing a bill in 1968 that gave the property to Jennings County. The park struggled for 20 years before finally evolving into today's popular destination.

The Jennings County Visitor Center is located in the William Read Home. In 1991 the Walnut Grove One-Room School was relocated to the property. Muscatatuck Park received a State Historical Marker in 1992.

In recent years, the park was able to renovate the historic Vinegar Mill site thanks to the Jennings County Community Foundation and Lilly Endowment, Inc. It also planted more than 90 mature trees after receiving the Hometown Indiana Urban Forestry Grant from the Indiana Department of Natural Resources Division of Urban Forestry.

Park in the large lot and walk to the William Read Home, a brick building that houses the Jennings County Visitor Center. If the center is closed, the small vestibule has maps and information about current events and local attractions.

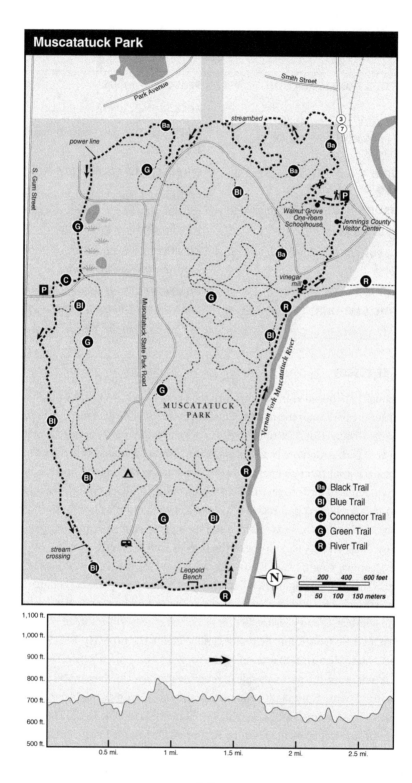

Muscatatuck Park

Park Avenue
Smith Street
power line
streambed
S. Gum Street
Ba
Ba
Ba
Ba
Ba
G
G
G
Bl
Walnut Grove
One-room
Schoolhouse
Jennings County
Visitor Center
P
3
7
C
P
Bl
G
G
vinegar
mill
R
R
R
Bl
Muscatatuck State Park Road
Vernon Fork Muscatatuck River
G
MUSCATATUCK
PARK
Bl
Bl
Bl
R
G
Bl
stream
crossing
Leopold
Bench
Bl
R

Ba Black Trail
Bl Blue Trail
C Connector Trail
G Green Trail
R River Trail

N

| 0 | 200 | 400 | 600 feet |
| 0 | 50 | 100 | 150 meters |

1,100 ft.
1,000 ft.
900 ft.
800 ft.
700 ft.
600 ft.
500 ft.

0.5 mi.   1 mi.   1.5 mi.   2 mi.   2.5 mi.

Walk back toward the parking lot and turn west to walk toward the Walnut Grove One-Room School, which was built in 1913. Follow the trail around to the back of the schoolhouse, down the hill, and at the junction turn right onto a compacted narrow footpath through the woods. Cross the footbridge and head uphill.

The trail zigzags through the woods amid dogwoods, sugar maples, and red oaks. Cross the waterway in an area with black slate at 0.3 mile. Some of these trails are shared with mountain bikers. Follow the well-worn trail to the right through the woods. Be wary of the multiple smaller trails that crisscross throughout the park.

The forest is primarily white and red oaks and sugar maples. To the left of the trail at 0.32 mile, before the path reaches a bend, is a great example of a shagbark hickory tree. The soil is sandy along this stretch through the upland woods.

Be careful of your step over the exposed rock and roots along the portion of the trail that is eroding. If it is wet out, the compacted soil is very slick. The tulip, pawpaw, and spicebush are abundant along this portion of the hike.

Crisscross the stream at 0.42 mile before following the trail (labeled blue, mountain bike, and brown) to the left. Shagbark hickory, sweet gum, red oak, elm, sassafras, dogwood, and sugar maple trees make up the canopy structure of the woods. Beneath are spring wildflowers such as mayapples.

The trail becomes a mowed path near the power line right-of-way in an area of younger woods with sweet gums and sugar maples. At 0.84 mile you'll see a small pond and wetland area complete with cattails and water lilies as well as leopard frogs and bullfrogs. Cross a small bridge over the wet area near the end of the wetlands at 1.1 miles. Watch for red-winged blackbirds along the cattail blooms, as well as wood thrushes working the edge of the woods.

Take the blue trail (connector) to the right, between the large white pine trees. Continue through the tulip and former white pine stand. This area sustained a lot of wind damage in 2008, and several large white pines were destroyed. The surge of new growth provides habitat for many songbirds and mammals.

At 1.2 miles pass the gravel parking lot, cross the road, and continue on the trail straight ahead. When the trail splits, follow the blue trail to the right. The forest transitions to a tulip and white pine stand with little understory and a lot of very straight trees. Cross the creek at 1.4 miles.

Head downhill over the exposed rocks and roots at 1.6 miles, and into a dense upland forest. The trail meanders uphill, and at 1.9 miles you'll find a Leopold bench at the intersection of several trails. Follow the signs for the blue and green trails straight ahead through the woods of spicebush, sugar maples, beeches, and oaks.

At 2 miles the trail leads down a steep hillside and then skirts the edge of the Muscatatuck River. Good footing on this section of the trail is difficult on a good day and nearly impossible if it has been raining. Be careful crossing a huge dip in the trail. To the left is a dolomite outcrop with moss-covered stone.

The low basin is filled with sycamore, box elder, and pawpaw trees. Continue following the trail along the river corridor over the exposed bedrock. This trail is a narrow, uneven path through boulders and dolomite outcrops.

At 2.4 miles a large chunk of rock has fallen, creating a cave-like area extending about 10 feet back from the edge. The trail skirts along the edge of the 60- to 80-foot-high cliff and over gnarly roots. Pass between a large boulder and the cliff and over the funky chinquapin oak. At this point in the hike, you might be wondering what state you are in since it doesn't look like Indiana due to the unusual-looking rocks, small caves, and lichens. Continue on the trail and cross the bridge at 2.6 miles. Continue straight ahead to the stone steps that lead to the Vinegar Mill, which never produced a drop of vinegar.

The stories go something like this: Mr. Read was building the original mill when he was interrupted by a curious hunter who asked what he was doing. In one account, Mr. Read replied, "If you stay long enough, you'll find out." And in the other story line, he replied, "Vinegar." Either way, Mr. Read was not only funny but also a cautious businessman who obviously didn't like people knowing what his plans were before he was done.

The Vinegar Mill shelter stands in what was once the location of the second stone-cutting mill. The first one was about 100 feet farther upstream. From the second floor of the shelter, you'll have a wonderful view of the river corridor.

At 2.7 miles the trail crosses the parking lot and road. Look uphill to the right and you'll see where it reenters the woods. Continue following the trail uphill into the woods and to the right to the Jennings County Visitor Center. Walk to the front of the building and to your vehicle in the lot.

Nearby Activities

Muscatatuck National Wildlife Refuge, Selmier State Forest, Hardy Lake State Recreation Area, Pennywort Cliffs Preserve, and Clifty Falls State Park and Clifty Canyon Nature Preserve offer plenty of additional hiking trails and are included in this book.

GPS Trailhead Coordinates and Directions

N38° 59.413'   W85° 37.092'

From the intersection of I-275 and US 50 on the west side of Cincinnati, follow US 50 West about 50 miles to North Vernon, Indiana. Turn left and head south on IN 3/7 for a little more than 1 mile. Muscatatuck Park is on the right side of the road.

45 Pennywort Cliffs Preserve

In Brief

Off the beaten trail, Pennywort Cliffs Preserve is a serene trek through the woods along an old road that passes in and out of existence. This hike is a peaceful escape from the world.

Description

If you are looking for a hike that isn't the least bit urbanized (except for occasional airplane noise), this is the hike for you. Pennywort Cliffs Preserve is 216 acres of woodland forest with three springs and a waterfall. This hike doesn't include the waterfall because you must go off-trail to reach it, which creates a host of problems (including damaging a fragile habitat and potentially getting you lost).

Finding the trailhead is an adventure in itself. It is easy to miss—repeatedly. The entrances to Pennywort are simple cut-ins through the standard overgrowth of edge species such as multiflora rose and poison ivy. This alone probably discourages less-adventurous hikers who would turn around and head for a trail system in a more civilized setting.

Pennywort Cliffs has no amenities. The trails are remnants of an old road system being commandeered by the surrounding woods and are laced with fine threads of silk from orb-weaving spiders.

Serene Pennywort Cliffs doesn't see a lot of hikers. At times the trails verge on woods and wander; that's why it's important to bring along a compass or GPS unit.

Yellow signs mark the nature preserve boundary, and, unless it has fallen, one is located near the south entrance. Park your vehicle off the edge of the road near the barn. Since this is a farming community, park as far off the road as possible to allow wide equipment to pass, but not too far or you'll need a tow.

Enter the preserve by way of the old road into the forest of American beech, dogwoods, pawpaw, and spicebush. The overgrown trail is passable. Watch for poison ivy along the edge of the trail as well as on the trail itself. And be relentless in checking for ticks. Unless the area has been recently mowed, plan on walking through tall grasses and stepping over fallen tree limbs along the trail.

The forest of mature red oak, beech, and shagbark hickory trees stretches 60–80 feet high. Typically, you would expect a woods with a dense, high canopy to be cool during the heat of summer, but the trees block most of the air movement, making for humid and sticky summer hikes.

LENGTH & CONFIGURATION 2-mile out-and-backs	**ACCESS** Daily, sunrise–sunset; free
DIFFICULTY Easy	**MAPS** USGS *Volga*
SCENERY Classified forest and springs	**WHEELCHAIR ACCESSIBLE** No
EXPOSURE Shaded	**FACILITIES** None
TRAFFIC Light	**CONTACTS** The Nature Conservancy, 317-951-8818; **tinyurl.com/pennywortcliffs**
TRAIL SURFACE Mowed path	**COMMENTS** Pennywort Cliffs Preserve is a wonderful place to enjoy the tranquility of nature; just be sure to bring along the insect repellent and a GPS unit or compass. The trail is not well marked or maintained.
HIKING TIME 2 hours	
DRIVING DISTANCE 1.5 hours west of Cincinnati	
SEASON Year-round	

The forest slowly transitions to one dominated by beech and tulip trees just 350 feet into the hike. The forest structure is an extraordinary textbook example of what a forest should look like. Visit during spring to see wildflowers such as Virginia bells, trillium, and jack-in-the-pulpit in full bloom.

Near 650 feet, the trail passes through an area with ferns on both sides. It doesn't look like much of a trail at 0.14 mile, but when the trail splits, take the trail to the right labeled SW (faintly marked on a tulip tree). Immediately, you'll pass through another large area of ferns near several enormous American beech trees.

The trail is bordered with aromatic spicebush. Spicebush berries were used by pioneers as a substitute for allspice. When the leaves are crushed they smell like lemon-scented furniture polish. In fact, you can steep the twigs in hot water to make a tea. If you decide to try wild edibles, make sure you consult at least two good identification books and two good wild edible cookbooks.

In the wet depressions along the trail, look for animal tracks. White-tailed deer, raccoons, opossums, and wild turkeys are common occupants of this protected forest. At the trail junction at 0.22 mile, the trees are faintly labeled S and F. Follow the trail labeled S to the right.

At the next trail junction at 0.28 mile, follow the trail labeled SW to the right. This trail passes through a wonderful beech-maple forest and ends at the enormous fallen beech tree at 0.36 mile. This is a great opportunity to investigate the root structure of this giant tree. The ground that the beech tree once shaded is now open to full sunlight, and several sweet gum trees are growing in this new opening.

Retrace your steps to the previous intersection with the tree labeled SW and turn right. Follow this trail down to the open area with white oak trees. This is an

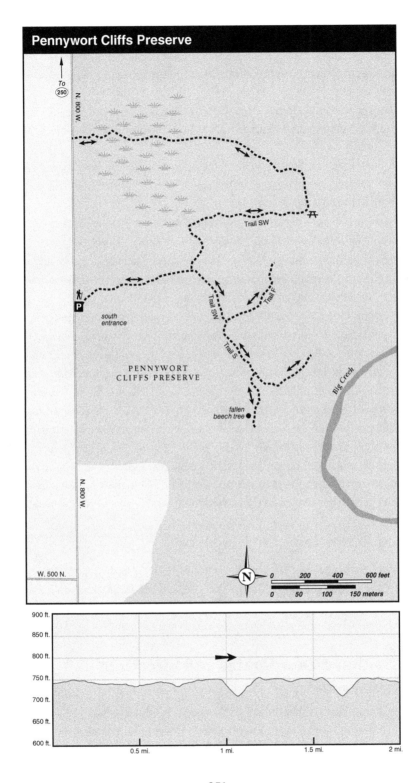

Pennywort Cliffs Preserve

To 250

N 800 W.

Trail SW

Trail SW

Trail F

Trail S

south entrance

P

PENNYWORT CLIFFS PRESERVE

fallen beech tree

Big Creek

N 800 W.

W. 500 N.

N

| 0 | 200 | 400 | 600 feet |
| 0 | 50 | 100 | 150 meters |

900 ft.
850 ft.
800 ft.
750 ft.
700 ft.
650 ft.
600 ft.

0.5 mi.   1 mi.   1.5 mi.   2 mi.

enjoyable spot to attract birds by calling "pssh." Retrace your steps to the intersection and turn right.

Follow the trail to the intersection with the trees labeled s and f at 0.65 mile into the hike. Turn right onto the overgrown F Trail and be careful to not get into the stinging nettles.

Continue on this trail until you reach the open area underneath a very large sugar maple tree. This is a nice place to sit, relax, and do absolutely nothing—which is harder to do than you'd think.

Retrace your steps back to the intersection of the S and F Trails and turn right onto the SW Trail, which isn't well marked but should look familiar since you're retracing your earlier steps. At 0.92 mile pass the trail that brought you in from the road. Continue quietly on the trail downhill. You may surprise a white-tailed deer or at the very least see a variety of Neotropical migrants. Use the "pssh" sound to attract songbirds.

As you continue down the hillside, you enter a breathtaking cathedral of enormous sugar maple and tulip trees in this low-lying area. At 1.1 miles, cross a wet area with some exposed stones. This is a good spot to look for black-and-yellow millipedes.

Continue on the trail to the picnic bench in the open area surrounded by very large sassafras trees. Continue uphill and follow the trail to the left through the forest of dogwood, beech, sugar maple, tulip, and black cherry trees. Parts of this heavily rutted trail have standing water, and the route passes through what appears to be a wet woods. Beware of deer trails. Stay to the left to head to the road and back to your vehicle.

When you reach the country road, turn around and retrace your steps to the intersection with the sign for sw—this was the first trail intersection you encountered on this hike. Turn right and retrace your steps to the trailhead and your vehicle.

Nearby Activities

Muscatatuck Park, Muscatatuck National Wildlife Refuge, Hardy Lake State Recreation Area, Selmier State Forest, Clifty Falls State Park, and Clifty Canyon Nature Preserve are also great places to hike and are included in this book. If you're looking for a bite to eat, Madison, Indiana, has plenty of hometown restaurants.

GPS Trailhead Coordinates and Directions

N38° 48.885'   W85° 32.227'

From Madison, Indiana, travel north 7.7 miles on IN 7. Turn left onto IN 250. Travel 3.4 miles and turn south onto County Road N 800 W. Travel south 1.4 miles; the preserve is on the east (left) side of the road across from the barns.

46 Selmier State Forest

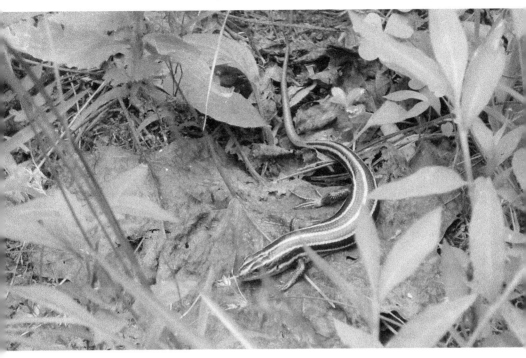

Only young five-lined skinks have the blue tail.

In Brief

Selmier State Forest includes a pleasant stroll along the West Vernon Fork of the Muscatatuck River, through pine stands and mixed-hardwood forests. If you look closely you can still see some of the damage that occurred in 2008 from a shearing windstorm and Hurricane Ike.

Description

Selmier State Forest is Indiana's smallest state forest. Mrs. Frank Selmier donated 355 acres on behalf of her husband. From 1921 to 1934, Mr. Selmier planted pine, black locust, black walnut, sycamore, and tulip trees throughout the property. In fact, most of this property is in Indiana's Classified Forest program.

Nestled near the West Vernon Fork of the Muscatatuck River, Selmier State Forest has several incredible river overlooks. Once you enter the state forest, continue on the

LENGTH & CONFIGURATION 3.7-mile balloon	**ACCESS** Daily, sunrise–sunset; free
DIFFICULTY Easy	**MAPS** USGS *Butlerville;* Selmier State Forest map
SCENERY Forest, river corridor, and ponds	**WHEELCHAIR ACCESSIBLE** No
EXPOSURE Mostly shaded	**FACILITIES** None
TRAFFIC Light	**CONTACTS** Selmier State Forest, 812-346-2286; **in.gov/dnr/forestry/4818.htm**
TRAIL SURFACE Gravel roads, access lanes, and mowed paths	**COMMENTS** Wear hunter orange during hunting seasons for white-tailed deer, turkey, squirrel, and raccoon. Go to **in.gov** and search for hunting seasons for current dates. A map for the self-guiding nature trail is available at the office.
HIKING TIME 3 hours	
DRIVING DISTANCE 1.5 hours east of Cincinnati	
SEASON Year-round	

road to the first turnoff to the right. Park and then walk around the gates to begin the hike on the trail heading west, away from the road you came in on.

Immediately upon entering this trail you'll come to a bench and several numbered markers for the self-guided tour. Follow the gravel lane back under the canopies of tulip, American beech, and sugar maple trees. At number 13 is a white oak tree and at number 12 are a tulip and some beech trees.

Continue on the gravel lane. White pines, dogwoods, sweet gums, American beech, and spicebush line the trail's edges. Pass by the small white pines and pawpaw trees at 0.17 mile. Soon tulip trees begin to dominate the forest. At the trail junction at 0.25 mile, follow the trail north. The White Pine Trail is marked with a trail signpost amid the beech trees.

Pass through the white pines, being careful to avoid the poison ivy along the edges of the trail. The orange blossoms of jewelweed also border the trail. The jewelweed seedpods are hydrostatically charged, so when pressure is applied to the seedpod it explodes. Kids love these bursting seedpods, which feel like wriggling worms in your hand.

A bench is adjacent to a large tulip tree at number 3 and several small pawpaw trees. The trail passes downhill over several railroad-tie steps. An old dam area at 0.35 mile still contains water, and it's easy to see fish swimming in the clear water below.

The trail continues uphill. Turn right at the trail junction near the benches. The forest includes a variety of hickories, tulip, and black cherry trees, and red and white oaks.

Pass the pond to the left of the trail at 0.52 mile. Several wood duck nesting boxes are placed around the pond. Wood ducks typically nest above water in the hollows of

Selmier State Forest

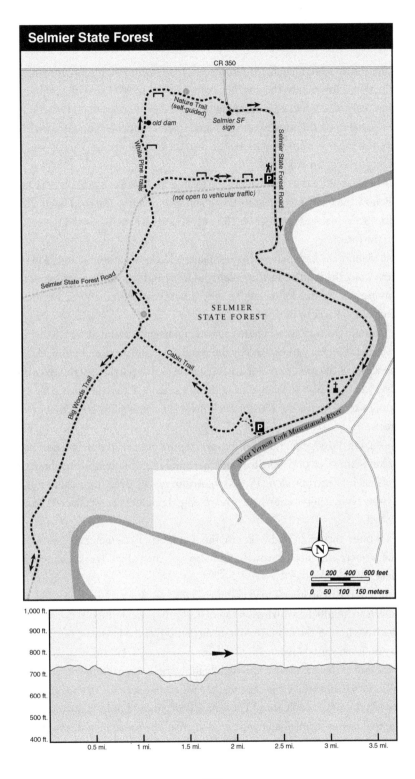

CR 350

Nature Trail
(self-guided)

old dam

Selmier SF
sign

White Pine Trails

Selmier State Forest Road

P

(not open to vehicular traffic)

Selmier State Forest Road

SELMIER
STATE FOREST

Cabin Trail

Big Woods Trail

P

West Vernon Fork Muscatatuck River

N

| 0 | 200 | 400 | 600 feet |
| 0 | 50 | 100 | 150 meters |

1,000 ft.
900 ft.
800 ft.
700 ft.
600 ft.
500 ft.
400 ft.

0.5 mi.   1 mi.   1.5 mi.   2 mi.   2.5 mi.   3 mi.   3.5 mi.

trees. After the ducklings hatch, the female calls to them and they jump from the nesting box to the water. Amazingly, the ducklings can fall close to 300 feet without injury.

Adult male wood ducks are stunning with iridescent chestnut and emerald as well as ornate patterns on their feathers. The females are a buff chestnut color with brilliant white around the eye. Wood ducks make a distinct call: the males a "jeeb," and the females an "oo-eek, oo-eek."

The bench before the trail reaches the main gravel road is a nice place to take a break. Follow the trail onto the gravel road and hike down to the road lined with tall sycamores, redbuds, and hornbeam. The only sounds are the birds and the rustling of leaves in the forest.

At 0.75 mile, the lane passes over a small creek. Look for animal tracks in the sandbars. Along the road's edges are plenty of ferns and wild ginger. Pass your vehicle at 0.85 mile and continue following the main gravel road with the West Vernon Fork of the Muscatatuck River to the left.

Near 1 mile the trail (gravel road) curves and begins to lead downhill through an area of shagbark hickory trees. Pass by the stand of large American hemlocks.

The views of the river corridor are incredible. Some portions of the river bottom appear very flat and easy to wade during the dry season. The river flows over a large, flat dolomite area. Across the Muscatatuck River is an enormous collection of sycamore trees.

Look along the edges of the river for several piles of stacked stones. These are remnants of Mr. Selmier's work, as he had multiple buildings and ponds throughout the area.

Pass the cliff outcrops along the river corridor where large stones have tumbled into the waterway. Theses enormous square-edged boulders are scattered throughout the riverbed.

At 1.4 miles turn right and walk into the Summerfield Cemetery. The area behind the fence is the resurgence of growth. Look for evidence of wild turkeys and white-tailed deer.

Return to the main gravel road and turn right. Nearby is a large, cave-like rock with American hemlocks growing on top of it. Pawpaw, sugar maple, sycamore, and box elder trees border the road. Do not go farther down the lane past the private-property boundary markers.

At the end of the gravel road and slightly to the right is a parking area at 1.7 miles. The trailhead is behind the cable rope that blocks vehicle access. Walk around the rope and between the sugar maple trees. The Cabin Trail winds uphill, away from the river.

The trail passes through an open wooded area. The forest includes sugar maple, tulip, and pine trees with plenty of understory ferns. Wild turkeys scratch through the leaf litter. It looks like someone went through the woods with a rake. Watch the surface of the trails for evidence of this behavior as well as turkey scat.

At the T-intersection with Big Woods Trail at 2.1 miles, turn left onto Big Woods Trail. The trail leads through white pine, American beech, tulip, and red oak trees. At the end of the trail at 2.6 miles, near the farm field, turn around and retrace your steps.

Pass Cabin Trail to the right at 3.2 miles. Immediately after this is a small pond on the left. Look for skinks and box turtles sunning in the open area. White pines and sassafras dominate this portion of the trail.

Pass several more trails to the right and left of the main trail before reaching the intersection with the Nature Trail and the gravel road at 3.5 miles. Just before the intersection is another large area of jewelweed.

Turn right on the gravel lane and retrace your steps to your vehicle.

Nearby Activities

Muscatatuck Park, Muscatatuck National Wildlife Refuge, Hardy Lake State Recreation Area, Versailles State Park, and Clifty Falls State Park and Clifty Canyon Nature Preserve offer multiple hiking opportunities.

GPS Trailhead Coordinates and Directions

N39° 01.994'   W85° 35.882'

From I-275 and US 50 on the west side of Cincinnati, follow US 50 West 50 miles to North Vernon, Indiana. Turn right and follow IN 3/7. At the split take IN 3 to the right. Travel 1.5 miles north and turn right onto West County Road 350 North. Drive 2 miles to the gravel-road entrance to Vawter Road into Selmier State Forest on the right side of the road.

47 Shrader-Weaver Nature Preserve

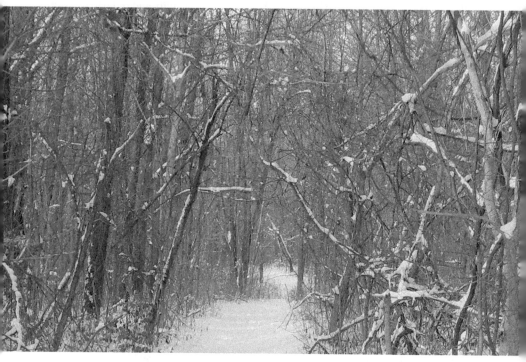

Hike the trails at Shrader-Weaver Nature Preserve throughout the year.

In Brief

Although there are many grand old trees in this unique sanctuary, the serene nature of the quiet woods qualifies Shrader–Weaver Woods as exceptional. Visit in spring for the wonderful wildflowers, and remember everything in Shrader–Weaver Nature Preserve is protected.

Description

This small nature preserve is about one hour from Cincinnati and 7 miles northwest of Connersville in Fayette County, Indiana. Nestled into rural farmland near the small town of Bentonville, Indiana, the Shrader–Weaver Nature Preserve is a wonderful trail far off the beaten path, which means it has light traffic and very little ambient noise. In

LENGTH & CONFIGURATION 2-mile modified figure eight	**ACCESS** Daily, sunrise–sunset; free
DIFFICULTY Moderate	**MAPS** USGS *Connersville;* trail-marker guides available at trailside sign-in stations.
SCENERY Old-growth forests, succession, wetlands	
EXPOSURE Mostly shaded	**WHEELCHAIR ACCESSIBLE** No
TRAFFIC Generally very light except during spring	**FACILITIES** None
	CONTACTS Indiana Department of Natural Resources, Division of Nature Preserves, 317-232-4052; **tinyurl.com /shraderweaver**
TRAIL SURFACE Dirt	
HIKING TIME 1–1.5 hours	
DRIVING DISTANCE 2 hours from Cincinnati	**COMMENTS** Everything in Shrader–Weaver Nature Preserve is protected. Spring is best for bird-watchers and wildflower enthusiasts. Winter is great for solitude seekers.
SEASON Year-round, but best in spring, fall, and winter	

fact, at times it is so peaceful and calm that you can hear your own heart beating. The terrain is easy to traverse, making it a great winter hiking destination.

In all fairness, I am slightly biased as I grew up in this area and enjoyed hiking in the Weaver Woods with my mother and brother when I was young. But after you experience the sheer beauty of the woods and the perfect stillness, I bet you'll be a bit biased too.

The preserve was a gift to the people of Indiana from Laz and Edith Weaver, who donated their 108-acre historic property as well as Philip Shrader's 1830 home located on the site. They donated the property to The Nature Conservancy, which then transferred it to the State of Indiana.

For the botanist, Shrader–Weaver Nature Preserve is a delightful slice of history. The preserve hosts a 28-acre old-growth forest, an incredible diversity of wildflowers, a successional forest, and a seep spring. For the nature nut, the mixture of habitats brings a delightful array of songbirds and woodpeckers as well as white-tailed deer, foxes, rabbits, squirrels, and raccoons.

Spring is the best time for wildflower and songbird enthusiasts, and the winter months are best for wildlife watchers who enjoy seeing animal tracks in the snow as well as hearing the occasional snort and stomp of a deer.

To begin the hike, turn off North County Road 450 West and into the parking area directly off the road. The gravel lane leads to a private residence. The parking area for this hike is between the gravel lane and the signage for Shrader–Weaver Nature Preserve.

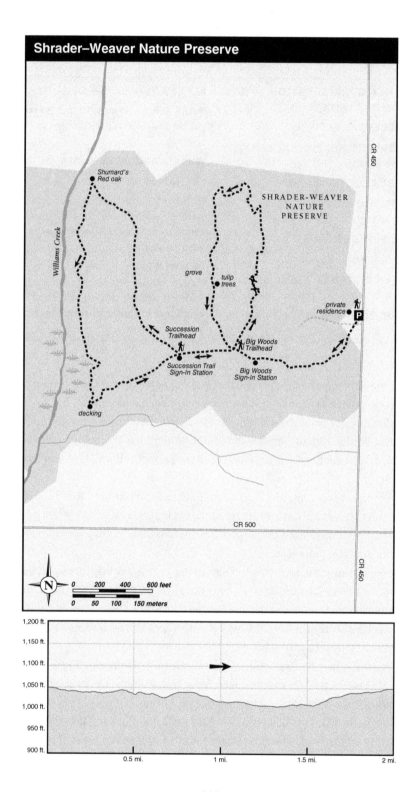

Shrader–Weaver Nature Preserve

Shumard's
Red oak

Williams Creek

SHRADER-WEAVER
NATURE
PRESERVE

grove

tulip
trees

private
residence

P

Succession
Trailhead

Big Woods
Trailhead

Succession Trail
Sign-In Station

Big Woods
Sign-In Station

decking

CR 450

CR 450

CR 500

N

| 0 | 200 | 400 | 600 feet |
| 0 | 50 | 100 | 150 meters |

1,200 ft.
1,150 ft.
1,100 ft.
1,050 ft.
1,000 ft.
950 ft.
900 ft.

0.5 mi.   1 mi.   1.5 mi.   2 mi.

Take note of the rules and regulations sign, and be sure to closely follow the Leave No Trace principles. Look beyond the rules and regulations sign to the wood line to the south for a bright yellow trail marker. Enter the woods at this main trailhead. The earthen trail is wide enough for two people.

Big Woods Trail and the connector path to the Succession Trail are at 0.2 mile. Sign in at the Big Woods station and grab a copy of the self-guided tour (under the board for the sign-in sheets) to interpret the natural information at numbered posts along the trail. To begin the Big Woods hike, proceed to the right to the Big Woods trailhead.

Except for one steep hill, the trail path is wide and winds gently through the woods. The self-guided tour is a nice addition to understanding the history and nature of the area. Please refer to it for supplemental information about the nature preserve.

While you're likely to see or hear woodpeckers in the old-growth forest, several other residents—such as screech, barred, and great-horned owls—may go unnoticed. The sugar maple and American beech forest is common in the Greater Cincinnati area, but the sheer age of trees in the Big Woods makes this a unique hike. A great example of a beech tree is at trail marker 2; notice how the bark is gray and smooth. Look around: a fierce competition rages between the beech and sugar maple saplings as they fight for survival under the dense canopy of the older trees.

Oak species in the Shrader–Weaver Woods include bur, swamp white, white, red, and chinquapin. Near trail marker 6, the forest changes and now is dominated by tulip poplar trees.

Walk toward the footbridge and note the enormous bur oak at marker 7. This massive tree and several others along the trail are roughly 200 years old. The path winds uphill for a short while and passes a few black cherry trees. A black cherry tree's bark is very dark and looks as if someone glued burned potato chips to the bark.

Take a journey back in time 0.2 mile into the Big Woods Trail. A fallen tree provides a great exploration of decay and the life that comes from it. Various cut trees allow you to see a slice of history when you stop to count the number of rings. Each ring represents one year of growth. Years with good growing conditions are wider than years when the tree was under stress. The trail heads up a slight hill, with the edges of adjacent farm fields visible as the trail curves through the old woods.

The path soon passes through a forest of American beech, sugar maple, black walnut, green and white ash, black cherry, tulip, and red elm trees of various ages. After 0.4 mile, the trail bends sharply and heads down a steep hill to a footbridge over a gully area littered with glacial boulders.

American hornbeam, also known as blue beech or ironwood, joins pawpaws, dogwoods, spicebush, and a multitude of saplings to complement the diverse understory. When the trail joins with the connector, turn right and enjoy the walk under the cathedral-like canopy of the large oak, tulip, and maple trees.

Sign in at the station and grab a tour guide to the Succession Trail. The clearly marked trailhead is to the right of the sign-in station. This area is going through succession from an agricultural field (1970) to the early succession or pioneer species you see today. The most common are box elder, black cherry, red elm, and tulip trees, as well as hackberry and sugar maple.

About 150 yards into Succession Trail, the path climbs uphill, goes downhill, and then flattens out into a slightly older stand of trees. Head uphill to an incredible bur oak tree at marker 3, about 0.4 mile into Succession Trail. At more than 5 feet in diameter and with an expansive branching pattern, the tree is about 200 years old, experts surmise.

Note the patchy bark of the white oaks throughout the area. The ground area to the right is a seep spring. Sycamores, white oaks, hackberries, American hornbeams, poison ivy, skunk cabbages, marsh marigolds, and jewelweeds thrive in the wet woods.

Cross the nice boardwalk deck that was built by David Sawyers and Troop 136 as an Eagle Service Project in 1989. Look for jewelweed and dogwoods. The trail climbs uphill past a thicket of multiflora rose and invasive species such as bush honeysuckle. Head downhill to the junction point, turn right, and take the main trail back to your vehicle.

Nearby Activities

If you're itching for more hiking, head to the Mary Gray Bird Sanctuary 7 miles south of Connersville, off IN 121. In Connersville you can find restaurants, grocery stores, and gas stations. The Whitewater Valley Railroad hosts several themed events throughout the year. And, in honor of my grandparents, Francis and Margaret Keller, stop in Kunkel's and grab a strawberry milkshake—just watch out for that ice cream headache.

GPS Trailhead Coordinates and Directions

N39° 43.207'   W85° 13.339'

From Connersville, take IN 1 North 5 miles. Turn west (left) onto Bentonville Road and drive approximately 4.5 miles. Turn south (left) on North County Road 450 West. The small gravel parking area and Shrader–Weaver Nature Preserve sign is less than 0.3 mile ahead on the west side of the road.

48 Versailles State Park

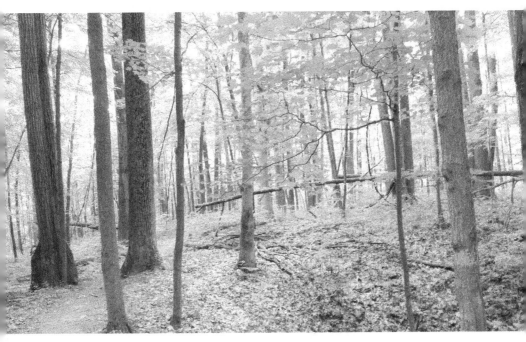

Sinkholes and old woods are prevalent at Versailles Sate Park.

In Brief

If you like fossils, you are going to love this hike. The 475-million-year-old Ordovician limestone, rich in fossils, is exposed in some locations. In those areas, one can easily see fossilized brachiopods, bryozoans, horn corals, and crinoids. Collecting fossils in the state park is not permitted. (Bummer.)

Description

Enter the park off US 50 and follow the signs to Oak Grove Shelter. The road to Oak Grove Shelter ends at a large parking lot. After parking, turn south and look at the open grassy area. The trailhead is near the edge of the fence posts that bar vehicle access to the Oak Grove Shelter. A signpost labeled Trail 1 marks the entrance to the hike. The trail is a single-person-wide, loose stone–covered path through the woods. After entering the woods, the trail proceeds downhill and over the top of large stones.

Be careful along this section of the hike as there are many trails that crisscross the area. Continue following this trail to the left when it meets with a trail intersection

263

LENGTH & CONFIGURATION 4.77-mile loop and figure eight	residents, $5 daily vehicle permit; out-of-state residents, $7 daily vehicle permit
DIFFICULTY Easy–moderate	**MAPS** USGS *Johnson;* Versailles State Park map
SCENERY Cliffs, sinkholes, waterways, woods, and Ordovician fossils	**WHEELCHAIR ACCESSIBLE** No
EXPOSURE Shade	**FACILITIES** Restrooms, drinking water, and picnic areas
TRAFFIC Light	
TRAIL SURFACE Soil and loose stone	**CONTACTS** Versailles State Park, 812-689-6424; **in.gov/dnr/parklake/2963.htm**
HIKING TIME 3.5 hours	
DRIVING DISTANCE 1 hour from Cincinnati	**COMMENTS** If you like bryozoans, brachiopods, horn corals, and crinoids, you are in for a treat. Collecting fossils in the park is not permitted. Be sure to see the covered bridge on the way into the park.
SEASON Year-round	
ACCESS Daily, 7 a.m.–11 p.m.; Indiana	

about 250 feet into the woods. Many spring wildflowers line this portion of the hike. Be careful of your footing over the slippery stones and loose-rock debris.

On this section of the hike, the sounds of cascading water and songbirds will drown out most modern noise. You'll come upon several small waterfalls around 470 feet into the hike. Be careful crossing the road at 0.18 mile. After crossing the road, look to the right to see where the trail continues.

The path enters the woodland under the high canopies of white oaks and sugar maples. The bark of larger white oaks has platy patches intermingled with distinctive shallow fissures. You can readily see the forest here because the woodland's understory is free of invasive honeysuckle. In spring a multitude of Neotropical migrants flit from tree to tree. Scarlet tanagers, indigo buntings, and Kirtland's warblers migrate to the tropics during the winter months and return here in the spring to raise their young.

Near 0.3 mile into the hike are several sinkholes that formed when the underlying limestone eroded, creating a collapse in the forest floor. These are just a few of the many sinkholes located through this park. If you're hiking with children, be sure to keep them safely away from the holes.

Throughout the park, many natural springs percolate through the forest floor. The combination of sinkholes and springs in the same location is thought to be evidence of a complex underground watercourse.

This portion of the hike looks like a sculpture garden because of the fallen trees and gnarled twists of thick grapevines. In the fall, deer actively seek out the small grapes. Wild ginger lines both sides of the trail as it heads downhill at 0.44 mile. In spring a variety of wildflowers, including wild geraniums, decorate the hillsides.

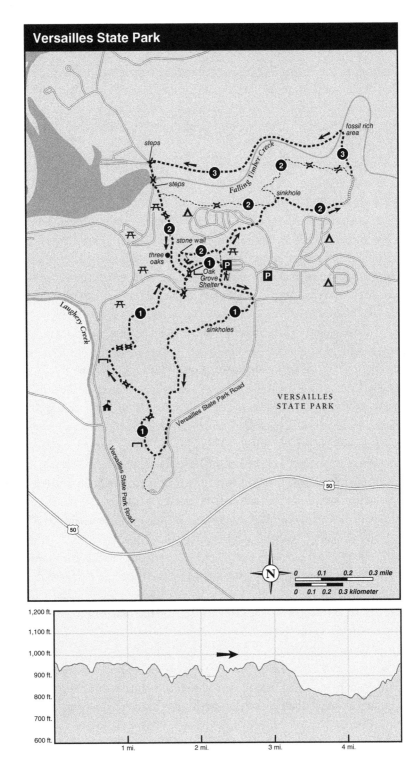

Versailles State Park

fossil rich area

steps

Falling Timber Creek

steps

sinkhole

stone wall

three oaks

Oak Grove Shelter

Laughery Creek

sinkholes

Versailles State Park Road

VERSAILLES STATE PARK

50

50

N

| 0 | 0.1 | 0.2 | 0.3 mile |

| 0 | 0.1 | 0.2 | 0.3 kilometer |

1,200 ft.				
1,100 ft.				
1,000 ft.				
900 ft.				
800 ft.				
700 ft.				
600 ft.	1 mi.	2 mi.	3 mi.	4 mi.

Cross a small stream at 0.57 mile and be careful to stay out of the poison ivy along both sides of the trail. Poison ivy is a beautiful, deep-green-colored plant with clusters of three leaves—hence the old warning "leaves of three; leave them be." Poison ivy might be a pain for humans, but several species of wildlife, including rabbits and deer, rely on it as a food source.

The forest structure changes near 0.68 mile, as the younger understory trees compete for sunlight. The forest is a place of quiet contemplation amid a battle for resources such as sunlight and water.

Trail 1 runs parallel to the Old Fire Road at 0.94 mile before returning to the woods. Several spur trails radiate from this trail. Just keep to the right and stay on the main trail.

At around 1.27 miles, you'll see several waterfalls. At the trail intersection at 1.47 miles, stay to the right and cross the footbridge. Enjoy a break on the bench at 1.57 miles before crossing a series of footbridges for the next 0.5 mile. Look for the bright red blooms of cardinal flowers along this portion of the hike.

The Oak Grove Shelter comes into view at 2.28 miles. This is a very easy area to get turned around in, as there are multiple trails that crisscross the area. (Just keep heading uphill to the Oak Grove Shelter.) When the trail intersects with Trail 2 (which is not labeled), take it to the west end of the Oak Grove Shelter area. The trail passes along the edge of a stone wall. Several spur trails radiate from Trail 2. Stay on the main trail, which parallels the Oak Grove Shelter playing field, parking lot, and picnic area.

Trail 2 crosses itself at 2.87 miles near another sinkhole. Continue on Trail 2 to the right. The forest is comprised of sugar maple, hackberry, and black cherry trees.

At 3.08 miles you'll pass a campground area on the left. The trail, which narrows to a single-person-wide deer path through the woods, sees more foot traffic because of its proximity to the campgrounds. During rainy weather, the next 0.2 mile will be very muddy. Trail 2 passes by another campground to your right.

Take Trail 3 when it connects with Trail 2 at 3.24 miles. This wide path leads down to the Fallen Timber Creek crossing at 3.4 miles. Watch the soil beneath your feet as you walk down the loose-stone path, because odds are there will be exposed bryozoans, brachiopods, corals, and crinoids. You can ogle the fossils, but collecting them at this state park is prohibited.

At the edge of Fallen Timber Creek, take a few moments to closely look at the rock debris. I have seen horn coral fossils that are 4–5 inches in length, as well as perfect specimens of brachiopods. If you can safely cross the creek, continue on Trail 3. The trail crosses the creek several times before exiting the beautiful woods and onto the road.

At 4.1 miles turn left onto the road and enjoy the views of the lake. Cross the bridge and turn left and take the steps back into the woods. Continue on the trail and at the T-intersection follow Trail 2 to the right. When you reach the trail split with three large oak trees growing together, take the trail to your left and weave your way uphill through the woods back to Oak Grove Shelter at 4.7 miles.

However, if the creek is out of its banks, retrace your steps back up the hill on Trail 3 to the turnoff to Trail 2. Cross the footbridge and continue on Trail 2, enjoying the view of the valley below. Cross another boardwalk at 3.89 miles before the trail begins to head downhill. Walk quietly along this portion of the path and you might be fortunate enough to see a wild turkey.

You'll see a closed-off area at 4.12 miles. Continue on the trail to the left, and in 0.1 mile, take the trail to the right. When the trail splits, take Trail 2 on the right side.

The trail passes near the campground at 4.2 miles. Carefully cross multiple small footbridges. Due to moist conditions, a thin layer of algae covers these footbridges, creating a slick surface. (Unfortunately, I discovered this the hard way.)

The trail exits into the campground and returns to the woods near the utility pole at 4.58 miles. For 0.1 mile, the trail heads down a steep hill over a series of railroad-tie steps and exposed bedrock. Be extremely careful on the steps and the bedrock, because if it is wet out everything is exceedingly slick due to the algae and the mud. Plus, the exposed roots and loose rocks make perfect toe catchers.

At the bottom of the hill, take the trail to the left. The small creek in this bottomland area provides the calming sounds of flowing water. Continue on Trail 2, and when it reconnects, follow the trail uphill.

Be aware this area is a lacework of user trails and the main trail is not well marked. To return to the Oak Grove Shelter, keep heading uphill and slightly left (north) while keeping an eye out for the Oak Grove Shelter, open grassy area, and parking area where you left your car.

Nearby Activities

Haven't worn you out yet? Head over to Muscatatuck Park, Muscatatuck National Wildlife Refuge, or Clifty Falls State Park to explore the excellent hiking trails. Versailles has a pumpkin show the last weekend in September and a bluegrass festival the first weekend of October. Crossroads Family Restaurant is a great place to have a sit-down meal.

GPS Trailhead Coordinates and Directions

N39° 04.559'   W85° 13.745'

From the intersection of I-275 and US 50 on the west side of Cincinnati, take US 50 West for 25 miles. The entrance to Versailles State Park will be on the north (right) side of the road.

49 **Whitewater Gorge:**
Cardinal Greenway

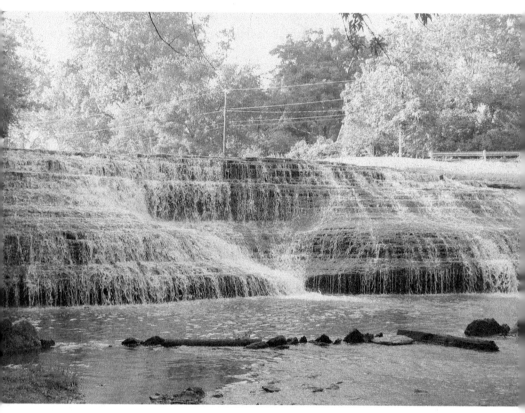

Whitewater Gorge Thistlethwaite Falls

In Brief

The Cardinal Greenway is a pleasant hike through the Whitewater Gorge area and cityscape of Richmond, Indiana. A side trail that leads through Springwood Lake Park takes you to Thistlethwaite Falls, well known for Ordovician fossils.

Description

The Cardinal Greenway is a rails-to-trails recreational pathway that, when completed, will cover 60 miles from Richmond to Marion, Indiana. The trail is paved and wide

LENGTH & CONFIGURATION 6.1-mile point-to-point	**SEASON** Year-round
DIFFICULTY Moderate	**ACCESS** Daily, sunrise–sunset; free
SCENERY Cityscape, forest, waterfall, Ordovician fossils, and West Fork of the East Fork Whitewater River	**MAPS** USGS *Richmond;* Cardinal Greenway trail map
EXPOSURE Mostly shaded	**WHEELCHAIR ACCESSIBLE** The Cardinal Greenway trail; sections that lead off of the main trail not accessible
TRAFFIC Moderate–heavy	**FACILITIES** Water and restrooms at Springwood Lake Park
TRAIL SURFACE Paved, mowed, and soil	**CONTACTS** Cardinal Greenways, 765-287-0399; **cardinalgreenways.org**
HIKING TIME 5 hours	**COMMENTS** Take the side trail through Springwood Lake Park to incredible Thistlethwaite Falls.
DRIVING DISTANCE 1.5 hours northwest of Cincinnati	

enough for a vehicle to access, although only foot and bicycle traffic is permitted. The out-and-back to Thistlethwaite Falls is partially paved, but not down to the falls.

A variety of outdoor enthusiasts use Cardinal Greenways, including bicyclists, walkers, stroller-pushing parents, and senior citizens. This hike is written as a point-to-point hike, so either plan for an out-and-back of 12.2 miles or have someone drop you off at the trailhead so you can hike to your car.

From the parking lot off Industries Road, head south to the trailhead. The trail is bordered by a split rail fence. Immediately after entering the trail is a wetland area. On both sides of the trail, horsetail—also called bottle-brush and scouring rush—is abundant. The horsetail plant has long been used for sanding or scrubbing because of its stems' high silica content. Want to see for yourself? Take a tarnished penny and rub a folded piece of horsetail around the face. With just a few passes, the penny will be shining.

Several portions of this trail are sponsored by different organizations that help maintain it. Some areas have a lot of honeysuckle growing up on both sides of the trail, along with a few locust trees. During this section of the hike, you're most likely to hear the sounds of industry, but don't fret; farther along, you'll hear only the sounds of nature.

At 0.86 mile, take the trail that leads to the left, downhill, over a small bridge, and into Springwood Park. To get there, follow the road to the right toward Springwood Lake, which is well known for the variety of waterfowl and shorebirds that frequent it. Expect to see Canada geese, mallards, grebes, trumpeter swans, and blue herons, as well as kingfishers.

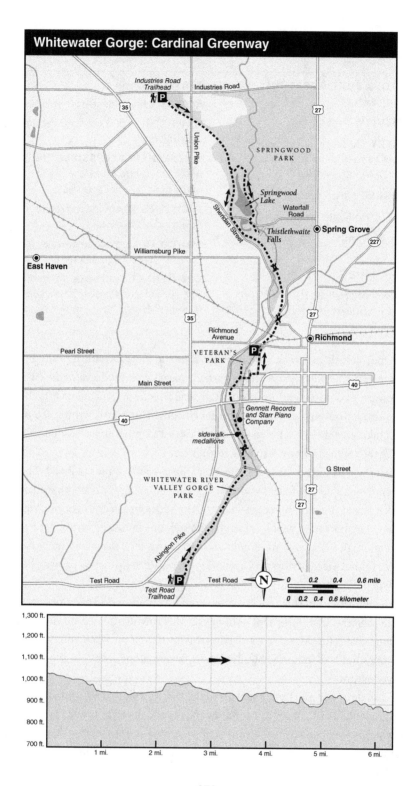

Whitewater Gorge: Cardinal Greenway

Industries Road Trailhead

Industries Road

35

27

Union Pike

SPRINGWOOD PARK

Sheridan Street

Springwood Lake

Waterfall Road

Thistlethwaite Falls

● Spring Grove

227

● East Haven

Williamsburg Pike

35

Richmond Avenue

● Richmond

27

VETERAN'S PARK

Pearl Street

Main Street

40

Gennett Records and Starr Piano Company

40

sidewalk medallions

G Street

WHITEWATER RIVER VALLEY GORGE PARK

27

27

Abington Pike

Test Road

Test Road

Test Road Trailhead

N

0   0.2   0.4   0.6 mile

0   0.2   0.4   0.6 kilometer

1,300 ft.
1,200 ft.
1,100 ft.
1,000 ft.
900 ft.
800 ft.
700 ft.

1 mi.   2 mi.   3 mi.   4 mi.   5 mi.   6 mi.

The lake is surrounded by bald cypress trees, which have feathery-looking leaves and produce knees—knobby roots poking up along the water's edge. Continue on the road to the park's entrance. Cross Waterfall Road and walk toward the chain-link fence. Follow the trail to the left toward the waterway.

Continue on the path down to the West Fork of the East Fork Whitewater River. As you get closer to the waterway, the incredible Thistlethwaite Falls becomes visible at 1.5 miles. This falls is created from the water eroding the Ordovician fossil-rich limestone and shale.

The falls are named after the Thistlethwaites, who in the mid-1800s built a dam; several mills, including lumber, grist, flour, and paper mills; and a lock to regulate the flow of water over the falls. The land near the falls is extremely rich in Ordovician fossils. Expect to see some incredible samples of horn coral, but don't take any home, as fossil collecting is not permitted.

Do not follow the path for the Whitewater Gorge Trail along this watercourse. It's not maintained, and in some areas is hazardous even for experienced hikers. Retrace your steps through Springwood Park and back to the paved trail at 2.2 miles. Turn left and continue on the trail.

Pass through an area with several trees of heaven. Their blooms are unmistakable, since they smell like stinky, sweaty socks. The trail crosses Waterfall Road at 2.5 miles. Continue on the path, and at 3.1 miles cross over the river via a concrete-and-steel bridge.

Pass a large parking lot, and over the next 0.4 mile, crisscross the river and road below via several bridges. At 3.8 miles you'll reach the trailhead for Cardinal Greenway near D Street. Walk to the street and take a right onto North Third Street. Turn right onto North A and at the next street turn left onto North Second Street. Then turn right onto Johnson Street. Follow Johnson downhill to Veterans' Memorial Park.

Continue on the trail by heading south, keeping the river to your right, and pass the substation. The trail passes by where the Gas Company Building used to be located. The paved trail goes under US 40 and continues to the old Gennett Records building.

Whitewater Valley Gorge Park is where Starr Piano Company and Gennett Records once thrived. This area was once home to several buildings that specialized in manufacturing pianos and records.

Here was the "cradle of recorded jazz" that contributed to the creation of country, blues, and jazz music. Continue along the sidewalk embedded with several medallions of famous recording artists, including Hoagie Carmichael, Jelly Roll Morton, Gene Autry, and Louis Armstrong, who recorded under the Gennett label.

Continue on the sidewalk to the trail and boardwalk. At 4.7 miles, the trail passes over the river before entering the woods of dogwood, ash, sugar maple, and box elder trees.

Pass the steps leading up to SW G Street at 4.9 miles and remain on the paved trail. Pass the access road at 5.1 miles with several large cottonwood trees near it.

Through the branches of ash, sugar maple, hackberry, red and white oak, and sycamore trees, you'll see the river valley to the left of the trail. The hillside to the right has plenty of unique rock outcrops, small streams, and small waterfalls. The side of the trail shows the characteristic layers of Ordovician shale and limestone. Enjoy a moment on one of the benches scattered along the trail.

Continue following the trail to the open area with picnic tables. A large boulder designates the dedication of the Whitewater Gorge Trail to the founding members of the Society for the Preservation of Resources, which worked to preserve the Whitewater Gorge for public use. The trail borders the wood line and ends in the parking area off Test Road.

Nearby Activities

Shrader–Weaver Nature Preserve, Mary Gray Bird Sanctuary, and the Brookville Lake area offer plenty of hiking and outdoor activities. Well known as Antique Alley, Richmond also has plenty of shopping and dining choices. When you are in the area, I highly recommend dining at Little Sheba's Restaurant in Richmond.

GPS Trailhead Coordinates and Directions

N39° 51.730'   W84° 54.719'

From I-275 and US 27 on the west side of Cincinnati, follow US 27 for 50 miles to the north side of Richmond, Indiana. Turn west onto Industries Road. In 1.25 miles turn left into the parking area for the Cardinal Greenways.

50 Whitewater Memorial State Park

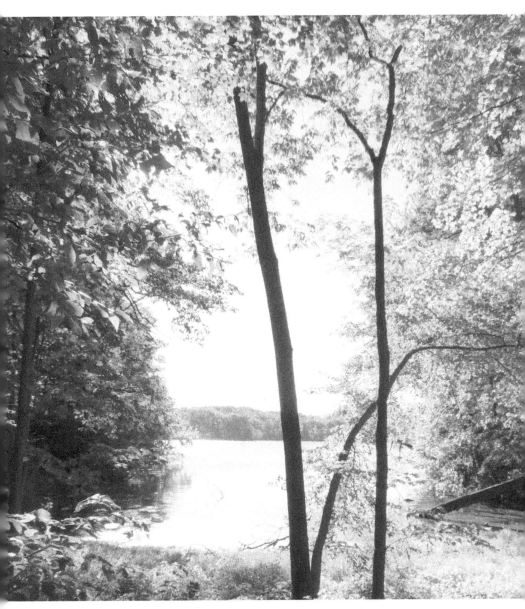

Lakeside views are plentiful at Whitewater Memorial State Park.

LENGTH & CONFIGURATION 4-mile balloon	residents, $5 daily vehicle permit; out-of-state residents, $7 daily vehicle permit
DIFFICULTY Moderate	**MAPS** USGS *New Fairfield;* Whitewater Memorial State Park map
SCENERY Woods, seep springs, and lake	
EXPOSURE Mostly shaded	**WHEELCHAIR ACCESSIBLE** No
TRAFFIC Moderate	**FACILITIES** Restrooms and water at main office; latrines
TRAIL SURFACE Soil and exposed rocks and roots	
HIKING TIME 3.5 hours	**CONTACTS** Whitewater Memorial State Park, 765-458-5565; **in.gov/dnr /parklake/2962.htm**
DRIVING DISTANCE 1 hour northwest of Cincinnati	**COMMENTS** Check **in.gov** for current advisories. Spend the day at Whitewater Memorial State Park hiking, boating, swimming, or even horseback riding.
SEASON Year-round	
ACCESS Daily, sunrise–sunset; Indiana	

In Brief

Nestled into the hillsides of Whitewater Memorial State Park, the trail passes through two great nature experiences: the Hornbeam Nature Preserve and Red Springs. Portions of the trail are rugged, and if the lake is high the Lakeshore Trail to the Observation Deck might be impassable.

Description

In 1949 Whitewater Memorial State Park was established as a living memorial to the men and women who served in World War II. Encompassing a 200-acre lake and 1,700 acres of woods, the park's many amenities include a beach, marina, campground, cabins, seasonal guided horseback rides, and plenty of trails.

From IN 101, enter the park and follow the main drive past the docks and to the parking area on the west side of the dam. Park, cross the road, and look for the entrance to Red Springs Loop to the right.

After entering the woods, the trail splits. Continue on the crushed-gravel Red Springs Loop to the right. Dogwood, elm, large redbud, basswood, locust, and ash trees along the trail provide ample shade for hikers and plenty of nesting spots for songbirds.

At 0.1 mile the trail heads downhill, then passes by upland hardwoods of sugar maple and oak, as well as the wildflower larkspur along the trail's edges. In spring this is the spot to enjoy the display of the season's wildflowers.

Be careful of your footing over the exposed roots along the single-wide footpath. To the left is a ravine. At 0.15 mile to the left is Red Spring Marsh, which is fed by the

Whitewater Memorial State Park

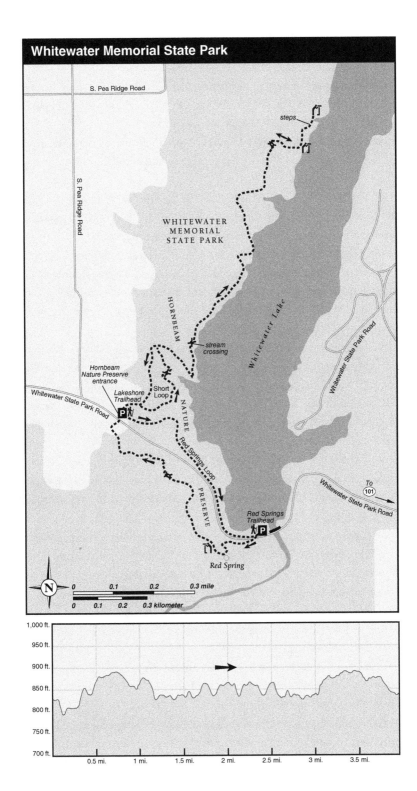

spring that flows year-round from the hillside. The rusty-red color stems from the iron and minerals in the water. The year-round spring and marsh provide a unique habitat for plants and wildlife, including an array of songbirds.

Pass the large red oak to the left. At 0.21 mile is the overlook of the springs from an observation deck. Allocate extra time to sit and enjoy the view of the springs and watch for wildlife.

Return to the trail and weave through the upland forest. The understory canopy is about 20–30 feet up, and the top canopy is 60–90 feet up. This is a nice, open forest that allows you to see readily for some distance through the trees.

You'll see a small creek to the left at 0.3 mile. The birds in this area couldn't seem to care less about human disturbance and are easy to spot as they go about their day. In 400 feet you'll pass through a grove of American beech trees and trillium. The bark of the American beech is smooth and an almost shiny gray color. Early spring is the best time to see trillium in bloom.

The trail heads downhill, with the creek to your left. At 0.4 mile cross the stream on the footbridge and continue uphill. The forest is dense with pawpaw and spicebush.

Enter the woods dominated by beech, sugar maple, and ash trees. At the top of the hill, at 0.5 mile, the forest is tulip and sugar maple trees with a high canopy of 70–80 feet. Near the fallen trees, keep an eye out for Carolina wrens, nuthatches, and brown creepers hunting for insects.

At 1 mile you'll pass several red and white oaks. The trail transitions to a mowed path that leads to the road. Cross the road and parking lot and head to the left of the entrance to Hornbeam Nature Preserve, which Red Springs Loop passes through. (Do *not* follow Red Springs Loop at this point.) To get to the Lakeshore Trailhead, follow the mowed path to the right and into the prairie, which is undergoing succession.

The trailhead for Lakeshore Trail is edged with plenty of redbuds and tulip trees. Lakeshore Trail was redesigned in the fall of 1998 due to flooding and beaver activity. Expect to see white-tailed deer as well as the occasional coyote.

At 0.8 mile, follow the trail to the right and enter Hornbeam Nature Preserve. In the cove area at 1.4 miles, cross over the footbridge. The view of the lake is very picturesque from this vantage point.

The trail leads uphill and past several hornbeam trees. At the intersection at 1 mile, follow the Lakeshore Trail to the right. This trail leads to a secluded observation deck. Use the flat stones to cross the stream.

The trail skirts along the edge of the lake. Follow the spur trail at 1.2 miles to the point, where you can enjoy watching waterfowl activity. Return to the main trail to continue on the Lakeshore Trail. Cross the small stream via a footbridge at 1.3 miles.

This area is fairly cool because of the breeze off the lake. Cross the gravel flood-plain at 1.5 miles. If there has been a lot of rain, this spot will most likely be impassable due to flooding.

Over the next 0.1 mile, wild ginger lines the edges of the trail, which leads into another sandy floodplain thick with poison ivy. The trail is extremely eroded. Be exceedingly careful as rolling an ankle is easy on this portion of the trail.

The trail passes through a stand of pine trees. The forest structure then transitions into sugar maple, beech, shagbark hickory, and tulip trees. The trail heads downhill to another stream crossing.

Cross over the footbridge at 1.8 miles in the bottom of a gorgeous valley. It's worth the time to sit and enjoy the serenity.

At 2.1 miles, stairs lead down to an observation deck. Watch your feet over the uneven rise and tread of the steps. Take advantage of the deck to watch and listen for birds. When you are done enjoying the solitude, retrace your steps along the Lake-shore Trail.

When you reach the intersection with the Short Loop at 3.1 miles, take the Short Loop Trail to the right. In 0.1 mile, the trail crosses a stream. This area is littered with fossil-rich flat stones, but don't pick them up. Fossil collecting is forbidden in the state parks and nature preserves.

If you are hankering for a good fossil hunt, the cut-through area along US 27 about 1 mile south of Richmond, Indiana, includes horn coral, brachiopods, cephalo-pods, and crinoids. A cut-through is where the hill has literally been cut through to allow the road to pass through at a safe grade. The cut-through exposes layers upon layers of rocks rich in Ordovician fossils. See the Introduction for more information on fossil hunting.

The Short Loop Trail is a flat and even grass path through the woods. At the next intersection at 3.3 miles, follow the trail straight ahead. In the grassy area, take a left and keep heading left to catch Red Springs Loop at 3.4 miles. Red Springs Loop passes through Hornbeam Nature Preserve—it was the trail you passed by earlier.

Hornbeam Nature Preserve is a dedicated state nature preserve with 81 acres of mixed-hardwood forest, including several large American hornbeam trees. You might know the American hornbeam by some of its more common names: blue beech, musclewood, and ironwood. The bark of the tree is a pale gray-blue and looks similar to striated muscles. Hornbeam Nature Preserve is well known for its spring wildflower display. Your best chance of seeing it is early to mid-spring. The trail skirts the edge of the road for a bit before ducking back into the woods and exit-ing into the parking lot.

Even in the heat of summer, Red Springs Loop through Hornbeam Nature Preserve is a cool retreat. Continue on Red Springs Loop until you reach the parking lot and your vehicle.

Nearby Activities

The Whitewater Memorial State Park is part of the Brookville Reservoir recreational area and offers a wide variety of activities, including more hiking trails. If you are looking for the trail less traveled, try Shrader–Weaver State Nature Preserve or Mary Gray Bird Sanctuary trails near Connersville, Indiana.

GPS Trailhead Coordinates and Directions

N39° 36.181'   W84° 58.265'

From the west side of Cincinnati at the intersection of I-275 and US 27, follow US 27 North 34 miles to Liberty, Indiana. In Liberty, turn left and head south on IN 101. Travel 1.7 miles to the Whitewater Memorial State Park entrance.

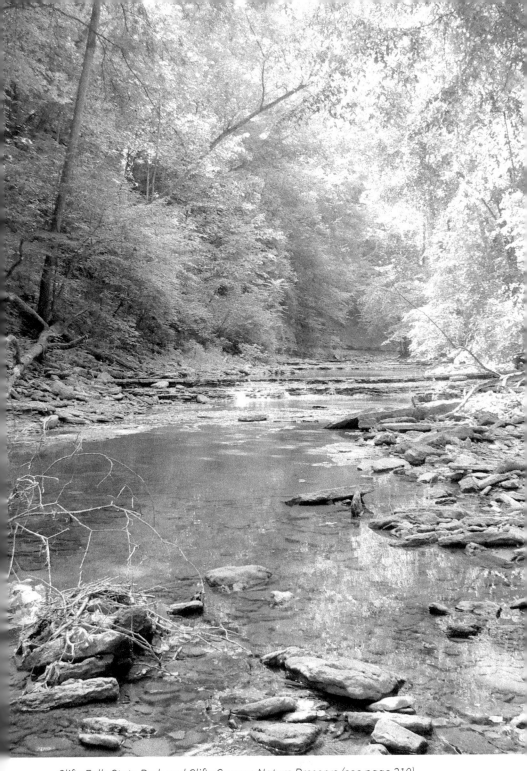

Clifty Falls State Park and Clifty Canyon Nature Preserve (see page 210)

KENTUCKY

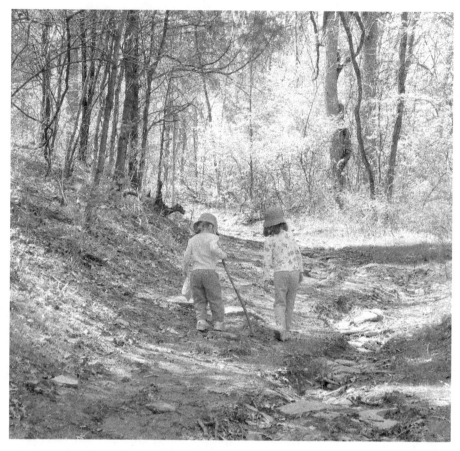

Big Bone Lick State Historic Site (see page 282)

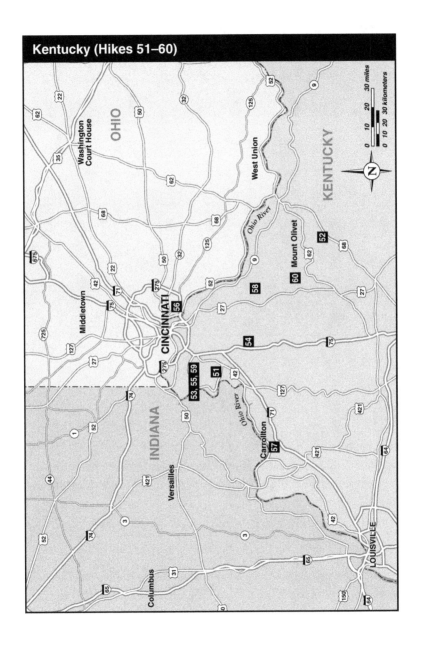

Kentucky (Hikes 51–60)

OHIO

Washington Court House

22
62
50
32
52
125
9
35
62
KENTUCKY
West Union
68
68
Ohio River
Mount Olivet
52
62
68
675
50
9
60
42
22
125
32
58
27
71
275
52
56
27
75
Middletown
54
75
725
127
27
275
53, 55, 59
51
42
74
125
421
50
Ohio River
71
1
52
421
57
421
64
44
Versailles
INDIANA
Carrollton
3
42
52
74
3
75
65
LOUISVILLE
31
65
150
Columbus
65
0
64

0 10 20 30 miles
0 10 20 30 kilometers

N

281

51 Big Bone Lick State Historic Site

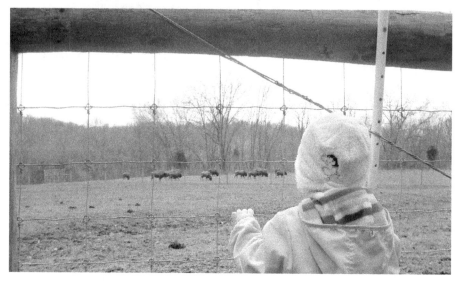

A herd of bison

In Brief

Once tread upon by mastodons, ground sloths, mammoths, and bison, Big Bone Lick offers a chance to take a trip back in time. The museum, outdoor museum, nature center, bison herd, and trails at Big Bone Lick State Historic Site provide glimpses into the unique history of this area.

Description

Once you enter Big Bone Lick State Historic Site, follow the signs to the office and nature center, and park in the lot. Between the nature center and the museum is a large kiosk. Follow the concrete ramp to the large kiosk and take the paved trail down to the loop-shaped Big Bone Lick Creek Trail. When the trail splits, take the trail to the right.

This was known as the Land of Big Bones due to the skeletal remains of mammoths, mastodons, and ground sloths that visited here for the rich mineral springs and swamps, then subsequently perished.

282

LENGTH & CONFIGURATION 5.7-mile loop	**MAPS** USGS *Rising Sun* and *Union;* Big Bone Lick State Historic Site Facilities map
DIFFICULTY Easy–moderate	**WHEELCHAIR ACCESSIBLE** Big Bone Creek Trail
SCENERY Woods, sulfur springs, bison herd, and lake	
EXPOSURE Sun and shaded	**FACILITIES** Restrooms and water in office and museum area
TRAFFIC Moderate	**CONTACTS** Big Bone Lick State Historic Site, 859-384-3522; **parks.ky.gov/parks /historicsites/big-bone-lick**
TRAIL SURFACE Paved, soil, and gravel	
HIKING TIME 3–4 hours	**COMMENTS** The museum has a few fossils, but unfortunately much of the fossil wealth of this area has been lost over time. The bison herd is interesting to watch. You may not have cell phone coverage on portions of this hike.
DRIVING DISTANCE 45 minutes south of Cincinnati	
SEASON Year-round	
ACCESS Daily, sunrise–sunset; free	

Beginning in the 1700s, as news spread around the world about the enormous fossil discoveries in the Land of Big Bones, fossils were removed by the wagonload and the area was slowly picked clean of its unique past. Over a period of 200 years, its history was lost.

People also used this place to collect salt, with early accounts placing American Indians here in the 1600s. In the late 1790s, commercialization of salt manufacturing resulted in as much as 60 bushels of salt per day being manufactured by collecting the water from the springs and boiling it down.

At 0.1 mile from the beginning of the hike, several side trails lead to the springs. In the 1830s–1850s, when epidemics of yellow fever and cholera swept through the Southern states, wealthy Southern families visited and bathed in the foul-smelling sulfur springs for its purported medicinal benefits, making this area a popular tourist attraction.

Cross the bridge over a small stream. This area was affected by vast glacial melt-waters that pushed through the area, creating new waterways.

The paved trail ends and a raised boardwalk begins at 0.59 mile. In the springtime, this portion of the trail is flooded, making it a perfect spot to look for tadpoles.

Continue following the trail until you return to the split. Retrace your steps up the hill and toward the nature center. Directly across from the nature center, up the grassy hillside, and to the right of the enormous oak is the trailhead for Gobbler's Trace/Bison Herd. Cross the road and follow the trail to the right to reach the bison herd. You'll soon enter a clearing with fencing in front of you, and on the other side of the fencing are bison.

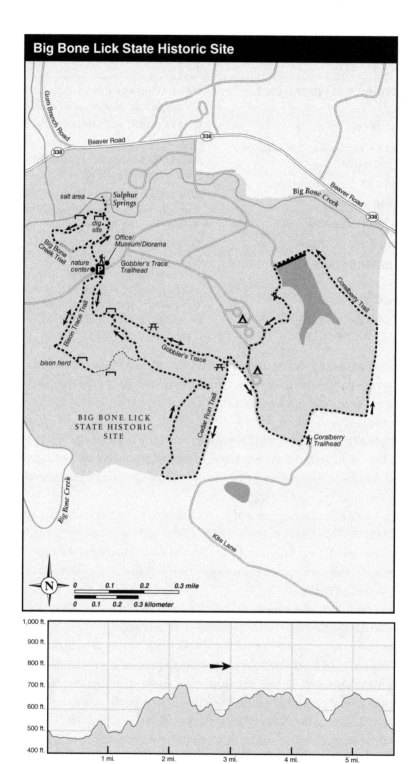

Big Bone Lick State Historic Site

Gum Branch Road

Beaver Road

338

338

Beaver Road

Big Bone Creek

salt area

Sulphur Springs

dig site

Big Bone Creek Trail

Office/Museum/Diorama

nature center

P

Gobbler's Trace Trailhead

Coralberry Trail

Bison Trace Trail

Gobbler's Trace

bison herd

Cedar Run Trail

Coralberry Trailhead

BIG BONE LICK STATE HISTORIC SITE

Big Bone Creek

Kite Lane

N

0   0.1   0.2   0.3 mile
0   0.1   0.2   0.3 kilometer

1,000 ft.
900 ft.
800 ft.
700 ft.
600 ft.
500 ft.
400 ft.

1 mi.   2 mi.   3 mi.   4 mi.   5 mi.

Bison and many other large mammals were once common in the Big Bone Lick area because the minerals, salts, and grasses provided vital nutrients.

After taking your time to watch the bison herd, retrace your steps to the junction with Gobbler's Trace. Follow Gobbler's Trace up the rock-covered path. This portion of the trail is an ankle twister as it leads uphill over several heavily eroded areas. Continue on this trail to a bench in the shade at 1.6 miles. Allow yourself a moment to enjoy the surrounding woods while taking a break. After the bench, continue to the trail intersection at 2 miles; turn right and follow Cedar Run Trail.

This single-person-wide trail parallels the property line as it leads down a steep hill with several large stones, crosses a creek, and then heads back uphill. The trail meanders through the woods, crossing several streams, before reconnecting with the Gobbler's Trace Trail at 3 miles.

Take Gobbler's Trace Trail to the right until it reaches the Cedar Run Trail intersection again. This time, take a left and follow Gobbler's Trace Trail to the campground and the Coralberry Trail.

When you enter the campground, follow along the fence line to the right, pass the footprint of the old water tower, and continue to the Coralberry Trailhead. On Coralberry Trail, keep following the fence line. This forest hosts several species of migratory songbirds; take a few moments to quietly listen to the birdsongs. This is a good spot to practice your skills of attracting birds by using the "pssh" sound.

Follow the main Coralberry Trail that parallels the fence. Avoid taking the side trails. Several portions of this trail are eroded, so be careful not to twist an ankle—you still have a ways to go.

At 4.6 miles the trail crosses the dam. Turn left and cross the dam. At the end of the dam continue straight ahead and immediately turn left after crossing a small footbridge. The trail is parallel with the lake.

Follow the trail (marked with red) slightly uphill on an old access road. Turn left off the access road and cross the footbridge. Enter the upland woods on a small footpath. In springtime, be on the lookout for wildflowers—in summer and fall, poison ivy.

Stay on this trail until it intersects with itself. Take the trail to the right, which will lead you to the campground. Exit the woods near the pavilion. When you reach the road turn left and follow it to the intersection. Turn left and follow the road to the footprint of the old water tower. Follow the trail to the fence line and retrace your steps along Gobbler's Trace Trail to the nature center.

Nearby Activities

Boone Cliffs State Nature Preserve, Middle Creek Park, Dinsmore Woods State Nature
Preserve, and Curtis Gates Lloyd Wildlife Management Area offer more hiking. The
Florence Mall has plenty of shops, plus restaurants to tempt your taste buds.

GPS Trailhead Coordinates and Directions

N38° 53.032'   W84° 45.167'

From Cincinnati, take I-75/I-71 South to Exit 175/KY 338. Turn right onto KY 338/
Richwood Road and follow it 4.2 miles through several turns. When KY 338 joins US
127 South/US 42 West turn left onto KY 338 North/US 127 South/US 42 West and in
0.5 miles, turn right onto KY 338 North/Beaver Road. The entrance is 2.8 miles ahead
on your left.

52 Blue Licks Battlefield State Resort Park

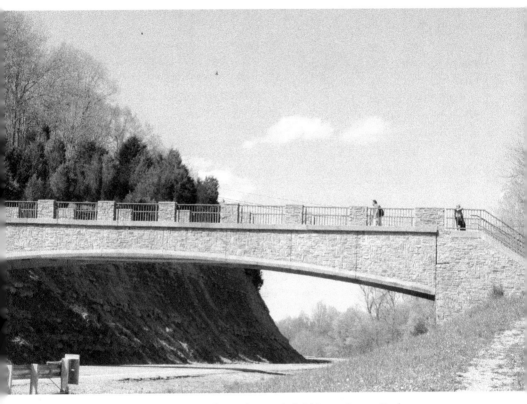

Bridge crossing over US 68 at Blue Licks Battlefield State Resort Park

In Brief

Whether you're a history or nature nut (or both), Blue Licks Battlefield State Resort Park offers excellent hiking trails that lead you through different habitats and also takes you back in time to when battles raged over territory, salt, and freedom.

Description

Kentucky's fifth state park, Blue Licks Battlefield State Resort Park, began in 1927 when local residents donated 32 acres. This ground has seen many battles, including

LENGTH & CONFIGURATION 3.1-mile loop	**MAPS** USGS *Cowan;* Blue Licks Battlefield State Resort Park map
DIFFICULTY Easy–moderate	**WHEELCHAIR ACCESSIBLE** No
SCENERY Woods, prairie, historic sites, and river	**FACILITIES** Restrooms and drinking water at the lodge and near the nature center
EXPOSURE Shaded and full sun	
TRAFFIC Light–moderate	**CONTACTS** Blue Licks Battlefield State Resort Park, 859-289-5507; **parks.ky.gov /parks/resortparks/Blue_Licks**
TRAIL SURFACE Soil, gravel, and exposed stone	
HIKING TIME 3 hours	**COMMENTS** Plan to spend at least 3 hours enjoying the many historical features along the hike. Budget enough time to enjoy a meal at the lodge and explore the Pioneer Museum. Includes Licking River, Savanna Loop, and Heritage Loop hikes.
DRIVING DISTANCE 2 hours south of Cincinnati	
SEASON Year-round	
ACCESS Daily, sunrise–sunset; free	

an August 19, 1782, conflict referred to as the Last Battle of the American Revolution, in which an estimated 70 Kentuckians died. This is also the site of many frontier wars between American Indians and early settlers. More detailed information about the battles waged on this ground is found in the Pioneer Museum and at kiosks along the trails.

After multiple expansions via the Kentucky General Assembly, the park now includes more than 1,000 acres. After you enter the park, follow the signs to the nature center and the Pioneer Museum and Gift Shop. Park in the area directly in front of the Pioneer Museum. Walk west toward the restrooms and concrete staircase and head down the hill to the William J. Curtis shelter.

Directly behind the William J. Curtis shelter house to the south is the trailhead for Licking River Trail. Daniel Boone and pioneers used this area as an escape route after the Battle of Blue Licks. The trail enters a forest of red and white oaks and sugar maple trees. Be careful of your footing over the stone steps and exposed roots.

The trail leads downhill and opens onto a road at 0.23 mile. Turn left and walk along the road. The Licking River is to the right. Pass through the parking lot at 0.4 mile and continue on the Licking River Trail. Cross the bridge over a small creek and continue on the trail uphill through the dedicated nature preserve by following the trail to the left. A meadow is to your right.

At the trail intersection at 0.75 mile, near the campground, follow the Savanna Loop Trail to the right. The nature preserve forest is open hardwoods with sugar maples, oaks, and a few red cedar trees.

Blue Licks Battlefield State Resort Park

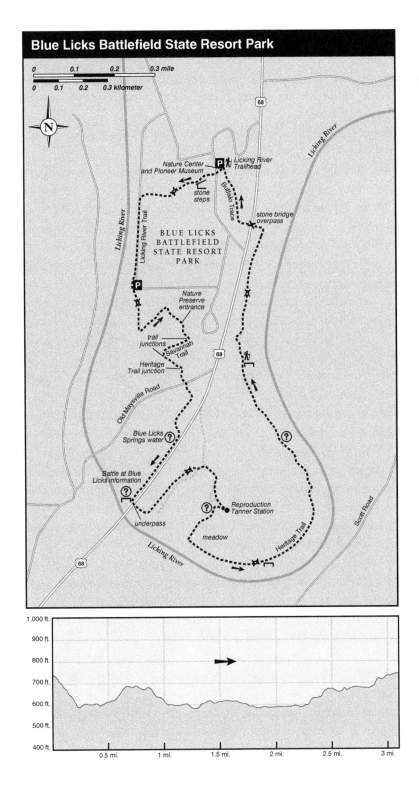

0   0.1   0.2   0.3 mile

0   0.1   0.2   0.3 kilometer

N

68

Nature Center
and Pioneer Museum

Licking River
Trailhead

P

stone
steps

Licking River

Buffalo Trace

stone bridge
overpass

Licking River Trail

BLUE LICKS
BATTLEFIELD
STATE RESORT
PARK

Licking River

P

Nature
Preserve
entrance

trail
junctions

Savannah
Trail

Heritage
Trail junction

68

Old Maysville Road

Blue Licks
Springs water   ?

Battle at Blue
Licks information   ?

?

Reproduction
Tanner Station

?

underpass

meadow

Heritage Trail

Scott Road

68

Licking River

1,000 ft.

900 ft.

800 ft.

700 ft.

600 ft.

500 ft.

400 ft.

0.5 mi.   1 mi.   1.5 mi.   2 mi.   2.5 mi.   3 mi.

Turn left onto the Heritage Trail and out of the nature preserve at the trail intersection at 0.87 mile. Be careful of your footing over the loose stone as you continue on this path heading downhill.

The boardwalk begins at 1.1 miles near Blue Licks Springs. The springs attracted mastodons, ground sloths, bison, and other animals in search of salts.

As they did on the acreage that is now Big Bone Lick State Historic Site in northwestern Kentucky (see previous profile), American Indians and early settlers who lived in this area collected salt by boiling off the water. In the mid-19th century, the water was bottled and used for medicinal purposes. This area was also the home of the Arlington Hotel, where wealthy Southern aristocrats visited during the summer months. By the 20th century, the spring dried up, as did the businesses and tourism that revolved around it.

At 1.3 miles a bench and kiosk await near the location of the historic Last Battle of the American Revolution. Here, Kentucky pioneers unsuccessfully fought an overwhelming force of American Indians and British soldiers. The battle was one of the greatest defeats in pioneer history. Blue Licks Battlefield State Resort Park hosts an annual reenactment of the historic Battle of Blue Licks, as well as demonstrations of American Indian and pioneer life.

Continue on the trail, passing under US 68 and following the gravel path downhill through the red cedars and grasses. Cross the footbridge at 1.5 miles. Head left when the trail exits onto the access road. Turn right when you reach the T-intersection with the gravel access road. Follow this road to the Tanner Station.

The reproduction of the Tanner Station pioneer outpost is impressive. Six-inch-thick cedar trees sunk into the ground create its fortlike fence. Inside the fence structure is a two-story building created with poplar that is open for you to explore. If it is open, be sure to check out the second floor.

This building is representative of trading posts typically found throughout the Licking River Valley. Tanner Station was built over the top of a spring and used to make and store salt. At the time, salt was a much-needed commodity that people would readily kill over; the station was therefore heavily guarded, and the second floor has many vantage points to shoot from.

After Tanner Station, return to the bench and continue to your left on the Heritage Trail. The trail tracks along the edge of the Licking River to the east. The river is easily seen and heard at various locations along the trail.

Continue on the trail into the meadow area with relatively little shade. Cross the footbridge at 1.9 miles, and in 0.1 mile, you'll find a bench to enjoy the view of the meadow and woods. Watch out for the abundant poison ivy growing under the canopy of box elders.

At 2.3 miles, the valley stretches out to the left of the trail. The area near where US 68 crosses over the Licking River is where people and animals have been crossing the river for thousands of years.

The trail leads out of the meadow area and into the woodlands at 2.4 miles. Ohio buckeye, hackberry, and basswood trees shade the path. This is a welcome relief, especially in the summer, from the full sun in the open meadow.

At 2.6 miles are a bench and a trailhead sign near the parking area. Continue on the trail on the north side of the parking area. This is an asphalt path between US 68 and the woods. Cross the footbridge at 2.8 miles.

Head uphill to the stone bridge that allows you to safely cross over US 68. The area to the right is a nature preserve. The endangered Short's goldenrod is located in the park. This rare plant was named after Dr. Charles W. Short, an amateur botanist. It is also the first plant in Kentucky to be placed on the U.S. Fish and Wildlife Service's endangered species list.

At the trail intersection, turn right onto the Buffalo Trace Trail. This trail is the remains of an ancient buffalo path or trace. In fact, most of US 68 in Kentucky and Ohio closely follows the well-worn path of the buffalo.

Follow the stone path under the redbuds. The trail exits the woods near the backside of the nature center. Continue around to the front of the building to the parking area and your vehicle.

Nearby Activities

Quiet Trails State Nature Preserve is indeed quiet and just a few miles north of Blue Licks Battlefield State Resort Park. Blue Licks's Pioneer Museum provides a glimpse into the life and times of the area, including mastodon bones and American Indian and pioneer artifacts. The park also provides an active schedule of events throughout the year.

GPS Trailhead Coordinates and Directions

N38° 25.921'   W83° 59.591'

From Maysville, Kentucky, follow US 68 West for roughly 20 miles to the entrance of Blue Licks Battlefield State Resort Park on the west side of the road.

53 Boone Cliffs State Nature Preserve

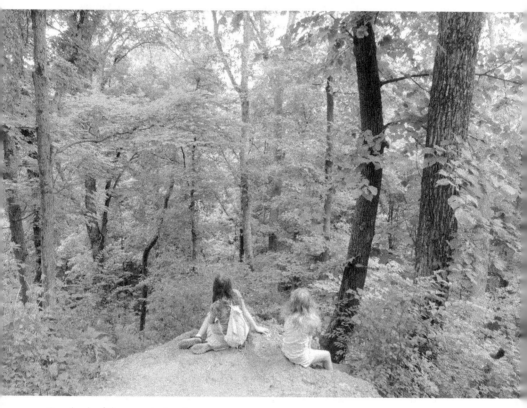

Overlook of the wooded valley

In Brief

Boone Cliffs State Nature Preserve is a fun hike with plenty of geological discoveries as well as incredible woodland overlooks. The trail weaves through the upland forest and provides several places to sit and enjoy the peace of the forest.

Description

From the small parking area, walk uphill toward the large kiosk sign. The narrow trail begins to the left of the kiosk. Boone Cliffs State Nature Preserve encompasses 74 acres of upland woods and incredible conglomerate cliffs.

LENGTH & CONFIGURATION 1.7-mile loop	**SEASON** Year-round
DIFFICULTY Moderate	**ACCESS** Daily, sunrise–sunset; closed during hunting season; free
SCENERY Upland woods, Kansan glacier age conglomerate cliffs, and natural springs	**MAPS** USGS *Rising Sun*
EXPOSURE Mostly shaded	**WHEELCHAIR ACCESSIBLE** No
TRAFFIC Moderate–heavy	**FACILITIES** None
TRAIL SURFACE Soil, exposed rocks and roots	**CONTACTS** Boone County Parks, 859-994-2117, **boonecountyky.org/parks /parkinfo/boonecliffs**
HIKING TIME 1.5 hours	
DRIVING DISTANCE 40 minutes south of Cincinnati	**COMMENTS** The overlook is absolutely incredible, so plan to sit and enjoy the view for a while. No pets are allowed.

The underlying geology was created when the glaciers met an equalization point, which means the glaciers advanced at the same rate that the warmer temperatures melted them. The Kansan-age conglomerate is a sedimentary rock created from the glacial wash deposit of rocks, silt, and minerals. It looks a lot like chunky concrete. Then, glacial meltwaters and (over time) natural springs carved a path through the conglomerate. Farther into the hike is the Boone Cliffs Overlook, which offers a spectacular view of the valley.

Spring-fed creeks flow into Middle Creek, and the wet ground provides a fertile spot for sycamores and ferns to flourish. The fragile habitat and conglomerate cliffs cannot withstand off-trail use, so don't stray from the path.

Shagbark hickory, sugar maple, and elm trees, plus an abundant understory of spicebush, greet you upon entering the woods. Continue on the trail to the edge of the creek, being careful of your step, as the creek has eroded some portions of the trail. In other spots you'll need to make your way around fallen trees. Turn right and enter farther into the calcareous mesophytic (calcium carbonate and well-balanced supply of moisture) old-growth forest.

The trail follows a shelf along the hillside before taking a sharp right and heading up a steep hill over a series of steps created from split logs secured with rebar. Be wary of the occasional orphaned piece of rebar sticking up, ready to grab the toe of your boot.

The trail passes more sugar maple and tulip trees, as well as American hornbeam. Lush spicebush, bright yellow in the fall, carpets the entire area.

At 0.18 mile, the trail leads to the right of a fence and through an area populated by spicebush as well as ash and pawpaw trees. Within 100 feet of the fence is a small grove of pawpaw trees. The fruit of a pawpaw is edible, but because this is a nature

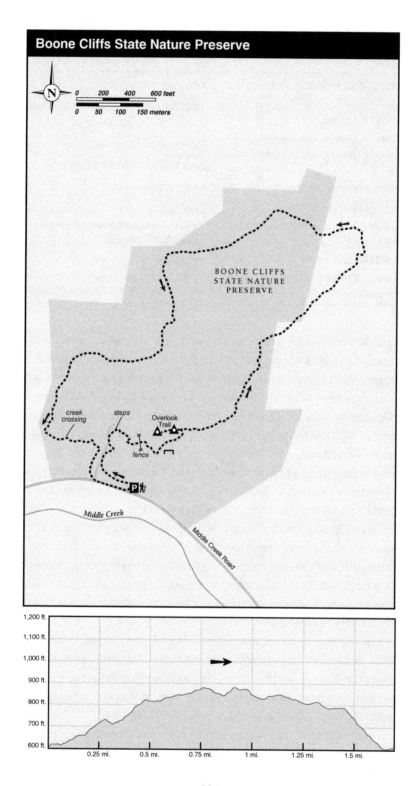

Boone Cliffs State Nature Preserve

0   200   400   600 feet

0   50   100   150 meters

BOONE CLIFFS
STATE NATURE
PRESERVE

creek
crossing

steps

Overlook
Trail

fence

P

Middle Creek

Middle Creek Road

1,200 ft.
1,100 ft.
1,000 ft.
900 ft.
800 ft.
700 ft.
600 ft.

0.25 mi.   0.5 mi.   0.75 mi.   1 mi.   1.25 mi.   1.5 mi.

preserve, you're not allowed to collect the fruit. Pawpaw tastes similar to a banana, which is amazing because the leaves smell like lemon-scented furniture polish mixed with diesel fuel.

Near 0.23 mile you'll see a bench where you can sit, catch your breath, and enjoy the scenery. A little more than 100 feet ahead is the first conglomerate rock outcrop. The concrete-like formation of sedimentary rock has different sizes and types of rocks embedded in it.

When the trail splits at 0.26 mile, follow Overlook Trail to the left to the overlook, a little less than 200 feet ahead. From there, the view of the valley some 60–80 feet below is astounding. Sit and relax as you enjoy the vista through the treetops from this high vantage point. Retrace your steps and keep looking left to the drop-off for more great views.

Back at the trail intersection, continue straight ahead and into a forest with white and red oaks. To the left of the trail is a large ravine. Stay on the authorized trail to the left and pass the closed trail at 0.42 mile.

Beautiful specimens of American beech and sugar maples tower overhead. Watch your step over the exposed roots as the trail leads downhill and into the open woods. At the bottom, massive beech trees shade the forest floor, where ferns flourish in this wet valley. Cavities in the beech trees provide safe nests for squirrels and owls—albeit not in the same hole.

The trail leads back uphill through the forest of beech, tulip, and sugar maple trees. A well-placed bench is located at 0.54 mile. This is a wonderfully quiet spot to sit and enjoy the sights and sounds of the mature woods.

Continue on the one-person-wide trail, passing by sassafras, pawpaw, spicebush, and ferns. In fact, at 0.59 mile, a large grove of sassafras and pawpaw trees crowds the trail. Farther along, you'll pass several black cherry trees near 0.69 mile.

The valley to the left is filled with older sugar maple, tulip, and oak trees with canopies some 60 feet high. Later, you'll see several downed trees at 0.83 mile. This new opening in the canopy allows more sunlight to reach the forest floor. A stiff competition will erupt as the young trees flourish and begin to fight for sunlight and water.

Red oaks, tulip poplars, and sugar maples provide you with ample shade and the songbirds with plenty of cover. The tulip poplars have a distinctive gray-patterned bark and grow straight. Pioneers used tulip poplar for a variety of purposes, including housing construction. While tulip poplar trees were noted to be 190 feet tall and 10 feet in diameter back then, you'd be lucky to find one more than 150 feet tall and 3–4 feet in diameter now. In fact, if you find one, you should contact the appropriate state's big tree registry.

Another bench at 1.1 miles provides a place to enjoy the forest before you head back to your to-do lists. Continue on the trail while enjoying a view of the valley of tulips and box elder trees to the left. At 1.2 miles, the trail passes a black cherry tree. At the top of the hill are several downed trees; this area also will experience a surge of new growth in the next few years.

From the trail, several ridges are visible at 1.3 miles. The views from this ridge line are incredible, especially in the fall when the leaves are vibrant red, orange, and yellow.

The trail leads downhill at 1.4 miles over a series of large steps and exposed roots. It goes around a bend and continues downhill through a forest of sugar maple, syca- more, and chinquapin and white oak trees.

The trail crosses a small creek before exiting onto the road at 1.7 miles. Turn left and walk to your vehicle.

Nearby Activities

For more hiking and history, Dinsmore Homestead and Dinsmore Woods State Nature Preserve, Big Bone Lick State Historic Site, and Curtis Gates Lloyd Wildlife Management Area are great places to visit. For shopping or a bite to eat, head to the Florence Mall.

GPS Trailhead Coordinates and Directions

N38° 59.604'   W84° 47.079'

From Cincinnati, follow I-75 South and take Exit 181. Turn right and head west 5 miles on KY 18 to Burlington. Continue on KY 18 for 6 miles to Middle Creek Road. Turn left onto Middle Creek Road and travel 1.9 miles to the small paved parking area on the north side of the road.

54 Curtis Gates Lloyd Wildlife Management Area

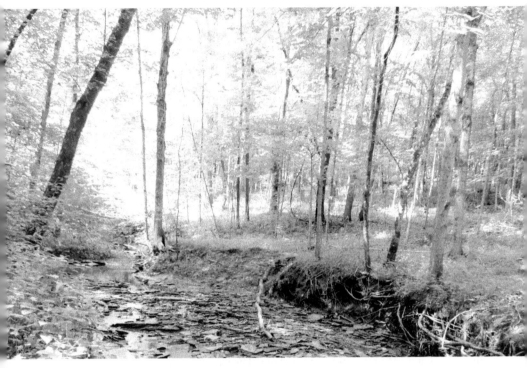

North Fork of Grassy Creek

In Brief

Old-growth forest, ridges, ravines, wildflowers, North Fork Grassy Creek, and a humorous monument await you at Curtis Gates Lloyd Wildlife Management Area. This hike and the incredible forest through which it winds might have been harvested if not for the foresight of Curtis Gates Lloyd, for whom the wildlife management area is named.

Description

Known for being kind as well as quirky, Curtis Gates Lloyd studied mycology (mushrooms) and traveled the world. His research was published in more than 5,000 papers. Lloyd wrote a 24-page will that protects the old-growth forest here and is the reason that we can enjoy walking among such grand trees today.

LENGTH & CONFIGURATION 1-mile loop	**MAPS** USGS *Walton;* Curtis Gates Lloyd Wildlife Management Area map
DIFFICULTY Easy	**WHEELCHAIR ACCESSIBLE** No
SCENERY Hardwoods	**FACILITIES** None
EXPOSURE Shaded	**CONTACTS** Curtis Gates Lloyd WMA, 859-
TRAFFIC Light	428-2262; **tinyurl.com/lloydwma**
TRAIL SURFACE Soil	**COMMENTS** Imagine two tracts of
HIKING TIME 1 hour	old-growth forest that have never been
DRIVING DISTANCE 45 minutes south of Cincinnati	logged. Hiking is permitted throughout the wildlife area, but you should be aware that this area is open to hunting except
SEASON Year-round	for the 250 acres surrounding the ranges,
ACCESS Daily, sunrise–sunset; free	clubhouse, and old-growth woods.

Wildflowers, old-growth trees, and hundreds of bird species fill the wildlife area. You are welcome to hike along any of the dirt roads and wander the woods. Just remember the area outside of the old-growth forest hiking trail, clubhouse, and lake is open to hunting.

The wildlife management area totals 1,179 acres. Included is the 250-acre tract encompassing the clubhouse, shooting ranges, and old-growth forest. Lloyd is quoted as saying, "There has never been an axe to them," and his trust agreement for land stipulates that nothing gets cut or hauled out. The land was originally the Lloyd Library and Botanical Park and Arboretum and, according to his wishes, his final resting spot. When he passed away in 1926, his body was cremated and the ashes were spread over the land.

Curtis Gates Lloyd was the youngest of three brothers. The older brothers, John Uri and Nelson Ashley, were actively involved in the study of pharmacy. All of the brothers owned the Lloyd Brothers Pharmacy. John Uri developed botanical preparations, and Nelson Ashley co-owned the Cincinnati Reds. Nelson Ashley also introduced concrete grandstands.

Curtis Gates's passion was the study of plants. In 1886, when he met local mycologist A. P. Morgan, Curtis Gates focused on the scientific study of mushrooms. He left the family business to travel the world in pursuit of his studies and became well respected for his contributions.

The Lloyd brothers developed the Lloyd Library and Museum in Cincinnati, which is open to the public. Curtis Gates also developed a recreation center in Crittenden.

Curtis Gates Lloyd Wildlife Management Area

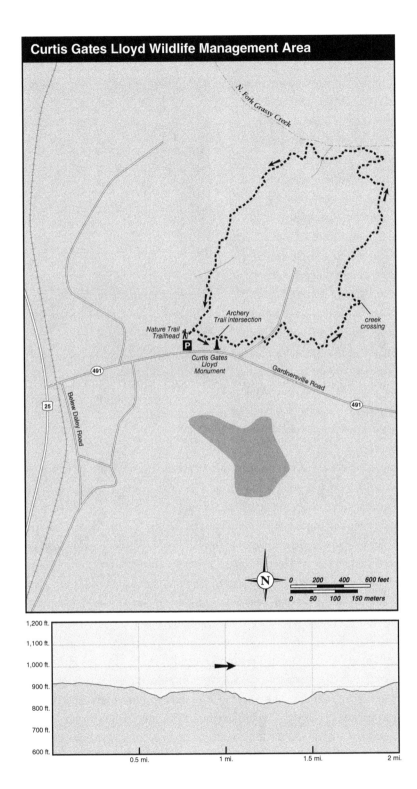

His quirky sense of humor and take on life can be seen along the trail at the monument. The trailhead is at the east end of the large parking area in front of the clubhouse. Walk to the picnic table resting atop of the concrete pad at the edge of the woods. Step onto the trail and into an impressive forest.

The trail leads through one of Kentucky's oldest tree stands. At the intersection 30 feet into the hike, take the trail to the right and up a slight hill. Watch out for stinging nettles during the summer months. When you brush past the plant, sharp, tiny spines covering the leaves and stems penetrate the skin and release histamine and formic acid. The result is an itchy rash relieved with hydrocortisone creams and cool compresses.

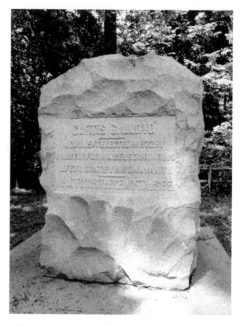

Curtis Gates Lloyd's monument to himself

Stinging nettles also have a long history of medicinal purposes, including pain relief, but before you take matters into your own hands—don't. Consult with a doctor knowledgeable in the field of botanical medicine.

Hackberries and sugar maples dominate the woods. Hackberries are elm trees and easily identified by their characteristic bumpy, corky bark. The trees begin to get much larger in diameter 260 feet into the hike. In the spring, look for the chartreuse-colored leaves of mayapples covering the forest floor. Pass by several large oak trees to the right of the trail. At 281 feet, pass the amphitheater and Archery Trail to the left.

This wildlife restoration area is funded by federal aid through the purchase of hunting equipment. Via the Pittman–Robertson Act, an inherent tax is included on the price of hunting equipment. The funds are collected by the U.S. Fish and Wildlife Service (USFWS), and states can apply for funding for projects under the guidelines of the USFWS Wildlife and Sport Fish Restoration Program. This program has helped restore and protect vital wildlife habitat. The incredible story behind the program is that hunters, state wildlife management agencies, and hunting equipment manufacturers asked to be taxed so the funds could be used to benefit both game and nongame species.

Stay on the trail to the right and head to the large stone monument inside the split rail fence.

The large stone monument between the edge of the trail and the road is an example of Curtis Gates Lloyd's sense of humor and take on life. On the enormous stone is the inscription "Curtis G. Lloyd—Born in 1859–Died 60 or more years afterwards—The exact number of years months and days that he lived nobody knows and nobody cares." On the other side: "Curtis G. Lloyd—Monument erected in 1922 by himself, for himself, during his life, to gratify his own vanity.—What fools these mortals be!"

Continue on the trail behind the monument. Unfortunately, invasive bush honeysuckle is present on this beautiful property. Under the canopy of basswoods, pawpaws, redbuds, and sugar maples, the trail weaves through the woods. At 524 feet into the hike, you'll come up on a hillside filled with wild ginger.

Enter a pleasant stand of trees with a high canopy and lots of wild ginger. Cross over the path and continue on the trail straight ahead. At 0.14 mile, the forest transitions abruptly from one with no understory saplings to one filled with saplings under the canopy of basswoods and sugar maples.

At 0.2 mile, pass the Archery Trail again and follow the Nature Trail to the right. The trees labeled 4, 17, and 19 are white oaks. The trail heads downhill at 0.23 mile. Cross the small ravine at 0.26 mile. Step down the flat stones and cross the creek bed at 0.38 mile.

This area is abundant with birds, and the air is filled with the delightful calls of wood thrushes, woodpeckers, vireos, and more. The labeled trees are red and white oaks and shagbark hickories. A sugar maple sapling arches overhead before the trail heads downhill. Ash, oak, and hickory trees fill this area.

Throughout this section of the hike, grapevine grows into the canopy. At 0.56 mile, you'll see some excellent examples of basswood trees.

At 0.58 mile, the trail curves by large red oak trees. The hillside begins to slope to the right and the trail leads through a ravine dominated by sugar maples. The understory is pawpaws.

At 0.62 mile, tree 10 is a white oak with the characteristic trunk of platy bark with flat patches of bark. Tree 21 at 0.63 mile is a shagbark hickory. A variety of wildlife, including wild turkey, white-tailed deer, and squirrels, relies on the mast (nuts) produced from hickories and oaks.

To the right of the trail is North Fork Grassy Creek. In the creek bed are several deep pools in the oxbows. Quietly watch birds and mammals as they frequent this water source.

Pass the large sycamore tree (at 0.7 mile) on the bank of the creek. The large roots of this tree snake down into the streambed and help stabilize the surrounding soil.

Cross a small steam at 0.72 mile and walk along the floodplain. The creek is to the right, and tracks of raccoons, deer, and opossums are commonly seen along its silty shores. After 0.74 mile, the trail heads uphill among shagbark hickories.

Fragrant spicebush and sassafras trees line the trail at 0.83 mile. Nearby, three tulip trees grow together in a clump. Cross the drainage area at 0.86 mile. Along the edges of the trail are spicebush, sassafras, tulip poplar, and sugar maple trees.

Cross the stream at 0.88 mile. Grapevine crisscrosses over the top of the trail, and at 0.92 mile you'll reach an enormous tulip tree. Continue on the trail, and at the junction turn right and head back to the picnic bench and parking area.

Nearby Activities

Boone Cliffs State Nature Preserve, Dinsmore Homestead and Dinsmore Woods State Nature Preserve, and Kincaid Lake State Park provide more hiking trails through beautiful woods. The Florence Mall area has plenty of dining and shopping opportunities.

GPS Trailhead Coordinates and Directions

N38° 46.371'   W84° 35.987'

From Florence, Kentucky, travel south on I-75 and take Exit 166. Turn east on KY 491. When KY 491 and US 25 join, turn south and travel through Crittenden. After 1 mile, turn east on KY 491/Gardnersville Road, cross the railroad tracks, and turn north into the shooting range/parking area. Park in the east corner near the picnic bench.

55 Dinsmore Homestead and Dinsmore Woods State Nature Preserve

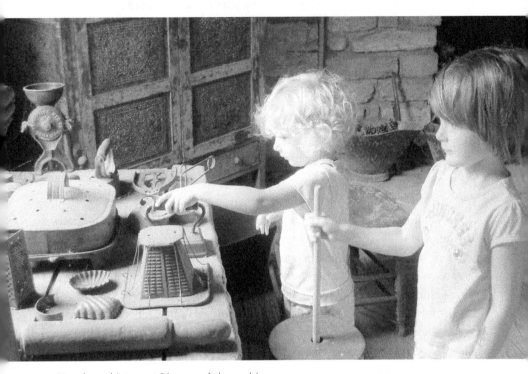

Hands-on history at Dinsmore's log cabin

In Brief

Dinsmore Homestead is also home to Dinsmore Woods State Nature Preserve, which is managed by Boone County Parks. Plan extra time to explore the homestead, cabin, garden, outbuildings, and cemetery.

Description

Dinsmore Homestead is on the National Register of Historic Places. Mrs. Martha Breasted, a Dinsmore descendant, donated this early-19th-century site and the surrounding 107 acres to The Nature Conservancy in 1985.

LENGTH & CONFIGURATION 1.83-mile balloon	**ACCESS** Daily, sunrise–sunset; closed during hunting season; free
DIFFICULTY Moderate, but plan for a rugged hike due to possibility of fallen trees	**MAPS** USGS *Lawrenceburg;* **arcgis.boone countygis.com/flex/BooneParks**
SCENERY Dinsmore Homestead, log cabin, cemetery, forest, and ravines	**WHEELCHAIR ACCESSIBLE** No
EXPOSURE Mostly shaded	**CONTACTS** Dinsmore Homestead, 859-586-6117; Kentucky State Nature Pre-
TRAFFIC Light	serves Commission, 502-573-2886;
TRAIL SURFACE Soil and exposed rocks and roots	**dinsmorefarm.org** or **naturepreserves .ky.gov/naturepreserves/Pages/dinsmore. aspx**
HIKING TIME 2 hours	
DRIVING DISTANCE 40 minutes south of Cincinnati	**COMMENTS** Finding the trailhead and staying on the trail is difficult because trail maintenance is minimal. You'll likely have
SEASON Year-round	to work around downed trees.

The homestead was converted into a museum that provides a glimpse into daily life in the early 1800s. In fact, the museum looks as if you've stepped back in time and are walking through a family's home—and they might just be in the other room. Tours are available Wednesday, Saturday, and Sunday and begin on the hour 1–4 p.m. or by appointment.

More information about the history of the Dinsmore Farm is at **dinsmorefarm .org.** Julia Dinsmore (1833–1926), who inherited the land, kept a daily journal and was a published poet. Her accounts of daily life during this time period serve as invaluable glimpses into the past.

The forest on this property is primarily an unaltered old-growth hardwood forest composed of sugar maple and white ash trees, as well as white, red, Shumard, and chinquapin oaks. This area is also well known for wildflowers in the springtime, including larkspurs, spring beauties, and wood poppies.

Walk behind the home to the log cabin. This is fun to explore with small children, as there are a spinning wheel, cooking implements, and other items from this time period.

Continue walking up the hill behind the home toward the Wine House. The hill-sides were once a well-maintained vineyard during the 1800s and early 1900s. Pass the Wine House and continue uphill through the pawpaw trees and spicebush. At the top of the hill under the canopy of tulip trees are the buffalo clover recovery zone, the Dinsmore Cemetery, benches, and the trailhead for the Dinsmore Woods State Nature Preserve. The cemetery is to the left, surrounded by a stone wall. From the hilltop where the cemetery is, one could see the Ohio River and into Indiana.

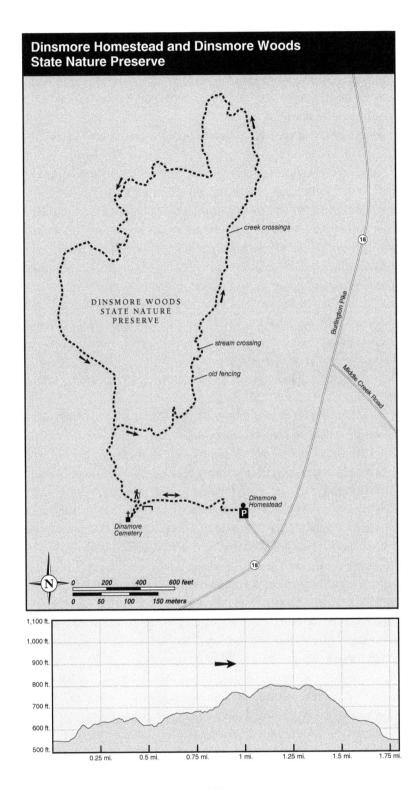

Dinsmore Homestead and Dinsmore Woods
State Nature Preserve

DINSMORE WOODS
STATE NATURE
PRESERVE

creek crossings

stream crossing

old fencing

Dinsmore
Homestead
P

Dinsmore
Cemetery

Burlington Pike

Middle Creek Road

18

18

N

| 0 | 200 | 400 | 600 feet |

| 0 | 50 | 100 | 150 meters |

1,100 ft.
1,000 ft.
900 ft.
800 ft.
700 ft.
600 ft.
500 ft.

0.25 mi.   0.5 mi.   0.75 mi.   1 mi.   1.25 mi.   1.5 mi.   1.75 mi.

The nondescript entrance to Dinsmore Woods State Nature Preserve is to the right, along the edge of the woods. Walk on one of the small footpaths through the tall buffalo clover to the trailhead.

The wood sign for the preserve, near a large, fallen tree, nearly blends into the surrounding area. The trail is directly to the right of the sign. Trail maintenance is minimal, so you may encounter several downed trees on the path. Cross the trees, if it is possible and safe, rather than going off-trail through this fragile habitat.

When you enter the woods, pass through an area of pawpaws and spicebush under a canopy of American beech and some enormous tulip trees. This is a beautiful forest with light trail traffic. If you are seeking solitude, here's your chance to find it—well, except for the occasional airplane noise from the Cincinnati/Northern Kentucky International Airport.

At 0.32 mile, when the trail splits, follow the trail to the right. Watch for the green trail medallions to help stay on the correct trail rather than accidentally following a well-worn deer path.

A multitude of songbirds challenges your identification skills. Listen for red-eyed vireos, chickadees, nuthatches, wrens, and wood thrushes, plus many more. You'll pass both red and white oaks. Some have grapevine growing up into their canopies.

The forest is now composed of tulip trees, a few hickories, and Ohio buckeyes. As the trail leads downhill into a low-lying area at 0.49 mile, basswoods, locusts, sugar maples, hackberries, pawpaws, and spicebush comprise the forest structure. Hackberries, part of the elm family, are easy to identify because of their distinctive bumpy or bubbly looking bark.

At 0.54 mile, the trail heads downhill and appears to end before turning sharply to the left and back uphill. You might need to cross downed trees along this section of the trail. If you can't cross over the top of the tree remember to never go under a fallen tree—the risks are just too great. Evaluate if the root or the crown end is the shortest distance and begin to work around the tree. If you are going along the root end be careful of the hole created from the root ball. Go slowly, always keep the trail in view, and return to the trail as soon as possible. Cross over the stream and take notice of the impressive sycamore trees.

The trail winds along a shelf on the hillside. Sugar maple, tulip, and oak trees cover the hillside to the left, while grapevine covers it to the right. Look for signs of wild turkeys, such as areas on the forest floor that appear to be raked and scat that looks like a curled section of gray-colored caulking with white flecks.

Several honey locust trees are to either side of the trail at 0.67 mile. Pawpaws and sugar maples begin to dominate the forest structure at 0.84 mile.

Reach the flat stone at the top of the hill and continue along the ridge of sugar maple and Ohio buckeye trees. The trail leads into an open, flat area at 1.4 miles, with plenty of hackberry trees. Then it heads downhill through a forest with pawpaw and sugar maple saplings.

When the trail rejoins itself, continue straight ahead. Follow it to the trailhead, then turn left to get to the path that leads downhill to the homestead and your vehicle.

Nearby Activities

Boone Cliffs State Nature Preserve, Big Bone Lick State Historic Site, Fort Thomas Landmark Tree Trail, Middle Creek Park, and Curtis Gates Lloyd Wildlife Management Area are all great places to hike nearby. The Florence Mall area offers plenty of shopping and dining.

GPS Trailhead Coordinates and Directions

N39° 00.046'   W84° 48.788'

From Cincinnati, take I-75/71 South. Take Exit 181/KY 18 West for 11.3 miles. The preserve is on the north side of the road. Turn right and park in the gravel lot.

56 Fort Thomas Landmark Tree Trail

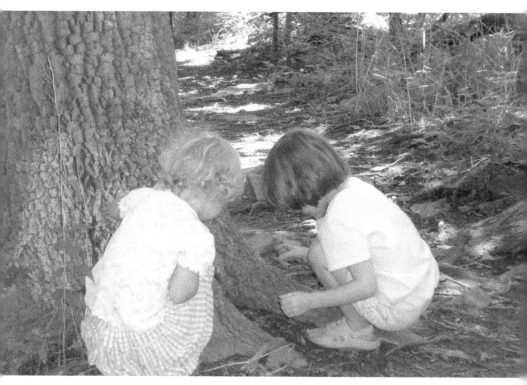

Exploring the leaf litter critters at the base of a tree

In Brief

Located just a few minutes away from Cincinnati, the Fort Thomas Landmark Tree Trail includes trees more than 100 years old. This quiet hike weaves through the ridges and valleys of northern Kentucky.

Description

Fort Thomas was named after General George H. Thomas, who earned the nicknames of the "Rock of Chickamauga" and "Hammer of Nashville" during victorious Civil War battles. Construction of the fort on 111 acres began in 1890 and was completed seven years later.

LENGTH & CONFIGURATION 1.1-mile loop	**ACCESS** Daily, sunrise–sunset; free
DIFFICULTY Moderate	**MAPS** USGS *Newport*; Fort Thomas Landmark Tree Trail map/tree guide available at the kiosk on the trail
SCENERY Oak-dominated forest, ravines, and ridges	
EXPOSURE Mostly shaded	**WHEELCHAIR ACCESSIBLE** No
	FACILITIES None
TRAFFIC Moderate–heavy	**CONTACTS** The City of Fort Thomas, 859-441-1055; **kentuckytourism.com /outdoor-adventure/trail/landmark-tree -trail/99**
TRAIL SURFACE Soil with exposed rocks and roots	
HIKING TIME 1 hour	
DRIVING DISTANCE 30 minutes south of Cincinnati	**COMMENTS** This is a fun hike to take children on to improve their tree identification skills. Some of the hills are steep and eroded and may provide a mildly challenging hike.
SEASON Year-round	

Nearby, at the corner of Douglas Street and KY 1120, is the iconic 90-foot-tall Stone Water Tower, which supplied an average of 15,000 gallons of water per day in the late 1800s. The water tower also serves as a memorial to the 6th Infantry officers and soldiers who fought and died in Cuba during the Spanish–American War. The cannons flanking the tower are from Spanish ships captured in Havana Harbor.

The Fort Thomas Landmark Tree Trail, created in 1993 by the Fort Thomas Tree Commission, boasts several trees that are more than 100 years old. You'll find the trailhead near the bench in the wooded area; the path leads downhill into the forest. Even in the heat of summer, this trail tends to stay cool because of the dense canopy.

Check the kiosk for information, a trail map, and an Updated Tree Trail Information printout. This is a good trail for practicing your tree identification skills as numbered markers identify 14 different species along the trail.

At 166 feet into the hike when the trail splits, go right. At the next trail junction, follow the trail straight ahead. Pass a Shumard oak to the right of the trail at 0.11 mile. The alternate leaves are teardrop shaped and have seven to nine lobes with bristles at the end of each tooth. Along this portion of the hike you'll see a lot of bush honeysuckle. The trail surface is eroded, so be careful of your footing over the exposed rocks and roots.

The trail splits at 0.12 mile near a picnic table. Follow the trail to the left, noting the shagbark hickory trees, which have distinctive peeling bark.

To the left of the trail are several large red oak trees and a fairly open forest floor. The trail heads downhill through a forest dominated by oak trees. Here, stop and listen

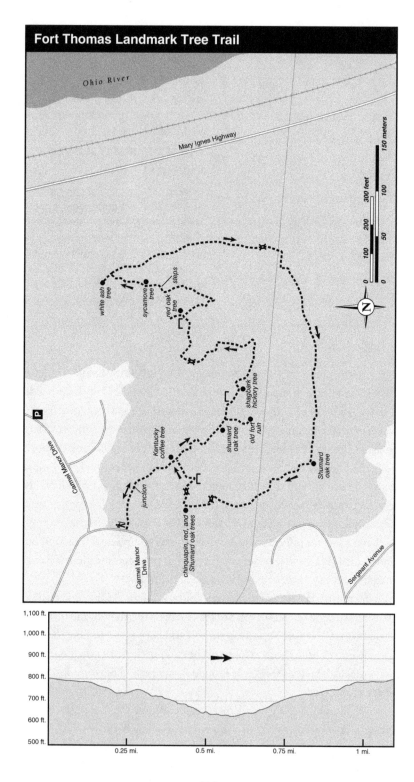

Fort Thomas Landmark Tree Trail

Ohio River

Mary Ignes Highway

150 meters

300 feet

100

200

50

100

N

white ash tree

sycamore tree

red oak tree

steps

Carmel Manor Drive

P

Kentucky coffee tree

junction

shagbark hickory tree

shumard oak tree

old fort ruin

Shumard oak tree

Carmel Manor Drive

chinquapin, red, and Shumard oak trees

Sergeant Avenue

1,100 ft.

1,000 ft.

900 ft.

800 ft.

700 ft.

600 ft.

500 ft.

0.25 mi.   0.5 mi.   0.75 mi.   1 mi.

310

for the songs of various songbirds, such as the red-eyed vireo's "Here I am. Where are you?" or the chickadee's song, which sounds similar to the creaking of a rusty swing.

The trail takes a hard left at 0.19 mile and continues downhill through the forest of white and red oaks, sugar maples, and elms. In spring, trillium, mayapples, and other wildflowers cover the forest floor near the 0.21-mile mark.

Cross a bridge over the small creek at 0.24 mile, in the bottom area. This pleasant woods is open and shaded by basswoods and oaks. The trail leads uphill. At the junction at 0.3 mile, take a break on the bench and a moment to enjoy the tranquility of the woods and hillsides.

Continue on the trail to the right, which leads downhill. At 0.38 mile, pass through a grove of pawpaw trees. Ohio buckeyes provide shade and wild ginger provides ground cover at 0.41 mile. As you head downhill be careful of the T-posts that once secured wood steps. The posts stick up out of the ground and the jagged edges are painted chartreuse to alert you to the danger of tripping. Also, be careful of the occasional wood tie with exposed nails.

Speaking of exposed, this trail is severely eroded in spots, making it difficult to hike over the exposed roots and rocks. Descend the steps at 0.43 mile and pass the enormous sycamore tree to the right of the trail. The tree's hollowed heartwood leaves a large, open area inside its trunk.

Pass through another grove of the odoriferous pawpaw trees at 0.46 mile. The crushed leaves smell like a combination of lemon-scented furniture polish and diesel fuel. Tree 11 at 0.51 mile is a white ash. Ash trees are susceptible to the emerald ash borer, a beetle that has decimated thousands of ash trees in North America and has done significant damage to ash tree populations throughout this region.

The forest is comprised of Ohio buckeye, sugar maple, and red oak trees. Tree 14 is a black walnut, which is unusual to find in the woods except in deep rich soils of bottomlands because black walnut trees prefer to stand alone in the field or yard.

Pass over the roots of the large red oak tree to the left of the trail. At 0.55 mile, cross a bridge by the ravine area to the left. The forest is dominated by sugar maples. In the valley, look for whitewash (owl scat) along the trail; if there is a lot of whitewash, it indicates a place where owls prefer to roost.

The valley area is insulated from urban noise and provides a tranquil retreat. The trail heads uphill at 0.61 mile. Cross the muddy area. The trail parallels the stream's edge.

Along the trail are several rocks with fossils. Pass by the hackberry trees at 0.66 mile and continue uphill over the railroad-tie steps and exposed roots. Cross the bridge to the left and continue up the steps. Be careful, as there are more exposed T-posts in this area.

Be wary of poison ivy growing along the edges of the trail. Cross another foot-bridge at 0.69 mile. The trail leads to the right before it reconnects with the main trail. Follow the main trail uphill to the left.

Pass by the chinquapin oak to the right at the top of the hill and enjoy another chance to sit and peacefully enjoy the beauty of the woods. At the next intersection, follow the trail to the left and retrace your steps to your car.

Nearby Activities

Newport and Covington, Kentucky, offer plenty of shopping and dining opportunities. California Woods Nature Preserve has great hiking trails and an incredible nature center. At Eden Park, you'll find several trails, as well as a reflecting pool, conservatory, and art museum.

GPS Trailhead Coordinates and Directions

N39° 03.802'   W84° 26.481'

From Cincinnati, take I-471 South to Exit 2 and follow US 27 South less than a mile, then turn left onto KY 1120. In 0.5 mile turn right onto River Road/Carmel Manor Drive. Follow Carmel Manor Drive to the entrance drive to Carmel Manor. Do not park on the manor's grounds. The small paved parking area is south of the driveway to Carmel Manor. Park and walk to the trailhead near the bench just inside the edge of the woods.

57 General Butler State Resort Park

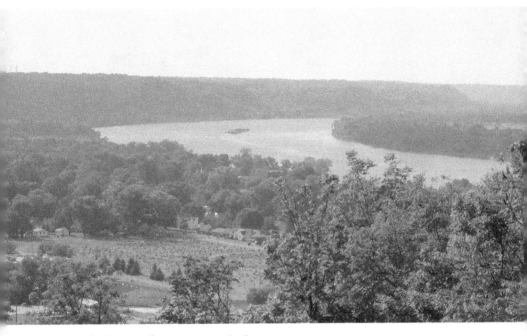

View of Ohio River from stone overlook

In Brief

General Butler State Resort Park offers more than 6 miles of trails through upland forests and a retired ski resort that provides excellent valley views. The Two Rivers Restaurant is an excellent place to grab a bite to eat.

Description

The park was named as a tribute to General William Orlando Butler (1791–1880) and the military history of the Butler lineage. Like his family, General William Orlando Butler was a dedicated public servant who was well known and admired throughout the nation.

He began studying law and then served in the U.S. Army during the War of 1812 against the British and American Indians. His history includes being captured by

LENGTH & CONFIGURATION 6-mile series of loops	**MAPS** USGS *Carrollton;* General Butler State Resort Park map
DIFFICULTY Difficult	**WHEELCHAIR ACCESSIBLE** No
SCENERY Woods and valley vistas	**FACILITIES** Water and restrooms at lodge
EXPOSURE Shade and full sun	
TRAFFIC Moderate	**CONTACTS** General Butler State Resort Park, 502-732-4384; **parks.ky.gov/parks**
TRAIL SURFACE Soil and mowed paths	**/resortparks/General-Butler**
HIKING TIME 3–4 hours	**COMMENTS** The view of the Kentucky and Ohio Rivers from the Stone Overlook is incredible, and the restaurant at the resort lodge is very good. Plus you can burn off dessert on the 6-mile hike up and down hills.
DRIVING DISTANCE 1 hour south of Cincinnati	
SEASON Year-round	
ACCESS Daily, sunrise–sunset; free	

American Indians, being imprisoned by the British at Fort Niagara, and serving as a congressman 1839–1843. In 1844, he received the unanimous nomination from the Democratic Party for governor of Kentucky but lost. He then fought for the United States in the Mexican War. In 1848, he ran for vice president of the United States but suffered another loss. Later, in 1861, Butler served as a member of the Washington Peace Conference, which tried to prevent civil war in America.

General Butler State Resort Park encompasses 791 acres, including a 33-acre lake. The Stone Overlook, built in the early 1930s by the Civilian Conservation Corps (CCC), offers incredible views of the confluence of the Kentucky and Ohio Rivers. Be sure to take advantage of one of the several opportunities to exit the trail and enjoy the breeze at the Stone Overlook.

Enter the park from KY 227 and follow General Butler Road through the park until you reach the left turn leading to the General Butler Mansion. Park and walk toward the mansion. This home now serves as the Butler–Turpin State Historic House. Built in the Greek Revival style in 1859, this antebellum eight-room home is open to the public. Original furniture pieces, military history, and family heirlooms are on display. Call 502-732-4384 for hours of operation. Outside are the Butler Cemetery and several gardens.

The Boy Scout Trail, a connector to the Fossil Trail, begins directly behind Butler–Turpin State Historic House. Immediately upon entering the woods, cross a small footbridge and begin walking uphill over exposed roots, parallel to a small creek. This area is full of white oaks, hackberries, box elders, and several large grapevines.

At 0.28 mile, the Boy Scout Trail crosses General Butler Road and continues uphill. At the trail intersection 470 feet ahead, turn north (left) onto the Fossil Trail

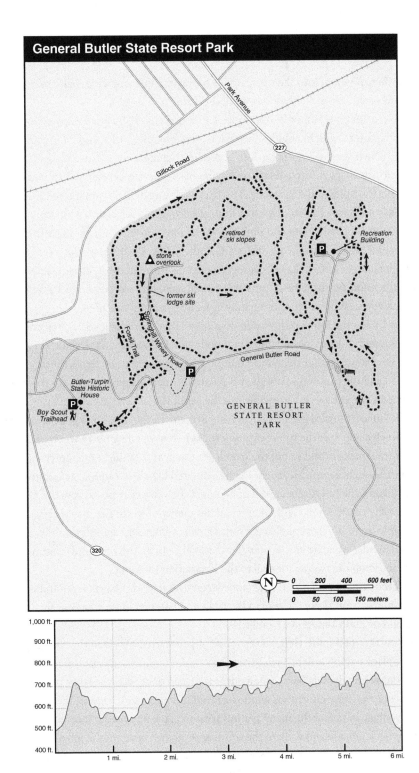

General Butler State Resort Park

Park Avenue

227

Gillock Road

retired ski slopes

stone overlook

former ski lodge site

Fossil Trail

Springhill Winery Road

Recreation Building

P

P

General Butler Road

Butler-Turpin State Historic House

Boy Scout Trailhead

P

GENERAL BUTLER STATE RESORT PARK

320

N

| 0 | 200 | 400 | 600 feet |
| 0 | 50 | 100 | 150 meters |

1,000 ft.

900 ft.

800 ft.

700 ft.

600 ft.

500 ft.

400 ft.

1 mi.   2 mi.   3 mi.   4 mi.   5 mi.   6 mi.

and continue downhill into the open woods of sugar maple and white oak trees. Numerous songbirds make their homes in this forest.

Cross the dry streambed at 0.54 mile. The sounds of the busy roadway echo through the forest, which includes box elders, sugar maples, oaks, and Ohio buckeyes. The trail, which goes down a steep hill, is slick during rain.

The forest changes into a dense collection of shagbark hickories and an understory of sugar maples and dogwoods. The bark of dogwoods (no pun intended) appears dry and cracked, like the earth during a drought. This contrasts sharply with the dogwood's delicate white and pink four-petal blossoms that appear in early spring.

This park was constructed by the CCC in the 1930s. The men working for the CCC built cottages and shelter houses, created trails through the dense forest, and planted trees and shrubs. One impressive accomplishment was creating 33-acre Butler Lake back when labor was predominately done by hand, not machine.

Near 1 mile, the forest is open and dominated by shagbark hickories, red and white oaks, and sugar maples. Amid basswoods and dogwoods on the right, three sycamore trees grow together to create a unique woodland structure. Cross the dry streambed and the trail soon flattens as it passes through stinging nettle, ash trees, and sugar maples with grapevine growing into the canopies.

At 1.3 miles, the trail goes around a hairpin curve to the left and then heads downhill at a steep angle over the top of exposed rocks before opening into a wet meadow.

The trail ducks in and out of the woods for the next 0.2 mile before entering a forest of spicebush, honeysuckle, sugar maples, and red oaks at 1.9 miles. At 2.2 miles, the trail leads downhill to a beautiful open forest. Be wary of exposed roots.

The valley area is lined with ginger and has plenty of white oak, hackberry, and sugar maple trees. A vernal pool at 2.3 miles is full of frogs and tadpoles. At the trail junction 0.1 mile after the vernal pool, leave Fossil Trail on the right and continue straight ahead on the connector trail to the Recreation Building.

Pass the remnants of several old stone structures near the 2.5-mile point, before the trail intersection. Take the trail to the right and enter an open area near the Recreation Building and Conference Center.

Follow the road south (left) to the lodge. If you started hiking in the morning, this is a great place to grab lunch. Two Rivers Restaurant on the lodge's bottom floor offers a filling buffet and dessert bar. Upstairs near the main desk, take the steps up to the large open area where enormous windows provide a panoramic view of the forest. Take advantage of one of the many seating areas to catch up on your journaling.

Step back outside and walk to the south around the corner of the lodge to the Woodland Trailhead. At the intersection follow the trail to your left. The trail is a narrow footpath with strategically placed flat stones over the mucky sections.

At the intersection at 3.2 miles, continue on Woodland Trail to the right. When the trail splits in 0.1 mile, follow the Fossil Trail connector to the left and cross the dry streambed. Cross the service road at 3.4 miles and continue on the Fossil Trail straight ahead.

Enter a forest dominated by shagbark hickories, sugar maples, white oaks, and plenty of honeysuckle. Near 3.5 miles, to the right of the trail is a hillside and valley below. The eroded trail heads back uphill over exposed rocks and roots. Pass the side trails leading to the Recreation Center and continue on the Fossil Trail to the right. Soon, near 3.7 miles, you'll pass several old concrete steps and a building foundation.

The trail comes out on what appears to be an old service road and continues downhill. Pass behind the area where the ski lodge used to sit and, at 4.3 miles, continue following the Fossil Trail by taking the trail to the right.

Ohio buckeyes, white oaks, and sugar maples dominate. Exit the woods at 4.6 miles into an open grassy area. Continue following the mowed trail through the grass while watching for birds of prey overhead.

The trail reenters the woods at 5 miles. Aromatic spicebush lines both sides of the trail, which leads uphill into a sugar maple–dominated forest. At 5.3 miles, when the trail splits, take the path to the right. It edges along a very narrow hillside shelf.

The hillside to the right is nearly straight down, so watch your step. Cross the footbridge at 5.5 miles. At the next trail intersection at 5.6 miles, take the trail to the right and cross General Butler Road at 5.7 miles. Follow the Boy Scout Trail down the hill, past the Butler–Turpin house, and to your vehicle.

Nearby Activities

Need to stretch your legs more to work off those tasty desserts? Clifty Falls State Park in Indiana offers more hills to climb and vistas to view. Plus, in Madison, Indiana, you can find a host of distractions to keep you busy while you are pondering your next adventure.

GPS Trailhead Coordinates and Directions

N38° 40.193'   W85° 09.960'

From Cincinnati, take I-71/75 South and then follow I-71 South. Travel 32 miles on I-71 South to Exit 44/KY 227 Carrollton/Worthville. Turn right onto KY 227 North and follow it toward Carrollton, Kentucky. Travel 1.7 miles to the entrance of General Butler State Resort Park on the southwest side of the road. Turn into the park and follow General Butler Road to the Butler–Turpin State Historic House and park in the lot.

58 Kincaid Lake State Park

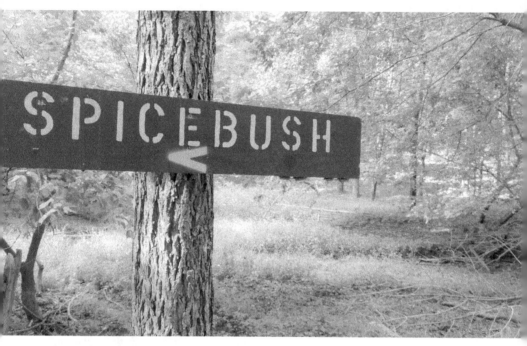

Look for deer bedding in this low-lying area.

In Brief

Kincaid Lake State Park is a wonderful family-friendly park encompassing 850 acres of Kentucky's rolling terrain. Multiple playground areas, a swimming pool, paddleboat rental, a recreation center, campground, and trails offer plenty of recreational opportunities. The 183-acre lake has fishing opportunities for both avid and novice anglers.

Description

Kincaid Lake State Park is located in the rolling hills of northern Kentucky. Enter the park and follow the road to the recreation center, which provides programming from Memorial Day to Labor Day. Programs include crafts and outdoor fun and games. Additional activities include a wide variety of playground equipment and a miniature golf course.

To begin the hike, follow the paved path to the right of the basketball courts from the recreation center. The trail enters a forest dominated by eastern red cedar trees.

LENGTH & CONFIGURATION 3.3-mile series of loops	**ACCESS** Daily, sunrise–sunset; free
DIFFICULTY Moderate	**MAPS** USGS *Falmouth*; Kincaid Lake State Park map
SCENERY Woods and streams	**WHEELCHAIR ACCESSIBLE** No
EXPOSURE Shaded	**FACILITIES** Restrooms and water at recreation center
TRAFFIC Moderate	
TRAIL SURFACE Soil with exposed rocks and roots	**CONTACTS** Kincaid Lake State Park, 859-654-3531; **parks.ky.gov/parks /recreationparks/Kincaid-Lake**
HIKING TIME 1.5–2 hours	
DRIVING DISTANCE 1 hour south of Cincinnati	**COMMENTS** This family-friendly park offers lots of activities to keep everyone engaged.
SEASON Year-round	

Follow the trail to the small shelter house at 0.16 mile. Pass through the shelter house and descend the steps. At 0.17 mile, when the trail intersects with another trail, take the trail to the right.

As the trail heads downhill, the forest transitions from a red cedar–dominated forest to hardwood forest with red and white oak, sugar maple, and hickory trees. When the trail reaches the bottom area at 0.26 mile, take the trail to the right, following the waterway.

Shagbark hickories dominate this portion of trail. The wetland area is located to the left of the trail at 0.28 mile. Along this portion of trail, keep an eye out for whitewash on the ground. This is an indication of owls in the area. Look at the nooks and crannies of the large white oak trees and see if you can spy one of the many large nests created from sticks. Owls are protected by the U.S. Fish and Wildlife Service, as well as by state laws. You're not allowed to collect any feathers, including the ones shed by the owls.

The trail heads uphill at 0.29 mile and the forest transitions back to red-cedar forest at 0.31 mile. At the intersection just down the hill from the shelter house you passed through earlier, turn right and take the trail back downhill. This time at the trail intersection in the bottom area at 0.35 mile, turn left near the stream. Follow the trail along the valley of hardwood forest.

The stream flows to your right, and a high canopy of sugar maple, Ohio buckeye, white oak, and shagbark hickory trees shade the trail. To the left is a hillside with several drainage areas flowing into the creek.

At 0.4 mile you'll reach a suspension bridge near the trailheads for the Ironwood and Spicebush Trails. Cross the bridge to follow the Spicebush Trail to the left. At this

Kincaid Lake State Park

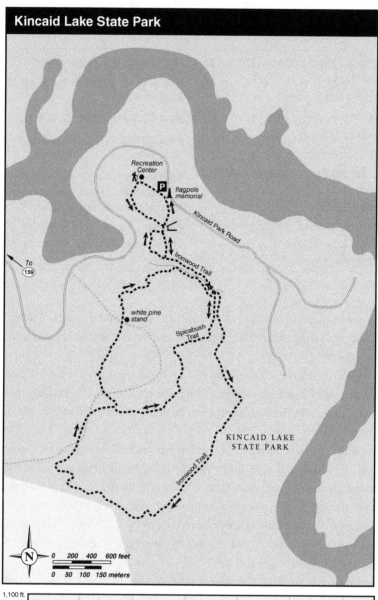

Recreation Center

P flagpole memorial

Kincaid Park Road

To 159

Ironwood Trail

white pine stand

Spicebush Trail

KINCAID LAKE STATE PARK

Ironwood Trail

N

0 200 400 600 feet

0 50 100 150 meters

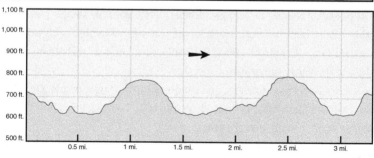

1,100 ft.

1,000 ft.

900 ft.

800 ft.

700 ft.

600 ft.

500 ft.

0.5 mi. 1 mi. 1.5 mi. 2 mi. 2.5 mi. 3 mi.

point a small creek will be to your left. Spicebush is a small footpath that meanders through the woodland area.

Large sycamore, elm, and Ohio buckeye trees, as well as enormous ropes of grapevine, bracket the trail. Two drainage areas combine to form the creek at 0.47 mile. Keep watch for white-tailed deer throughout this hike.

The trail takes a hard left at 0.53 mile and climbs over an eroded hillside for almost 0.1 mile. As the trail continues uphill, the hardwood forest transitions from sugar maples and oaks to eastern red cedars. The trail surface changes from soil and exposed rocks to a mowed grass path at 0.62 mile.

The trail intersects with the connector to Ironwood Trail and the continuation of Spicebush Trail at 0.76 mile. Follow Spicebush Trail to the right. Spicebush and Ironwood are looped trails. This portion of the trail is a grass-covered, vehicle-wide pathway through a relatively flat area. You'll see a few shingle oaks mixed in among the red cedars during this portion of the hike.

At the end of the roadway, the trail enters a planted white pine stand at 0.94 mile. The path leads downhill and in 0.1 mile turns right and leads into an upland forest of sugar maple, white oak, and red oak trees.

Keep following the trail to the right. As the trail heads downhill and gets closer to the waterway, spicebush covers the hillsides. The trail reaches the creek and follows the streambed to the bridge at 1.19 miles. Cross the bridge and this time proceed on the Ironwood Trail to the left of the bridge.

This is a single-person-wide footpath through the woods. In summertime, expect the edges of the trail to be lined with stinging nettles. The canopy trees are predominately Ohio buckeye, sugar maple, shagbark hickory, and white oak.

You'll come upon several small waterway crossings near the 1.3-mile mark. The trail leads uphill and into a younger forest, then heads downhill for about 100 feet to the creek, which it parallels before crossing it at 1.47 miles.

The trail leads back uphill. If you like ironwood (also known as American hornbeam or musclewood), then you're in for a treat at 1.74 miles because there's a small grove of ironwoods before the trail heads downhill.

The trail crosses the creek at 1.9 miles and enters a red-cedar forest. Continue following the trail to the right until it connects with the Spicebush Trail at 2.51 miles. Turn right and follow the Spicebush Trail downhill.

In the flat bottom area, continue following the trail as it turns right and parallels the stream. The forest is once again dominated by white oaks. Cross the bridge again at 2.64 miles.

Take the trail to the left and retrace your steps to the shelter house. Pass through the center of the shelter house and continue on the small footpath uphill. This leads into a mowed open area. Walk to the flagpole memorial. Then proceed to the parking area and your vehicle.

Nearby Activities

Florence Mall is a favorite shopping and dining location. Curtis Gates Lloyd Wildlife Management Area, Quiet Trails State Nature Preserve, and Blue Licks Battlefield State Resort Park offer additional hiking and wildlife-viewing opportunities.

GPS Trailhead Coordinates and Directions

N38° 43.473'   W84° 16.981'

From Cincinnati, take I-471 South to exit onto US 27 South. Drive south on US 27 for 19 miles, then turn east (left) on KY 177. Follow it for 4 miles and turn right onto KY 159. Travel 4.8 miles to the entrance of Kincaid Lake State Park on the left.

59 Middle Creek Park

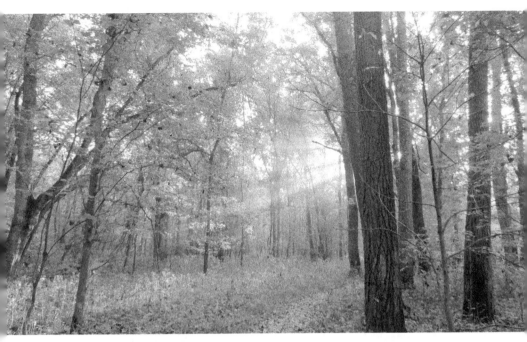

Early-morning hikers see more wildlife and fewer people.

In Brief

Hilly terrain will get your heart pumping. Escape from the chaos of daily life is granted, as there is virtually no cell signal. Enjoy this trek with a friend, as going solo is not a good idea. Due to an abundance of deer and old access trails, bring along a copy of Boone County Parks' Middle Creek map to aid in navigation.

Description

Do not do this hike solo. The hike is in an area with almost no cell signal and plenty of opportunities to get lost or roll an ankle. Even if you hike with a friend, let someone else know your plan and when you expect to return. Do not do this hike during hunting seasons, as private lands surround the park, and the park is closed then.

You must pay careful attention to where you are in the park. Print and bring a copy of the Middle Creek Park's map for added reference. Due to the rugged nature of the hike, as well as deer and old access trails that aren't on the map, people do get lost in this park.

LENGTH & CONFIGURATION 5.3-mile loop	**ACCESS** Daily, sunrise–sunset; closed during hunting season; free
DIFFICULTY Difficult	**MAPS** USGS *Rising Sun;* **boonecountyky**
SCENERY Forest and creeks	**.org/parks/ParkInfo/MiddleCreek/Middle**
EXPOSURE Mostly shade	**Creek.pdf**
TRAFFIC Light. Share the trails with horse riders.	**WHEELCHAIR ACCESSIBLE** No
	FACILITIES Latrine
TRAIL SURFACE Soil, exposed rock, gravel, and mowed	**CONTACTS** Boone County Parks, 859-334-2117; **boonecountyky.org/parks**
HIKING TIME 5–6 hours	**/ParkInfo/10**
DRIVING DISTANCE 40 minutes from Cincinnati	**COMMENTS** Limited to no cell phone reception. To help with navigation, bring
SEASON Year-round	the map from Middle Creek Park as well.

Now that we have all the scary bits out of the way, let's hike!

Middle Creek Park opened in 1993 and is comprised of 230 acres of forest with plenty of hills to climb and creeks to cross. To begin hiking, look for the entrance with the large sign. A gravel trail leads into a fairly dense forest of sugar maples and tulip poplars with ample grapevine.

Take Trail 1 down the railroad-tie steps. As you enter the valley area, a forest of white and chinquapin oaks, sycamores, and sugar maples begins to surround you and block out the ruckus of civilization.

Follow the main trail as it heads east, paralleling the creek to your right. Pass the horse trail that turns to the left; it leads back to the parking lot. Be careful of your footing around the walnuts along this section of the trail.

At 0.3 mile, enormous sycamore trees mark the point at which you cross the creek. The bench is a good place to sit and take in the peaceful surroundings. Do not continue on Trail 1, which splits to the right and left. Instead, follow Trail 6 uphill to the aptly named Mud Road. Pass Trail 4 and follow Trail 6 by taking a modest right and continuing straight ahead. If it has recently rained, expect plenty of mud.

Continue uphill over the exposed rocks and roots. Cross the small creek at 0.6 mile. Aromatic spicebush and pawpaws are shaded under a canopy of sugar maples, cottonwoods, and elms.

At the Trail 1 connection, turn right onto Trail 1. The trail levels off and heads downhill into a gorgeous forest of sugar maples, tulip poplars, and white oaks. Follow the hairpin turn at 1.26 miles to stay on Trail 1. (Do not take black Trail B.)

The open forest provides plenty of beauty to enjoy. Grapevine curls into the canopies while songbirds chatter amongst themselves. Pick your way carefully down the

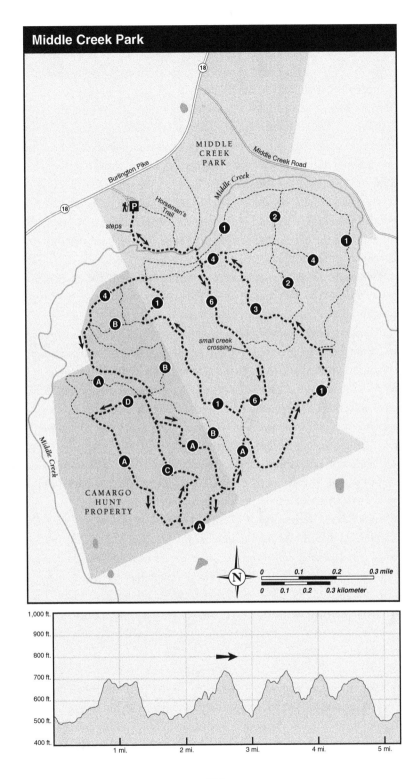

Middle Creek Park

MIDDLE
CREEK
PARK

18

Middle Creek Road

Burlington Pike

18

Middle Creek

Horseman's Trail

P

steps

1

2

1

4

4

4

2

1

6

3

B

1

small creek
crossing

B

A

6

1

D

B

A

A

A

C

A

CAMARGO
HUNT
PROPERTY

Middle Creek

A

N

0   0.1   0.2   0.3 mile

0   0.1   0.2   0.3 kilometer

1,000 ft.
900 ft.
800 ft.
700 ft.
600 ft.
500 ft.
400 ft.

1 mi.   2 mi.   3 mi.   4 mi.   5 mi.

hillside over the exposed rocks and roots. Be extra careful in the fall when leaves are on the compacted clay soil; it will be slick.

At the intersection at 1.42 miles, follow Trail 4 to your left and walk along a row of Osage orange trees. Sold as natural fencing, the saplings would be planted a foot apart and the branches woven together. This created a formidable barrier of thorny branches that grew thicker and stronger with each passing year. Due to the strength and beauty of the orange-colored wood, it also has a long history of being utilized for bows.

Over the next 0.2 mile, the trail passes through a stand of red cedar before exiting on the edge of a field. Turn left and walk along the edge of the woods. Pass by Trail 1 and continue along the edge of the property. To your right will be several clumps of red cedars and to your left the forest.

Continue walking this edge as it curves around to the right and heads downhill. When you reach the trail deeply rutted with the hoofprints of horses, turn left to follow it into the woods. This the yellow Connector Trail.

At 1.8 miles the trail weaves by the large fallen tree and edges closer to the creek. Continue on the trail as it pulls away from the creek. Step over the small drainage crossing and in less than 60 feet you reach an intersection. Turn right, go down the steep hill, cross the creek, go up the hill, and when you reach the larger trail (purple Trail A) turn left. At the 2-mile mark is the junction with Trail C; stay on Trail A to the left.

Take your time hiking along this serene trail. Turn right when the purple Trail A splits at 2.36 miles. Be wary of user-made trails. Stay on Trail A until you reach the gray Trail C junction at 2.6 miles; turn right and follow Trail C. The trail flattens out for a little bit for a nice break. At 2.72 miles Trail C takes a sharp left and heads down the steep hill. Watch your footing over the rocks.

In 0.2 mile, Trail C connects with Trail A. Follow Trail A straight ahead. Continue on the purple Trail A as it leads uphill. Pass the intersection with the Connector Trail that you came in on earlier and at the next intersection turn left onto the hunter green Trail D. At the trail junction with Trail A, turn left and follow Trail A.

The trail follows the ridgeline and then starts to head slowly downhill over a grass-covered path surrounded by tulip poplars, spicebush, sugar maples, and elms. Walk quietly and slowly along the edge of the trail and you'll likely surprise a flock of turkeys feeding in the grass.

When you reach the fence and gate you passed earlier for gray Trail C, make sure you pass through the gate to continue following purple Trail A to the right. When the purple Trail A splits at 3.78 miles, follow the trail to the right and cross the creek.

In 0.1 mile, pass the intersection with the black Trail B and continue following purple Trail A to the right. At the intersection with the blue Trail 1 in 0.1 mile, turn right and continue on blue Trail 1. Pawpaws line both sides of the trail under a canopy of sassafras, cottonwood, and basswood along this ridgeline trail.

Listen for the occasional stomp and snort of a white-tailed deer amid melodies of songbirds. Due to the horse traffic, portions of this trail are, for lack of a better term, choppy. The trail takes a sharp curve as is heads into a valley with red and white oaks, tulips, and sugar maple.

Climb the hill and take a break on the bench. Continue on the trail to the left labeled TO TRAIL 2 AND TRAIL 3. Pass the pond to the left and look for snakes, turtles, and frogs. Stay on Trail 3 passing the connector trail and Trail 2.

In 0.2 mile, the trail begins to descend. Watch for deer along this portion of the trail. When you reach the T-intersection with Trail 4, turn left and follow it along the edge of an old fenced roadway.

When you reach Mud Road and the intersection with Trail 1, take a right and in a few feet you'll see Trail 1. Retrace your steps back to your vehicle from this point.

Nearby Activities

Florence Mall and the Field & Stream store are right off of I-71/75. Looking for more hikes? Dinsmore Homestead and Dinsmore Woods State Nature Preserve and Boone Cliffs State Nature Preserve are also owned and managed by Boone County Parks and are literally across the road from Middle Creek Park. Big Bone Lick State Park has more leg-stretching opportunities.

GPS Trailhead Coordinates and Directions

N38° 59.872'   W84° 48.868'

From Cincinnati, take I-75/71 South. Take Exit 181/KY 18 West for 11.3 miles. The Middle Creek Park entrance is on the south (left) side of the road. Turn left and park in the gravel lot.

60 Quiet Trails State Nature Preserve

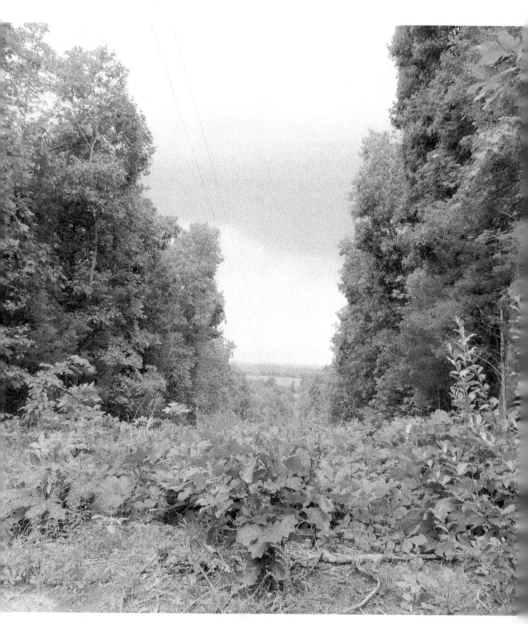

Beautiful vista at Quiet Trails right before the pond loaded with frogs

LENGTH & CONFIGURATION 1.9-mile balloon	**MAPS** USGS *Claysville*; Quiet Trails State Nature Preserve brochure
DIFFICULTY Moderate	**WHEELCHAIR ACCESSIBLE** No
SCENERY Woods, prairie, and river	**FACILITIES** None
EXPOSURE Shaded and full sun	
TRAFFIC Light	**CONTACTS** Kentucky State Nature Preserves Commission, 502-573-2886; **naturepreserves.ky.gov/naturepreserves** **/Pages/quiettrails.aspx**
TRAIL SURFACE Soil and mowed paths	
HIKING TIME 1.5 hours	
DRIVING DISTANCE 1.5 hours southeast of Cincinnati	**COMMENTS** Quiet Trails State Nature Preserve is a remote nature preserve that truly offers an opportunity to get away from it all.
SEASON Year-round	
ACCESS Daily, sunrise–sunset; free	

In Brief

Nestled into the rugged hillsides of Kentucky, Quiet Trails State Nature Preserve has more than 3 miles of trails that lead through woodlands as well as prairies. Trails cross over the top of the Kope Formation of Ordovician shales and limestones.

Description

Quiet Trails State Nature Preserve officially began in 1991 when Bill and Martha Wiglesworth donated 110 acres of land to the Commonwealth of Kentucky. During the 20 years the Wiglesworths owned the land, they actively worked to restore the natural land by planting native wildflowers, grasses, and trees. The purchase of an additional 55 acres of adjacent fields and forest brought Quiet Trails State Nature Preserve to a total of 165 acres of wooded hillsides, open prairies, and Licking River vistas.

Numerous butterflies, white-tailed deer, wild turkeys, chipmunks, squirrels, songbirds, snakes, turtles, frogs, and other wildlife are part of the mosaic of life that abounds in the solitude of Quiet Trails. In fact, more than 130 species of birds, 98 species of trees, and 100 species of wildflowers have been identified in this area.

Park in the lot, secure your vehicle, and at the north corner of the fence, look for a small pass-through near the padlocked gate. Be careful of the poison ivy around the base of the fence as you squeeze through and enter the trails.

Immediately, several trails intersect. Follow the Challenger Trail, a wide and deeply set trail (it feels more like an old roadbed), into the woods. You will see plenty of side trails throughout this hike—ignore them.

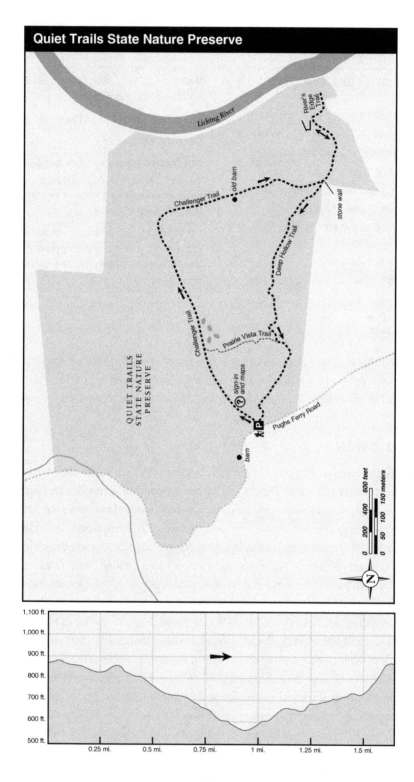

Quiet Trails State Nature Preserve

Licking River

River's Edge Trail

old barn

Challenger Trail

stone wall

Deep Hollow Trail

Challenger Trail

Prairie Vista Trail

QUIET TRAILS
STATE NATURE
PRESERVE

sign-in
and maps

Pughs Ferry Road

barn

600 feet
400
200
0

150 meters
100
50
0

N

1,100 ft.
1,000 ft.
900 ft.
800 ft.
700 ft.
600 ft.
500 ft.

0.25 mi.   0.5 mi.   0.75 mi.   1 mi.   1.25 mi.   1.5 mi.

The number of trails has been reduced, and you'll notice makeshift blockades of large limbs barring your access. However, also be aware that at some points along this trail you will need to go over or around fallen trees.

I highly recommend going around fallen trees or at least jumping far from the edge of a downed tree so as to avoid angering any snakes that may have tucked up under the curved edge.

Pass the sign-in and kiosk area with information about the variety of snakes that call Kentucky home (timber and pygmy rattlesnakes, copperheads, and cottonmouths) and don't bother opening the mailbox unless you want to see some spiders skitter about.

Overhead, songbirds and dragonflies zip by, while on the ground slower-moving critters enjoy the warm sunlight. Watch for box turtles (slow-moving rocks). Box turtles live on land and have very high, domed shells with dark brown and yellow colorations. Male box turtles typically have red eyes and a concave abdomen, while female box turtles have yellow-brown eyes and a nearly flat abdomen.

Stay on Challenger Trail, and after passing under the power lines, look to the right for the pond. Slowly and quietly sneak up on the ponds' inhabitants. You'll likely see bullfrogs and green frogs as well as the occasional turtle.

Expect to see multiple signs of turkeys, including feathers, scratching marks on the ground, and the characteristic cylindrical white-gray scat, which is shaped like the letter "J" or a question mark.

Watch for the distinctive large, mitten-shaped leaves of sassafras. Plenty of sassafras saplings fill the woods in the low-lying areas. Pioneers dug up the roots of sassafras trees, cleaned off the dirt, and steeped the roots in hot water to create a spring tonic to clarify their blood. In fact, the sassafras flavor was used to create the drink sarsaparilla, which was the inspiration for root beer. Sassafras leaves are dried and ground into a fine dust called filé powder, which is commonly used in Cajun cooking.

Continue on the Challenger Trail over an old stone access road. Enter a stand of red cedars and then pass by the barn on the right side of the trail. Don't risk your safety by entering the dilapidated structure.

At the intersection with Deep Hollow Trail at 0.8 mile, continue on Challenger Trail downhill to your left. Pass the stone wall and spur trail, as well as the old outbuilding, shelter house, and well. Look for delicate blue larkspur along the edges of the trail before reaching the large grassy area.

The Challenger Trail transitions with little fanfare to the River's Edge Trail. Follow the River's Edge Trail downhill. Sounds of the river percolate through the woods. The Licking River is soon visible.

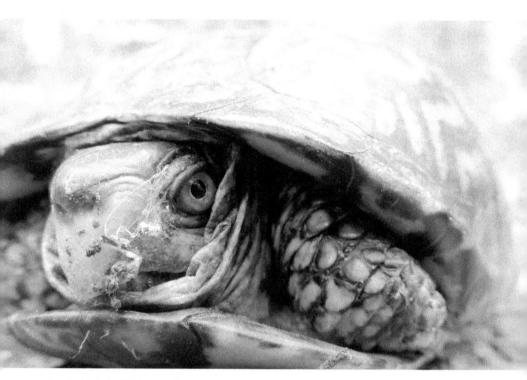

Box turtle is lookin' at you!

At the end of the trail, turn around and retrace your steps to Challenger Trail. Be sure to bypass the two spur trails near 1.9 miles and stay on Challenger Trail by following it uphill. You'll spot an old, vertically stacked stone wall near 2.1 miles. This wall is easier to see on your way back up the hill.

Immediately after the stone wall, you'll reach the intersection with Deep Hollow Trail, which you'll take to the left and follow through the upland woods of sugar maple and basswood trees. You'll be passing by several old trail connections. For the most part these are marked "closed" simply by the piles of limbs and logs.

The Deep Hollow Trail follows along a shelf in a beautiful forest comprised of red and white oaks, sugar maple, and hickory trees. At 1.4 miles, step across the creek on the flat stones.

Take your time along the Deep Hollow Trail to enjoy the serenity of this mature forest. The creek bed and hillsides are filled with moss-covered rocks and fallen trees.

On the left side of the trail, watch for the bridge to nowhere. The trail heads uphill and through a small grove of pawpaws and redbuds. Stay on the Deep Hollow Trail by staying to your left at the connection with the Prairie Trail. At 1.8 miles, pass under the power lines. You'll soon see the fencing that surrounds the parking area. Be careful of poison ivy as you make your way around the fence and back to your vehicle.

Nearby Activities

Blue Licks Battlefield State Resort Park offers reenactments, plenty of history, a lodge, a great restaurant, a campground, and wonderful trails. To the south is Buffalo Trace Preserve, owned by The Nature Conservancy (TNC). You must have permission from TNC to visit this preserve.

GPS Trailhead Coordinates and Directions

N38° 33.416'   W84° 13.631'

From Cincinnati, take I-471 South to Exit 1A/US 27 South. Follow US 27 South 39 miles. Turn left onto KY 1284/Sunrise–Richland Road. Travel 2.7 miles to the four-way intersection in Sunrise. Pughs Ferry Road is straight ahead. Pughs Ferry Road turns left in 0.7 mile and left again in 0.5 mile. After the last turn, travel 0.7 mile; the gravel parking area is on the right.

Appendix A: Outdoor Shops

Bass Pro Shops

basspro.com

300 Cincinnati Mills Dr.
Cincinnati, OH 45240
513-826-5200

Benchmark Outfitters

benchmarkoutfitter.com

9525 Kenwood Rd. #24
Cincinnati, OH 45242
513-791-WILD (9453)

Field & Stream

fieldandstreamshop.com

520 Clock Tower Way
Buttermilk Towne Center
Crescent Springs, KY 41017
859-331-0364

REI

rei.com/stores/cincinnati.html

2643 Edmondson Rd.
Cincinnati, OH 45209
513-924-1938

Roads Rivers and Trails

roadsriversandtrails.com

118 Main St.
Milford, OH 45150
513-248-7787

Appendix B: Hiking Clubs

American Discovery Trail Coordinators

Indiana
Jeff Edmondson
460 Maple St.
Zionsville, IN 46077
jeffret@indy.rr.com

Ohio/Kentucky
Don Burell
4994 Bonaventure Ct.
Cincinnati, OH 45238
513-922-3867
dbcinoh@fuse.net

American Hiking Society

americanhiking.org

Buckeye Trail Association

buckeyetrail.org

Cincinnati Parks Foundation: Hiking Club

hikecincyparks.com

Great Parks of Hamilton County: Walk Club

Designed for people age 55 and older who enjoy morning walks in the park for fitness. To register and find additional information, go to **greatparks.org/events/walk-club.** A valid Great Parks of Hamilton County vehicle permit is required to enter all the parks.

Sierra Club: Miami Group

miami.ohiosierraclub.org

Tri-State Hiking Club

tristatehikingclub.com

Appendix C: Hiking with Children and Outdoor Programs

Hiking with Children

Make it simple; keep it simple. Young children have short attention spans and anything (a hike, for example) that requires their long-term attention can bring out the whiny child lurking within. Start by setting the rules: walking only, stay on the trail, and don't touch green leaves until mom or dad identifies the plant.

Have the kids pick which trail to explore. Break the hike into small sections by looking for treasures. Look for opportunities about 20 feet farther along the trail to engage your kids, such as who can find the bench, does anyone see a fence, or what is that on the next sign? Think up things to find: a fallen leaf with round edges, a fallen leaf with pointy edges, an acorn, a buckeye, a dried cicada shell, a wildflower, or a tree with a fork. You get the idea.

Also, take a break and lie on the ground (if suitable) and watch the clouds or make a "pssh" sound to attract birds.

Start working on identification skills. Have your children create names for what they see and have them explain why. When the kids get a little older try some of the easy-to-use identification guidebooks. Some state agencies provide them free of charge. Some identification books use a dichotomous key (yes-or-no key); these are relatively inexpensive and small enough to tuck into a back pocket.

Packing List

➢ **SEE-BOXES** Small clear plastic boxes with a magnifying lens built into the cap. They are typically sold in nature center shops. You can put items inside of the box to examine more closely or use the lid as a handheld magnifying lens.

➢ **MINI-BINOCULARS** You'll find easy-to-use and inexpensive binoculars in sporting goods stores or departments.

➢ **KIDS' DIGITAL OR REUSABLE CAMERA** Show your child how to use the camera and then allow their artistic side to run free by letting them decide what to photograph.

➤ **BIRD, TREE, WILDFLOWER, ANIMAL, AND ANIMAL TRACK IDENTIFICATION BOOKS** Contact state wildlife, nature preserves, parks, and forestry agencies to see if they have free identification books and ask for them to be mailed to you. For the best regional identification guidebooks, shop at a nature center store.

➤ **SMALL NOTEBOOK AND COLORED PENS** Before the kids get tired, stop. Let them rest, draw pictures of what they see, and have a drink and a snack. My friend Bonnie's children have kept a journal since before they were able to write. She'd simply ask them what their most favorite part of the hike was and then they would write down in their journal exactly what they said. Years later, her children are able to enjoy reading through their adventures.

➤ **FOOD AND WATER** Dried fruit, beef jerky, nuts, clementines, apples, cereal, and breakfast bars. I also bring along a few lollipops and chocolate candies for when the kids are very tired toward the end of a hike—the idea of a treat helps to perk them up and the sugar gets them moving. Nalgene bottles are BPA free and made in the United States. The bottles come in a variety of sizes. I prefer the large 32-ounce screw top. For shorter hikes, this is all the water we need, and it eliminates the hassle of too many water bottles, which add weight and take up space. You can also look into a CamelBak, which is a bag with a tube attached to it housed in a backpack. You fill the bag with water or sports drink, carry it on your back, and drink by biting a valve to allow the fluid to flow out. This is great for longer hikes and when you need to have your hands free.

➤ **GALLON-SIZE RESEALABLE PLASTIC BAGS** Use them for compact trash removal by putting the trash into the bag, zipping it almost closed, squeezing out the remaining air, sealing it, and stowing it away in the backpack until the trash can be thrown away properly. Everything is trash—that includes the orange peel.

➤ **I ALSO BRING** a few tissues, antibacterial wipes, and a first-aid kit packed in resealable plastic bags.

Outdoor Programs

For more information on sharing the outdoors with your children, try the local grassroots movements of Leave No Child Inside—Greater Cincinnati and Great Outdoor Weekend:

Leave No Child Inside—Greater Cincinnati

lncigc.org

Great Outdoor Weekend

The last weekend in September is the Great Outdoor Weekend in the Greater Cincinnati area. It is a celebration of outdoor activities. All programs are free. For more details visit **cincygreatoutdoorweekend.org.**

Outdoor Programs (continued)

Adventure Summit

The Adventure Summit brings thousands of outdoor enthusiasts to Dayton, Ohio, for a weekend of outdoor skill, culture, and experience. Visit **theadventuresummit.com** for additional information.

Midwest Outdoor Experience

Midwest Outdoor Experience (formerly GearFest) is a multiday event, featuring outdoor activities, an exhibitor village, competitions, music, a craft beer garden and food, camping, and demos. Visit **metroparks.org/outdoorx** for additional information.

Paddlefest

The Ohio River Paddlefest is about more than kayaking and canoeing. Thousands of outdoor enthusiasts meet at Coney Island Park for a weekend of exhibits, presentations, classes, demos, gear swap, music, and fun. Visit **ohioriverpaddlefest.org** for additional information.

Stay Connected

Let's stay connected. Visit my website **cincyhikes.com** for information on trails, nature, hiking with kids, and outdoor adventures. Like **6060CincyHikes** on Facebook and share your trail photos with us.

Index

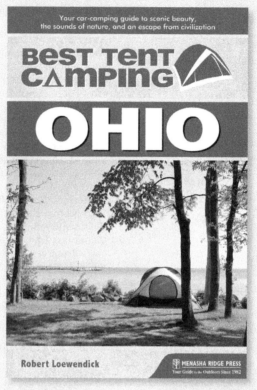
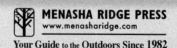

About the Author

In the woods or in a creek bed looking for fossils is where you can usually find **Tamara York,** if you are lucky and can keep up. She grew up exploring the woods near her grandparents' farm outside Connersville, Indiana. Her passion for the outdoors and goofing off brought her to Purdue University, where she graduated with a bachelor's degree in wildlife management. She and her husband have climbed Mount Katahdin in Baxter

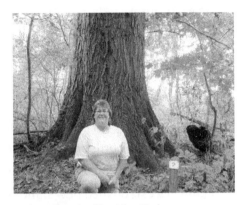

photographed by Allen York

State Park, Maine, and enjoy hiking with their daughters in state parks, wildlife areas, and forests in Ohio, Kentucky, and Indiana. Tamara is a trained and seasoned naturalist with more than 22 years of field experience and worked with the Indiana and Ohio Departments of Natural Resources before becoming a full-time freelance copywriter specializing in nature, outdoor recreation, travel, and the environment.

DEAR CUSTOMERS AND FRIENDS,

SUPPORTING YOUR INTEREST IN OUTDOOR ADVENTURE, travel, and an active lifestyle is central to our operations, from the authors we choose to the locations we detail to the way we design our books. Menasha Ridge Press was incorporated in 1982 by a group of veteran outdoorsmen and professional outfitters. For many years now, we've specialized in creating books that benefit the outdoors enthusiast.

Almost immediately, Menasha Ridge Press earned a reputation for revolutionizing outdoors- and travel-guidebook publishing. For such activities as canoeing, kayaking, hiking, backpacking, and mountain biking, we established new standards of quality that transformed the whole genre, resulting in outdoor-recreation guides of great sophistication and solid content. Menasha Ridge continues to be outdoor publishing's greatest innovator.

The folks at Menasha Ridge Press are as at home on a whitewater river or mountain trail as they are editing a manuscript. The books we build for you are the best they can be, because we're responding to your needs. Plus, we use and depend on them ourselves.

We look forward to seeing you on the river or the trail. If you'd like to contact us directly, join in at trekalong.com or visit us at menasharidge .com. We thank you for your interest in our books and the natural world around us all.

SAFE TRAVELS,

Bob Sehlinger

BOB SEHLINGER
PUBLISHER